QY 95

QY 95

CELLULAR PATHOLOGY
2nd edition

CELLULAR PATHOLOGY

2nd edition

Introduction to techniques and applications

D.J. Cook

*Senior Lecturer in Cellular Pathology, University of Portsmouth,
School of Pharmacy and Biomedical Science, Portsmouth, UK*

Scion

Second edition © Scion Publishing Ltd, 2006

ISBN 1 904842 30 5

First edition published in 1998 by Butterworth Heinemann (ISBN 0 7596 3111 2)
Reprinted in 2003 by Arnold, a member of the Hodder Headline Group

A CIP catalogue record for this book is available from the British Library.

Scion Publishing Limited
Bloxham Mill, Barford Road, Bloxham, Oxfordshire OX15 4FF
www.scionpublishing.com

Important Note from the Publisher

The information contained within this book was obtained by Scion Publishing
Limited from sources believed by us to be reliable. However, while every effort has
been made to ensure its accuracy, no responsibility for loss or injury whatsoever
occasioned to any person acting or refraining from action as a result of information
contained herein can be accepted by the authors or publishers.

Typeset by Phoenix Photosetting, Chatham, Kent, UK
Printed by Cromwell Press, Trowbridge, UK

Contents

Preface

It is nice to have the opportunity to produce a second edition of this book. Some things have changed but the popular structure of the book remains the same. Some of the changes are additions of new material, particularly in chapters 10, 12 and 17, whilst others are removal of older outdated material such as the references to stripping film in autoradiography where this particular product is, sadly, no longer produced. Chapter 10 on immunology techniques includes a range of newer techniques that have become popular since the first edition. Chapter 12 now introduces the changes to cytology screening in the UK where the use of fluid-based systems is replacing the traditional direct smearing and includes details of the Bethesda 2001 system for classifying cellular abnormalities. Some of the changes in chapter 17 relate to changes in legal requirements for safety in the laboratory. In the first edition safety was mentioned at many points in passing but there was no consideration of safety as a single topic. In this edition the individual references to safety remain embedded in the individual chapters but there is now a section purely on the organization and legal aspects of safety. Also changed in chapter 17 is a revised section mentioning the Human Tissue Act and introducing inter-laboratory quality control.

Other changes have occurred because of a change in publisher. The layout of the chapters has been improved and the learning objectives expanded. The contents list has been expanded significantly to help readers to navigate through the book more easily. The most important change is the inclusion of colour photographs in the book to help readers gain a better understanding of the subject in practice. So my thanks go to Jonathan Ray of Scion Publishing Ltd for encouraging the inclusion of the many colour photographs and also for his help in producing a new and better edition. My thanks also go to the copy-editor, Jane Hoyle, who checked my drafts and corrected my errors.

I am fortunate to be revising this edition at all. I began revising the material in the autumn of 2005 but then had a cycling accident at the end of November 2005. This fractured my skull and resulted in a subdural haematoma. The clot was removed at Southampton Neurological Centre and I was in Intensive Care on life support. Fortunately, I have recovered completely and so was able to complete the revisions in January 2006. I would like to thank the staff at Southampton Neurological Centre for their care and support. I would also like to thank Judy, my wife, and my children, Malcolm and Elaine, for their support and encouragement during my convalescence.

John Cook, Portsmouth, May 2006

Preface to the first edition

I was pleased when the opportunity to write this book arose. I have often thought that there was not a student oriented book on histological methods. I felt there was a need for a text covering the range of histological topics which was available at a price that undergraduates could afford.

The aim of this book is to be an introductory text for students studying biomedical sciences and it tries to cover the histological techniques used in the diagnosis of disease and in medical research. Many of these students will never become full time histologists and so do not need to know all the details of the techniques. They may, however, need to understand histological technique sufficiently to be able to read scientific papers that use histology, and to be able to communicate knowledgeably with histologists in their work. Cost has been kept down by not including all the detailed methods and the omission of experimental detail also allows the book to be shorter.

There are a number of very good laboratory books which are full of useful recipes telling you exactly how to prepare and stain histological sections. For students just beginning their study of histology these recipe books can be quite confusing. The reasons for using a particular technique can be lost in the details of how to actually carry out the stain. This book is intended to be different by being mainly a 'Why?' book rather than a 'How?' book. By that I mean that it attempts to explain the techniques available but does not attempt to give practical details. There are no protocols of methods which can be followed and practical details have been kept to a minimum. I hope to explain the uses of the methods, the advantage of doing one technique rather than another but without giving the full step by step instructions.

This does not mean that I think details are unimportant. On the contrary I think the details of a method are crucial to get a good result. It is just that for most students it is a distraction until they understand the overall concepts. I have referred to books in the recommended reading which are full of excellent recipes and invaluable detail of how the get the best results. I cannot thank the authors of these books enough for the help their books have provided over the years.

I was saddened during the writing of this book to find how many of the books I rely on have gone out of print. I have deliberately included quite a few of these out-of-print books in the reading lists in the hope that students will be able to find them in their libraries or obtain them through interlibrary loans. The number of currently available books on histological technique is sadly quite small and it seems that in each generation there are only two or three general histological method books in print at any one time. So I urge you to seek out these older books as they are still a mine of useful information.

I have taken the opportunity to extend the range of material covered compared to some laboratory manuals. I have included some techniques which are not currently used. Some are older methods that have been super-seded by newer and usually better techniques but I have included them both for simple historical interest and also because they sometimes have a useful theoretical point. I have also included some research techniques which are only used in relatively few laboratories either because of their interest or because they may become important in the future. I have also included optical illusions in microscopy as it is a particular interest of mine and I think the possibility of microscopists being fooled by what they think they see are not as well known as they should be.

I hope you enjoy the book and find it useful. I have certainly enjoyed putting it together.

J. Cook

Colour Plates

Chapter 2. Fixation and fixatives

Colour plate 1. The left-hand photograph shows a normal fixed piece of liver. The right-hand photograph shows a piece of liver left unfixed for 48 h before being processed but otherwise treated identically. The loss of structure and stainability is obvious. See page 10 for further information.

Formaldehyde	Bouin	Acetic acid
Glutaraldehyde	Mercuric chloride	Potassium dichromate	Zenker

Colour plate 2. Photographs of pieces of kidney fixed in different fixatives. All of the tissues were taken from the same kidney and processed identically. The effects of altering fixation are clearly seen in the staining reactions. Shrinkage effects can be gauged by observing the space around the glomeruli. See page 12 for further information.

Chapter 5. Cryotechniques

Colour plate 3. Frozen section of muscle showing a freezing ('waffle') artefact. The tissue at the bottom left shows holes where the tissue has failed to freeze properly and has been lost from the section. See page 56 for further information.

Colour plate 4. Large Gough and Wentworth section of a whole human lung. The tissue was frozen for support, sectioned (100 mm) using a large sledge microtome and then mounted on paper. The section shows large areas of black coal dust typical of a miner's lung. This type of section was used to determine lung damage in the assessment of compensation for pneumoconiosis in miners. See page 63 for further information.

Chapter 6. Staining theory

Colour plate 5. Simple haematoxylin and eosin-stained liver. The nuclei are visible as purple/blue round structures, the cytoplasm of the liver cells is pink and blood cells in the sinusoids have a more orange tinge. See page 68 for further information.

Colour plate 6. Van Gieson and trichrome methods. The left-hand photograph shows a van Gieson stain with red collagen and yellow erythrocytes. The Masson trichrome stain on the right shows yellow erythrocytes, red cytoplasm, especially of the Paneth cells, and blue collagen fibres. See page 90 for further information.

Colour plate 7. Silver impregnation techniques. The photograph on the left is a von Kossa stain on developing bone showing mineralization of the central bone; the bones at the top and bottom are not yet mineralized. The middle photograph is kidney stained to show reticulin fibres surrounding the convoluted tubules. The right-hand photograph shows cell borders in a simple squamous pavement epithelium. See page 93 for further information.

Colour plate 8. The use of silver impregnation to show astrocytes (left-hand image) and neurones (right-hand image). See page 93 for further information.

Chapter 7. Histochemistry: general considerations and the histochemistry of carbohydrates and lipids

Colour plate 9. The left-hand photograph shows salivary gland stained with alcian blue-/PAS for mucins. The pink-stained cells contain neutral mucin, whilst the blue-stained ones contain acid mucin. The right-hand photograph shows cartilage stained with toluidine blue demonstrating metachromasia. There is a colour shift from the blue colour visible in the soft connective tissue to purple in the cartilage matrix. See page 122 for further information.

Colour plate 10. Heart stained with oil red O and counterstained with haematoxylin and eosin. The hydrophobic lipid in the adipose tissue has stained strongly with the hydrophobic dye, whilst the cardiac muscle and fibrous connective tissue have failed to absorb the oil red O and instead are stained with the counterstain. See page 126 for further information.

Chapter 8. Histochemistry of nucleic acids, proteins and enzymes

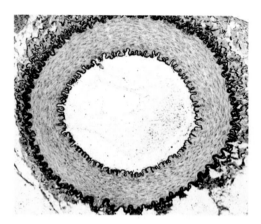

Colour plate 11. Cross-section of aorta stained with orcein to demonstrate the elastic fibres. See page 142 for further information.

Colour plate 12. Inflamed lung stained by the martius/scarlet/blue method. Fibrin stains red, whilst collagen stains blue. See page 142 for further information.

Colour plate 13. Liver stained using the Gomori method for phosphatase. The site of the enzyme appears black at the periphery of the liver lobules. See page 147 for further information.

Colour plate 14. Cross-section of voluntary muscle stained for succinic dehydrogenase enzyme. The dark blue fibres are the red-muscle fibres and are rich in mitochondria. The paler fibres are the white-muscle fibres and have fewer mitochondria. See page 150 for further information.

Chapter 9. Histochemistry of pigments, neuroendocrine amines and minerals

Colour plate 15. Cross-section of the lung of a cigarette smoker stained with the van Gieson method showing carbon deposited in the connective tissues. See page 159 for further information.

Colour plate 16. Asbestosis in a lung section stained using the Perls technique. The asbestos fibres have become coated with iron-containing pigments, which stain blue with Perls. See page 161 for further information.

Colour plate 17. Perls stain of kidney from a case of haemolytic anaemia showing deposits of iron-containing pigment in the convoluted tubules. The haemolytic disease has resulted in haemoglobin passing through the glomerulus and being reabsorbed by the cells of the tubules. See page 161 for further information.

Colour plate 18. Spleen stained using the Perls technique to show macrophages containing haemosiderin (a storage form of iron). See page 162 for further information.

Colour plate 19. Section of malignant melanoma with areas of brown melanin pigment visible on the left. See page 163 for further information.

Lipofuscin _____

Colour plate 20. Lipofuscin in heart muscle. In the haematoxylin and eosin stain on the left, lipofuscin indicated by the brown pigment is situated at the poles of the nucleus. On the right, the tissue has been stained with methylene blue to show the basophilia of the pigment. See page 164 for further information.

Colour plate 21. Argentaffin cells in the base of the crypt of Lieberkühn. See page 164 for further information.

Colour plate 22. Calcium in bone demonstrated by the von Kossa method of silver impregnation. The bones at the top and bottom show calcium deposits, whilst the middle bone shows no mineralization. See page 170 for further information.

Colour plate 23. Embryonic bones in a rat pup stained by the Dawson alizarin red method. See page 171 for further information.

Chapter 10. Immunological techniques

Colour plate 24. Anti-nuclear antibody shown by fluorescein-labelled anti-human immunoglobulin. See page 186 for further information.

Colour plate 25. Autoantibodies in the liver shown with peroxidase-labelled antibody and diaminobenzidene chromogen. The site of the autoantibody is shown by the brown deposit. See page 192 for further information.

Chapter 11. Autoradiography

Colour plate 26. Autoradiograph with black granules showing migration of the labelled compound from a blood vessel. There is also some retention of the drug in the endothelium of the vessel wall. See page 204 for further information.

Colour plate 27. The top photograph shows a longitudinal section of a rat that has been given a radioactive drug (an analgesic being tested for toxicity). The lower photograph shows an autoradiograph from this section using X-ray film. The dark areas in the autoradiograph show that the drug is mainly restricted to the lumen of the gut, with some being absorbed into the liver. See page 211 for further information.

Chapter 12. Exfoliative cytology and related techniques

Colour plate 28. Sampling devices for cytology. On the right is an Ayres spatula, which was the original device used in screening. This has a notched upper end that fitted around the neck of the cervix. The relatively short extension meant that it did not always sample the squamo-columnar junction so the Aylesbury spatula was developed with a longer beak. This is now available in both beechwood and plastic. The brush next to the plastic Aylesbury spatula is for endocervical sampling. On the extreme left is a commercially developed plastic 'brush' (Cervex brush), which has flexible plastic 'bristles'; this is also more effective than the Ayres spatula. See page 223 for further information.

Colour plate 29. This photograph of a cervical smear shows three superficial cells with pink cytoplasm and pyknotic nuclei. At the bottom is an intermediate cell with greenish cytoplasm and a larger nucleus. Also shown are a few neutrophil leukocytes with lobed nuclei. See page 229 for further information.

Colour plate 30. The two cells in the upper left of the photograph are intermediate cells with green-staining cytoplasm and large round nuclei. The cell at the bottom right shows a similar colour of cytoplasm but the nucleus is pyknotic, whilst the cell at the top right has pink-staining cytoplasm but a more open nucleus. This illustrates that the classifications and labels are not absolute and cells go through all stages; the changes in staining and nuclear morphology are not instantaneous and do not necessarily occur together. See page 229 for further information.

Colour plate 31. Parabasal cells stained with the Papanicolaou stain. See page 229 for further information.

Colour plate 32. Smear showing signs of inflammation. There are large numbers of neutrophil leukocytes with lobed nuclei and two plasma cells with characteristic clumps of chromatin at the margin of the nucleus. See page 230 for further information.

Colour plate 33. Cells from cervical smears displaying abnormalities indicative of pre-malignant or malignant change. See pages 242–245 for further information.

Chapter 13. Cytogenetics and molecular genetics

Colour plate 34. Tissue culture bottle containing red growth medium. See page 256 for further information.

Colour plate 35. Two tissue culture bottles. The bottle on the right is still at a reasonable pH but the more orange medium on the left shows a lowered pH. The colour change is due to the phenol red indicator incorporated in most media. See page 260 for further information.

Colour plate 36. Karyotype of a patient with Klinefelter's syndrome. The chromosomes are cut out of the photograph on the left and arranged in order to give the karyotype. See page 263 for further information.

Colour plate 37. Two cells showing Barr bodies. In the cell on the left, the nucleus shows a Barr body at the bottom right (at about '5 o'clock'), whilst the one on the right is visible at the top of the nucleus ('12 o'clock'). See page 267 for further information.

Chapter 14. Infective agents and amyloid

Colour plate 38. A multinucleated giant cell is shown in the centre of the image. See page 281 for further information.

Colour plate 39. Lung tissue stained with the auramine/rhodamine technique showing fluorescent bacilli from a case of tuberculosis. See page 285 for further information.

Colour plate 40. Kidney stained with Congo red for amyloid. The amyloid can be seen staining red in the two central glomeruli. See page 292 for further information.

Colour plate 41. Amyloid stained with Congo red viewed with crossed polarizers. The bright dichroic colour indicates the Congo red-stained amyloid. See page 293 for further information.

Chapter 15. Light microscopy

Colour plate 42. This shows three forms of microscopy applied to three unstained cheek cells. The top left image is routine brightfield microscopy, the right-hand image is darkground microscopy and the bottom left image is phase-contrast microscopy. See page 306 for further information.

Colour plate 43. Vitamin C crystals photographed using a polarizing microscope. See page 309 for further information.

Colour plate 44. The photograph on the left shows a conventionally lit cervical smear, whilst on the right is the same field of view using phase-contrast microscopy. In the centre of the right-hand field can be seen a Y-shaped clump of *Candida* yeasts. These are just visible on the left as a faintly stained structure. The ability of phase-contrast microscopy to pick out unstained or faintly stained material is clearly shown. See page 317 for further information.

The study of tissues and their diseases

Learning objectives
After studying this chapter you should confidently be able to:

■ **Describe the major types of artefacts in sections.**
  Loss of materials, gain of materials and distortion of tissue structure.

■ **Describe why several different methods are needed in histology.**
  Since tissues are altered, alternatives are needed to show which
  appearances are genuine and which are artefacts.

Ever since the microscope was invented somewhere around the beginning of the 17th century it has been used to magnify human cells and tissues. The great difficulty with the application of the microscope is that the tissues themselves are really quite featureless and uninteresting unless they are first prepared in some way to enhance the detail. This book is an attempt to explain the methods used in examining cells and to try to give a theoretical outline of the basis of the techniques.

1.1 WHAT IS CELLULAR PATHOLOGY?

I will begin with the words used to describe the topic itself. There are many words that have been used to describe the subject over the years and they all have some merit. The parent subject is **anatomy** (from the Greek meaning cutting up: *ana* = up and *tome* = to cut), which is the study of the organs and their shape, arrangement and structure. Anatomy is an ancient discipline. Ever since humans first started butchering animals, people must have realized that the body is made of different organs and that all of these organs have varying structures. Over many centuries, the study of anatomy catalogued and described the visible structure of the human body and laid the foundations of physiology by trying to explain the functions of each organ and how the organs interacted with each other (see *Box 1.1* for comments).

Box 1.1 Histology is complementary to other biological sciences

Histology does not exist in isolation but constantly interacts with other disciplines such as biochemistry and physiology. Many of the histochemical techniques used today are modifications of methods used originally in biochemistry. Biochemistry in turn depends on the information provided by histology to identify the sites where the biochemical events are occurring. The scientific disciplines are complementary. The main advantage of histology is its ability to localize materials and metabolic processes within the tissues and even within individual organelles in the cell. The main disadvantage of histology is the requirement that the materials being examined cannot be allowed to move and must be kept in their original site (*in situ*). The advantage and disadvantage are the same: the very thing that makes histology so useful also imposes its own problems. This is why histology needs the other disciplines and the other disciplines need histology. They are not competitors but allies in the scientific investigation of disease.

With the development of the microscope, the organs could be seen in finer detail and the discipline of **microscopic anatomy** was born. This is now normally called **histology**, the study of tissues and their structure. The term histology usually means the study of normal tissues, whilst the study of diseases in tissues is more correctly called **histopathology**, but fashions in science change and the more common term now is **cellular pathology**. This is a good name for the science since the basic structure of the human body is the cell and the basis of most human disease is also at the cellular level.

Tissues consist of cells and the study of the structure of cells is **cytology**, which can be used diagnostically. The prefix *cyto* can usually replace the prefix *histo* with the inference that the emphasis is on subcellular detail rather than on multicellular structures. Thus, we can have cytochemistry, immunocytochemistry, cytopathology and so on. In many cases the terms are simply interchangeable. Although this book is entitled *Cellular Pathology*, it is not limited to the diagnosis of disease and can be used equally as an introduction to normal histological techniques and/or research applications. There is no dividing line between the preparation of normal tissues and diseased tissues; the methods are the same, just the application is different.

1.2 PREPARATION OF TISSUES

One recurring feature of the investigation of biological materials is the problem of preparing the tissues. Ideally we would like to study living tissues but this is not always possible. Any method that alters the tissues making them more readily studied must also risk the possibility that the tissues are no longer representative of the living tissue. The only way to solve this dilemma is to have several quite different ways of studying the same problem so that any errors produced by one method are quite different to the errors introduced by the other methods. Anything that is always the same, regardless of how the tissue was prepared, can safely be assumed to be a feature of the tissue and not of the method of preparing the tissue.

The more preparative techniques we have, the better our understanding

To make sure we have got the right answers, we therefore need many different methods. The methods may not all be equally easy and they may not all be equally good, but we need them to make sure the methods we are using are valid. Some techniques have been very important historically but have been superseded by better and more reliable techniques. However, their influence may have been immense and so they should still be remembered.

It is also important to realize that you cannot do everything with one method. The large numbers of methods developed in histology often relate to just one or two problems. These problems may well recur in a different way, so knowledge of a variety of techniques may enable you to see how to overcome a modern problem using an older method. Thus, this book contains not only the currently important techniques but also some older or less popular ones.

Preparing tissues alters them

All of the techniques used in histological preparation have their own particular problems and all produce significant changes in the tissues. These changes in the tissues are known as **artefacts**. Artefacts are changes in the tissue brought about by the techniques used; they are errors introduced during the processing of tissues. The artefacts that can be produced are as many and as varied as the techniques that produce them. It would take several pages just to list all of the artefacts that can occur, but they can be grouped into three major types. Within each type there will be a variety of causes and a range of individual errors, but if we can understand the types of errors it often helps to recognize the errors and sometimes helps us to know how to avoid them.

Box 1.2 Artefacts

The term artefacts can also be spelt artifacts. They are both pronounced the same but I prefer the 'e' since it comes from the Latin *arte* (by art), although others disagree.

The most bizarre artefact I have had was a complete small spider in a stained section. During the drying of the section, a student had used a hotplate and put the section face up on the hotplate. A spider must have fallen onto it and was killed and dried down. The student never noticed, stained the section and then when it was being examined under the microscope there in the middle of the kidney was a spider.

Materials can be lost from the tissue during section preparation

The loss of materials is one of the commonest types of artefact. Sometimes it is not crucial if many materials are lost provided the important materials, and in particular the substance we are looking for, are retained.

If we take paraffin wax-processed tissues as an example, the materials that are lost from the tissues include:

1. All of the small water-soluble molecules. These are lost when we attempt to preserve the tissue by immersing it in a fixative. The materials lost include simple sugars (glucose, fructose, etc.), ions (sodium, potassium, chlorides, sulphates, phosphates, etc.), vitamins (thiamine, riboflavin, etc.), cofactors (ADP, NAD, etc.) and many others.
2. All of the lipids and lipid-soluble materials that are extracted by the alcohols, clearing agents and hot waxes used in preparing wax sections. The membrane lipids, steroid hormones and fat-soluble vitamins are lost as well as the simple adipose fats.

Thus, it is no use preparing a paraffin wax section to try and identify where NAD is located within a cell because it will all have disappeared. In paraffin wax sections, just about the only things that are retained are the proteins, some nucleic acids and a few other molecules. What is perhaps more surprising is how much information about tissue structure and function can be learned from such a depleted material.

Materials can be gained by the tissue during section preparation

This usually involves chemical additions to the structures. Any material prepared using aldehydes as preservatives will have extra aldehydes that were not there in life. Aldehydes form addition compounds (see Chapter 2) with at least some of the amine groups in proteins. If the preservation is done with mercury compounds instead of aldehydes, there will be a black deposit of mercury within the tissues that was not there before the fixative was added.

These chemical additions are an inherent part of the technique but there are also additions that can be less predictable. For example, during the handling of the tissues in the laboratory, the blocks may be placed on filter paper or handled with rubber gloves. Fibres from the paper or glove powder from the gloves may be transferred accidentally to the specimen and appear in the final preparation. These contaminants are artefacts since they were not there in the living body.

Structures can be altered or distorted during section preparation

The most common distortion is that tissues shrink during processing. Shrinkage in itself is not a serious problem provided everything alters to the same extent. As long as the shrinkage is regular, we can compare tissues with each other knowing that they will have been affected to the same degree. Unfortunately shrinkage is often irregular. Some materials shrink more than others and give a false impression. Take bone as an example. Bone consists of a very hard matrix containing a few scattered cells called osteocytes, which lie in small spaces in the bone called lacunae. In life, the whole of each lacuna is filled by the cytoplasm of the osteocytes. However, during sectioning, the soft tissue of the osteocyte shrinks much more than the hard matrix. As a result, in many sections of bone the osteocytes appear shrunken and a gap appears around the cells. This gap is an artefact of the processing.

All sections have some artefacts

Whenever a section is seen, there will be artefacts and the recognition of these is an important part of histology. It is also important to be able to avoid certain artefacts and so histologists need a range of methods that have different properties so that they can always manage to get a section that is useful. It may have other artefacts but the section will avoid the specific artefacts that would make it useless for a particular purpose. Thus, wax sections do not contain lipids but they do not have any ice crystal damage. Frozen sections retain the lipids but may show ice crystal damage. You must choose your method to suit your requirements.

Fortunately histological workers over the history of the subject have been very clever in approaching the problems in different ways and so most of what we now acknowledge as the structure of cells and tissues stands on a very firm base. But whenever the boundaries of a technique are extended, it is always correct to ask 'Is this real or is this just what has been done to the tissues?'

1.3 EVOLUTION OF HISTOLOGY

The preparation of tissues has been improving constantly and it seems likely that it will continue to improve in future. The earliest microscopists simply used whole mounts of small specimens with little or no use of dyeing. The earliest sections used free-hand sectioning but this gives only poor results and it was the introduction of the technique of embedding tissues in a solid medium and the use of dyes to enhance contrast and visibility that made histology into an accurate and reliable method.

The embedding techniques have been many and varied. Using these differing techniques, much of the tissue structure still remains very similar.

Box 1.3 Histology, science, art and craft

Histology is one area of science where there is a great deal of manual skill needed as well as scientific knowledge. The ability to cut sections is certainly crucial to obtaining acceptable results and a good microtomist needs a long apprenticeship. Staining requires skills in differentiation to get the optimal contrast in specimens. This has led to a certain amount of mystique in histology and the assertion that histology is more of an art than a science.

The results of histology are slides and these can certainly be aesthetically pleasing in an abstract way and are often used as illustrations and for covers of journals and magazines. But these images always reflect reality and are always based on scientific principles. Histologists do not actually create the results; they just bring out what is present in the tissues.

The other assertion is that histology is getting left behind. This again is not true. Histology may be involved with dyeing but it is not a dying art.

The appearances do change slightly, but by comparing techniques it is possible to determine the structure of the tissues as they would be inside the living organism. We can therefore also state with confidence that one technique will cause shrinkage, another will destroy some tissue components and yet another may alter the chemical nature of the tissues. Whenever a piece of tissue is to be investigated, the choice of the preparative technique will impose its own limitations and advantages. A single technique is never the best for every possible situation. You must know what you want to see and then choose the appropriate method. Thus, in this book there will be descriptions of several alternative techniques and a comparison of their advantages and problems.

Demonstration techniques are now more selective and specific

One of the major advances has been the improvement of demonstration methods. In the earliest years of micro-technique, the only method available to demonstrate structure was to use the few natural dyes that were available. These were often unreliable and the demonstrations were poor and the results did not keep well. The phenomenal increase in the number of dyes available following the synthesis of dyes (particularly from coal tar) made it possible to produce more selective methods and brighter colours. The use of many of these techniques is still an important part of micro-technique today. The development of the use of antibodies and histochemical techniques has allowed even more precision and it is now possible to identify and localize individual molecules and chemicals rather than just the vague staining of 'proteins'. Now there is a rapidly increasing use of nucleic acid techniques, which have unprecedented accuracy and can identify the actual genes and mutations of genes that are associated with many diseases. Where this will lead in the future is not absolutely clear, but histological micro-technique is certainly not a dead end with no significant further developments; rather, it is a lively and growing scientific discipline.

Histology is likely to change dramatically in the future

Histological techniques have not altered as much in the past century as those of other scientific disciplines such as biochemistry. A histologist from the late 19th century would probably adjust to working in a modern laboratory with little difficulty. He might need a little retraining in the advances that have taken place but at least he would understand the general concepts. Biochemistry, on the other hand, has changed dramatically and a 19th century biochemist would not recognize most of the instruments and techniques that are now routine. My feelings are that histological micro-technique will undergo a similar change in the coming years. It will be more important to understand the concepts behind the methods than to know the best recipe for a stain since many of the current techniques will become

Box 1.4 Histology is central to much modern research

Histology is still one of the most important research methods. A quick look in any major biomedical or biological journal will show that more than half of the papers will include some histological aspect. Histology can appeal to humans in a way that most scientific disciplines do not. Histology is essentially a visual science and human beings are highly visual, with the amount of information received and understood through vision being greater than all of the other senses combined. The display of a good histological preparation always appeals both aesthetically and intellectually since it is possible to see for oneself. No amount of tables or graphs can have quite the same impact as a good section.

obsolete and will be replaced. Only the underlying principles are likely to remain the same and will be as important in 50 years' time as they will be in 5 years' time.

This book, unlike the majority of textbooks on histological technique, is not a practical book full of recipes and methods, but aims to be an introduction to the concepts of tissue preparation. This does not mean that I think that the detail of the techniques is unimportant. I believe that the details and tips present in the laboratory recipe books are often quite fascinating in themselves and also are essential to anyone intending to work in a histological laboratory or use histology in a regular and practical way. The detail is always important when you come to actually prepare a tissue section, but when you are just beginning to learn about the subject the detail may get in the way of a deeper understanding. When you want to do histology, then you will need a laboratory manual, but I hope that having read this book first, you will be able to follow the method with understanding and not just an unthinking adherence to the recipe.

This book is also intended for people who are not themselves intending to become histologists but who will be working alongside histologists, who will need to talk to histologists and who will perhaps even make use of histology but without needing to do all of the preparation themselves. You may not need to know the minute-to-minute steps in preparing tissues, but if you are going to understand histology and histologists, then you need to understand their problems and their language.

Like all scientific disciplines, histology is absolutely enthralling to its disciples but can often seem boring and routine to non-histologists. I hope to try and bridge the gap between these extremes and show the fascination but without the tedious detail, to show the scope that histology can cover. If in the process I can make you think that histological methodology is worthwhile learning, then I will feel that the book has succeeded.

SUGGESTED FURTHER READING

Wallington, E.A. (1979) Artifacts in tissue sections. *Medical Laboratory Sciences* **36**, 3–61.

SELF-ASSESSMENT QUESTIONS

1. Outline what is meant by an artefact.
2. List the major types of artefact and give one example of each type.
3. Two sections are prepared by different methods to show the location of glycogen. The first section shows glycogen in hepatocytes (liver cells) evenly spread throughout the cells. The second shows glycogen present in the same cells but concentrated at one end of the cell.
   Can we conclude that hepatocytes contain glycogen?
   Can we conclude that glycogen is evenly spread in the hepatocytes?
4. Why is there no single method of tissue preparation that everyone agrees is the best?

Fixation and fixatives

Learning objectives
After studying this chapter you should confidently be able to:

■ **Describe why tissue removed from the body will change.**
Tissues can degenerate by three mechanisms. Putrefaction is destruction by micro-organisms, autolysis is degeneration by lysosomal enzymes and abnormal metabolism occurs in isolated tissues.

■ **Describe how fixatives stop post-mortem changes.**
Fixation is the attempt to stop tissue degenerating and preserve the tissue in a lifelike condition. Fixatives are usually enzyme poisons.

■ **List the properties of a perfect fixative.**
Fixatives penetrate tissues and kill cells quickly and evenly, prevent autolysis and putrefaction, do not alter the tissue adversely and prepare the tissue for sectioning. They must be economical, safe and easy to use.

■ **Discuss how different fixatives have special properties and uses in histology.**
All fixatives have drawbacks and advantages. Some are good for general structure, some are better for cytological detail and some for histochemistry. The fixative should be chosen to match the investigation.

■ **Describe how simple fixatives can be used in combination to improve preservation.**
Since all fixatives have drawbacks, there is no single perfect fixative. Using two or more fixatives in combination can sometimes improve preservation. Fixative solutions must also be mixed with salts and buffers to control osmotic pressure and pH.

2.1 TISSUE DEGENERATION

Human cells and tissues in the body can only remain alive because they are connected to the blood stream, which provides them with the oxygen and nutrients that they need and which also removes the toxic waste products of metabolism. If the blood circulation stops, or if the tissues are removed from the body during an operation, then the cells will be cut off from this essential life-support system. Once cells are deprived of oxygen for long enough, they will die. In histology we would like to see the cells looking exactly the same as they were in the living body so the tissue must be stabilized as quickly as possible. This is done by fixation.

Some effects of tissue degeneration can be seen in *Colour plate 1*.

Types of tissue change

The way in which tissues change can vary depending on the organ involved but we can identify three types of change that occur in all tissues:

1. The cells do not die instantly when the blood circulation stops but remain alive by drawing on their energy supplies and respiring anaerobically (see *Box 2.1*). This is a useful response since cells often get temporarily cut off from circulating blood; for example, lying for a long time on your arm in bed restricts the blood flow. When you move and allow the blood to recirculate into the area it results in 'pins and needles' due to the accumulation of waste products including lactic acid and carbon dioxide, both of which are acidic. If the cell was left without a blood supply for many minutes, the cells would die; this is the cause of bedsores. The affected cells would then be different to the state they were in before the blood supply ceased. They would have exhausted their store of glycogen and would be more acidic than normal tissues due to the lactic acid and carbon dioxide. Both of these can result in visible changes in the cell.

2. When the cells die, they begin to break down. The most important part of this breakdown occurs when the lysosomes release their enzymes into the cell cytoplasm. These enzymes include proteases, which destroy proteins, nucleases, which destroy nucleic acids, and lipases, which destroy lipids. This will eventually result in the complete disintegration of the cell and its contents. This process of self-digestion is called **autolysis**.

3. If bacteria or fungal spores alight on tissues, particularly dead tissues, they can begin to grow and this will result in microbial spoilage or **putrefaction**, which will drastically alter the structure of the tissues.

Box 2.1 Cell survival and cell death

The ability of cells to survive away from the body depends on their individual energy stores. Some cells have large stores of glycogen; examples include skin, muscle and heart tissue. Other cells have very little in the way of stored energy and are totally dependent on a regular supply of glucose, e.g. the neurones in the brain. Muscle and skin can therefore survive using their own supplies for considerable lengths of time, probably in excess of 20 min, but the brain will be permanently damaged in less than 2 min if totally deprived of a blood supply. Thus, it is safe to put a tourniquet around an arm or a leg to arrest bleeding but it is not safe to put a tourniquet around the neck for even a few seconds. This survival of some tissues allows the transplant of organs such as heart and kidney, which can be maintained in a healthy state *in vitro* and transported from one hospital to another.

Box 2.2 Putrefaction and rate of degeneration

Putrefaction is important in dealing with meat in everyday life since bacterial contamination can lead to food poisoning. Fortunately for butchers, the process is very slow so that, provided the meat is kept cool, it will not spoil by bacterial growth. Most tissues removed from the body are quite sterile and need to be contaminated by spores from the air before bacterial growth can even start. Autolysis is more rapid but is not a disadvantage for culinary meat; indeed, it is an advantage since it helps to tenderize the meat and improve the flavour. The traditional 'hanging' of meat for several days makes use of autolysis to improve its eating qualities. The different types and rates of change allow pathologists to estimate how long a body has been dead and this can be important in forensic pathology.

Putrefaction is not the most important change in histology

Collectively these changes are sometimes referred to as post-mortem changes. It is putrefaction that tends to be identified by most people as the most important form of change in pieces of tissue, but in histological terms this is a slow and therefore less important form of change than autolysis and abnormal metabolism (see *Box 2.2* for extra comments).

2.2 FIXATION

Fixation is an attempt to preserve the tissues in a lifelike condition (see *Box 2.3* for extra comments). Fixation must stop abnormal enzyme activity and metabolism, in other words kill the cells, and it must stop autolysis by inactivating the lysosomal enzymes. Most fixatives are therefore enzyme poisons. Destroying enzymes will also stop bacterial and fungal growth and so prevent putrefactive changes.

Fixation is usually achieved by immersing the tissues in a chemical solution; hence, it is referred to as chemical fixation, but it can also be achieved by heat. Bacteriologists have traditionally fixed their bacterial smears by passing them through the flame of a Bunsen burner. High temperatures destroy enzyme activity and so act as a form of fixation. This is not common in histology since it is difficult to control, but it has been

Box 2.3 Preservation of food

The process of fixation is not new. Preservation of meat for eating is an old technology. In food preservation, the processes can be slowed by removing water. In the absence of water, enzymes cannot act, metabolism is stopped and bacterial growth is greatly retarded. Water can be removed by simple drying in air, or by using salt to extract the water. Both will work with human tissue as well as with meat for food. The process is called mummification after the Egyptian mummies, which were dried using salts and preserved using oils and resins. However, the tissue becomes desiccated and shrunken, making mummification a poor method of preservation for histology. Although simple drying of tissues is not a good method by modern standards, some tissue structures can still be seen and identified in mummies over 5000 years old.

used for rapid fixation or in some histochemical investigations where the use of chemical solutions would interfere with the chemical reactions. Microwave ovens have made this form of fixation easier to apply and control and are probably the best way to heat-fix tissues. Microwave fixation is becoming increasingly popular for some applications. There is no cross-linking so later chemical fixation may be needed.

There are many chemicals that act as enzyme poisons but only a few are useful as histological fixatives. No fixative can perfectly preserve any tissue exactly the way it was in life, but some fixatives can give very good histological results for certain restricted purposes.

A perfect fixative needs several properties

Before considering some commonly used fixatives, it is useful to identify the properties that we would like to see in a perfect fixative.

A perfect fixative should:

- Penetrate tissues quickly and evenly; this makes all parts of the tissue look the same. If penetration is uneven, then the edges of the tissue will look quite different to the centre of the specimen.
- Kill cells quickly and evenly; the killing stops abnormal metabolism.
- Prevent autolysis.
- Prevent putrefaction.
- Not add any extraneous material to the tissue.
- Not swell or shrink the tissue.
- Prepare the tissue for later treatments such as staining and not prevent any later investigation that might be needed.
- Prevent desiccation and drying of tissue, which would cause shrinkage and distortion.
- Be safe to use (non-toxic, non-flammable).
- Be reasonably priced.
- Be convenient to use (shelf life, storage, etc.).

The first eight properties are related to how the fixative affects the tissues, whilst the last three are related to practical use of the fixative in the laboratory.

No reagent has all of these properties and fixation is always a compromise and is always less than perfect.

2.3 FIXATIVES

Commonly used fixatives

The following are a few of the common fixatives that are used for preserving tissues. Photographs of tissues treated with different fixatives can be seen in *Colour plate 2*.

Formaldehyde (HCHO)

This is a pungent toxic gas that is soluble in water. It is usually sold as a 37–40% solution of formaldehyde in water when it is called **formalin** (in the UK, formalin is a general term, but in some countries it is a trade mark). It is the most widely used fixative for routine light microscopy sections, when it is used as a 4% solution of formaldehyde. Note that 4% formaldehyde is made by diluting the formalin solution (i.e. 40% formaldehyde) using one part formalin to nine parts water (a 1:10 dilution) and it is often called 10% formalin. The terms formalin and formaldehyde are both still in common use but the concentrations are quite different. Thus, 10% formalin is the same strength as 4% formaldehyde. The use of formaldehyde concentrations rather than formalin concentrations is the more accurate and preferred method.

Formaldehyde is a very reactive chemical and undergoes several changes in storage. Formalin solutions are therefore usually impure and contain a number of contaminants, some added by the manufacturer and others formed during storage.

In aqueous solution, formaldehyde reacts with water forming methylene glycol:

$$HCHO + H_2O \rightarrow CH_2(OH)_2$$

Formic acid (methanoic acid) can be formed by oxidation of formaldehyde by the oxygen in air:

$$2HCHO + O_2 \rightarrow 2HCOOH$$

and also by the Canizzaro reaction:

$$2HCHO + H_2O \rightarrow HCOOH + CH_3OH$$

Methanol is also formed in this reaction. Methanol is deliberately added to formalin solutions by the manufacturers, partly to inhibit the Canizzaro reaction and also to prevent polymerization.

Finally formaldehyde polymerizes to form 'paraformaldehyde':

$$2nHCHO \leftrightarrow HO(CH_2O)_nH + (n-1)H_2O$$

This occurs especially in the cold conditions found in most chemical stores.

The paraformaldehyde does not harm the fixative except by reducing the formaldehyde concentration. Provided this is adjusted to take account of the loss, the final solution will still fix tissues very well. If the polymer formed is a short chain of less than eight formaldehyde molecules, then the paraformaldehyde remains soluble and will not be noticed, but if the chains are longer than eight carbons, it precipitates as a white powder. The paraformaldehyde will depolymerize if warmed or diluted. Depolymerization is more rapid if the solution is around neutral pH.

Thus, the commercial formalin solutions are really quite impure. The most important contaminant is the methanoic acid, which will affect the pH and the fixing properties. Acid formalin will, for example, produce a brown deposit around degenerating blood cells. This is an artefact and is therefore a nuisance. To prevent this occurring, only neutral formaldehyde solutions should be used and most laboratories normally use buffered formaldehyde as their routine fixative.

If greater purity is needed for critical applications, such as electron microscopy, then it is better not to use commercial formalin solutions. Instead, formaldehyde can be generated by depolymerizing paraformaldehyde. The paraformaldehyde is unadulterated and not contaminated in the same way as the commercial formalin solutions and is more reliable and purer.

Fixation properties of formaldehyde. Formaldehyde in solution is almost entirely in the hydrated form of methylene glycol and it is the methylene glycol that acts as the fixative. The glycol adds on to proteins, forming single and double additions.

$$CH_2(OH)_2 + R\text{-}NH_2 \leftrightarrow R\text{-}NHCH_2OH + H_2O$$

$$R\text{-}NHCH_2OH + R_2\text{-}NH_2 \to R\text{-}NHCH_2HNR_2 + H_2O$$

Single additions are easily reversed by washing in water for a few hours. Double reactions are more stable and produce methylene bridges.

These reactions occur slowly over a period of days, so formaldehyde is a slow-acting fixative and full fixation takes about a week, although adequate fixation occurs in 12–24 h.

As well as its main fixative properties, formaldehyde has several other advantages as a routine fixative. The effect of formaldehyde on tissues is to cause them to swell slightly; this means the organs remain soft and pliable. This soft fixation is good for dissection and for trimming of tissues into blocks for processing. Many other fixatives harden the tissue making trimming and dissection difficult or impossible. The tissue does, however, harden during processing, so the final paraffin block is very hard.

Formaldehyde is a very tolerant and forgiving fixative. Tissues cannot be overfixed and can be stored in formalin for many years. Many other fixatives can overfix the tissue and formaldehyde is often used to store tissues originally fixed in such fixatives.

Most fixatives alter the colour of tissues, often turning them a dull greyish colour. Formaldehyde is the only fixative that allows natural colour to be restored and so it forms the basis of all museum fixatives.

Formaldehyde is not perfect; it has its drawbacks. Cytoplasmic staining is duller after simple formaldehyde fixation than it is after many other fixatives. Formaldehyde is also toxic and causes formalin dermatitis and is a suspected carcinogenic agent (see *Box 2.4* for more details).

Glutaraldehyde

This is a bifunctional aldehyde that reacts more quickly than formaldehyde (it binds to 90% of NH_2 groups in 2 h; formaldehyde binds to only 70% of such groups in 7 days). It polymerizes very easily and glutaraldehyde solutions should be depolymerized before use. It is difficult to remove the glutaraldehyde from tissues and this makes histochemistry difficult; in particular, many aldehydes remain active since each molecule has two aldehyde groups and

---

Box 2.4 Formalin toxicity

Formaldehyde is a very dangerous chemical and should be handled carefully. Contact with the skin can result in an allergic reaction due to the formalin attacking skin proteins and modifying their structure sufficiently to make the body identify them as foreign. The immune system will then start attacking these proteins and this results in severe disease.

Always use protective gloves and clothing when dealing with formaldehyde.

Formaldehyde is also a respiratory poison and must only be used in a well-ventilated area. The ventilation must carry the fumes **away** from the face, so downward or backward ventilating systems are needed. Upward ventilation can actually pull the vapour towards the mouth and nose.

---

often only one is actually bound to the tissue so the second group remains active. These extraneous aldehydes prevent glutaraldehyde being a useful fixative when the periodic acid–Schiff reaction and other aldehyde-detecting reagents are being used. Glutaraldehyde inactivates all enzymes, thus totally preventing enzyme histochemistry. It also binds and masks many antigens, making immunotechniques difficult or even impossible.

Glutaraldehyde fixation gives excellent morphology but staining with acidic dyes is depressed. Like formaldehyde it is very dangerous if inhaled or in contact with the skin. Glutaraldehyde is widely used in electron microscopy.

Mercuric chloride

This is white crystalline solid soluble to about 7% in water. It is highly toxic as a cumulative poison, so small doses over a long period can gradually build up to a toxic dose.

Mercuric chloride fixes tissues by attaching to SH groups in proteins and it cross-links them forming a coarse coagulum of protein. Coagulating fixatives such as mercuric chloride leave relatively large fluid-filled spaces within the protein and allow rapid penetration of reagents into the tissues through these channels. Staining is not depressed since mercuric chloride does not block the NH_2 groups in the same way as the aldehyde fixatives and the cytoplasm stains brightly with acid dyes. The coagulation, however, leaves the tissue excessively hard and shrinks the tissue considerably. For this reason, it is never used alone and only in association with other softer fixatives.

Mercuric chloride leaves a black precipitate (mercury pigment) in tissues, which interferes with the appearance and needs to be removed. The pigment is easily removed with iodine, which converts it to mercuric iodide, followed by sodium thiosulphate (often referred to as 'hypo'), which removes the mercuric iodide.

Mercuric chloride is used less often nowadays because of its cost, toxicity and the difficulty of disposing of the waste fixative (see *Box 2.5*).

Osmium tetroxide

This is very expensive (up to £180,000 per kg), so is usually restricted to fixing very small pieces of tissue. It is a powerful oxidizing agent and adds on to double bonds and in so doing it blackens them. Since most lipids

---

Box 2.5 Problems with the use of mercury salts

Mercuric chloride was previously called 'corrosive sublimate'. The 'corrosive' refers to the fact that it attacks virtually all metals (including gold), so care is needed when using mercuric chloride as it will corrode jewellery (including wedding rings), scalpels and metal forceps. It will corrode metal piping, so prolonged disposal down laboratory sinks has been known to rot metal waste pipes and result in the flooding of laboratories.

Mercury and its compounds should not in any case be disposed of down the sink as it is toxic to sewage bacteria and will contaminate the effluent from sewage works.

---

contain double bonds it fixes lipids, and is the only fixative that really does so. For this reason it is widely used to fix lipid membranes for electron microscopy.

Fixation in osmium tetroxide makes proteins lose their acidophilia. It is volatile and can react with the cornea resulting in blindness. It must be handled only in fume cupboards.

Osmium tetroxide is widely used in electron microscopy as a fixative and stain for membranes, but is rarely used as a light microscopy fixative.

Acetic acid (ethanoic acid)

Although the correct chemical name is ethanoic acid, this is rarely heard in histology laboratories and the older, less systematic name of acetic acid is used universally. Unlike all of the preceding fixatives, acetic acid is a non-additive fixative and does not bind to any chemical groups in the tissues. Its main effect is to denature nucleic acids as a result of the pH change. It does not fix proteins and causes them to swell (especially collagen) and it effectively destroys mitochondrial staining.

Acetic acid is widely used to improve nuclear staining since it preserves DNA very well without blocking any dye-binding sites. The poor cytoplasmic staining from the loss of protein is an advantage in some types of work, e.g. chromosome studies where poor cytoplasmic preservation leaves the chromosomes more easily observed against a clear background. If a good cytoplasmic fixation is achieved, the cytoplasm will stain strongly and this will obscure the fine chromosome structure.

Acetic acid has often been included in fixative mixtures to combat the shrinkage of other fixatives (see *Box 2.6* for extra comments).

Alcohols (methanol, ethanol, propanol, butanol, etc.)

These are also non-additive fixatives and denature proteins and nucleic acids by removing their bound water and replacing it with the alcohol. This alters the shape of molecules (tertiary structure) without altering the reactive groups. Thus, alcohols preserve the chemical reactivity of many cellular materials and are popular in histochemical investigations.

The tissues do shrink considerably and may become overhard and brittle if long alcohol fixation is used. Alcohol is therefore less commonly used for fixing blocks of tissue, but is common for fixing smears or fresh sections (e.g. cryostat sections; see Chapter 5) where it is less of a problem if the cells become brittle as no further sectioning is needed.

Alcoholic fixation is probably more widespread than is acknowledged because a poorly fixed specimen is often processed unknowingly. The alcohol used in processing then acts as the fixative for any unfixed parts of the block.

Other fixatives

Many other chemicals have fixative properties, and fixatives in reasonably common use include picric acid, potassium dichromate and chromic acid. They all have some useful characteristics but their properties will not be dealt with in detail here.

Practical fixative solutions

Although the simple fixatives are the major component of most practical fixative solutions, they are rarely used as pure solutions and are usually made up with other compounds. These other components are often very important to the final result but are not directly involved in the fixation. They are used to control the environment around and within the tissues whilst fixation occurs.

The various types of additive can be grouped into three classes:

1. **To control tonicity (osmotic pressure).** Living cells are osmotic systems and will shrink in hypertonic solutions (high salt concentration) and swell and even burst in hypotonic solutions (pure water or low salt concentration). Blood plasma and cell cytoplasm have a tonicity of about 340 mOsm and this is said to be isotonic. The final tonicity of many practical fixatives is made hypertonic at around 400–450 mOsm. This is to ensure that, even when the fixative is removed by binding to tissues during the fixation process, the residual solution is still isotonic and will not cause cellular lysis due to osmotic imbalance. If the fluid became hypotonic before fixation was achieved, the cells might absorb water by osmosis resulting in swelling and eventual lysis.
2. **To control pH.** The use of buffers is preferred. Many buffers can be used including phosphate, Tris and cacodylates. The choice of buffer is controlled by other components. Phosphate buffers will precipitate if calcium or magnesium ions are added, whilst Tris and barbiturate buffers will react with aldehyde fixatives.

Box 2.7 Fixation by non-histologists can be done badly

Unfortunately fixation is often left to people who are not histologists. These include operating theatre staff who all too often mistakenly believe that the most important form of tissue breakdown is bacterial decay and so put tissues into antiseptics or disinfectants. These will certainly kill bacteria, but they do little else to preserve the tissues. Whenever possible, either do the fixation yourself or make sure that the person who does it understands what is needed; otherwise poor fixation and poor preservation will be the result.

I have personally received specimens from operating theatres in antiseptic solutions such as Savlon with dreadful results and even once in Domestos solution, which certainly killed the germs but did little to enhance the tissue preservation. I also received one specimen from a general dental practitioner in gin. This gave adequate preservation but I would not recommend it as a general fixative.

---

3. **Other additives for specific reasons.** For example, calcium is sometimes added to help preserve phospholipids, ammonium bromide is said to enhance the fixation of nervous tissue (particularly neuroglia) and detergents are used to remove membrane lipids and aid penetration of the fixative and other reagents such as lectins.

Physical conditions also play a major role and the temperature, volume and duration of fixation can also be critical.

Short fixation is common in histochemistry, especially when fixing frozen sections (2 min at 4°C, for example). Prolonged fixation in most reagents will result in overfixation and the tissue may become unusable. Even formaldehyde, which is often used for long-term storage of specimens, slowly alters the tissue, e.g. the ability of the tissue to stain with acid dyes becomes diminished.

The volume of fixative should be very large compared with the volume of tissue (20 times is a safe margin) since the fixative gets depleted or diluted by the tissue. This is often overlooked with very large specimens, which may be crammed into too small a container that is then topped up with fixative. A large ovarian cyst (whose total volume may be a litre or more) may arrive in the laboratory with less than 100 ml of fixative poured over it (see *Box 2.7*).

If the specimen is large and penetration is likely to be poor, the block should be cut into pieces small enough for diffusion of the fixative to reach all parts in a reasonable time. Alternatively the fixative can be perfused into the blood vessels and pumped through the vascular channels so that it reaches all parts of the tissue very quickly.

Compound fixatives

Since every simple fixative has deficiencies, many people have tried to improve fixation by using more than one fixative in a solution. The intention is to use the good properties of one fixative to counteract the bad properties of the other components.

For example, Zenker's fixative is based on mercuric chloride but has acetic

> **Box 2.8 Preservation in history and art**
>
> Fixation is usually associated with science, but Damien Hirst achieved notoriety by using animals in formaldehyde as examples of modern art. He exhibited a sheep in formaldehyde titled 'Away from the Flock' at the Serpentine Gallery in 1994, which was reputedly sold for £25,000. The mummified remains of the pharaohs have been icons of history for generations and the embalmed body of Lenin is an important tourist attraction in Moscow. Thus, preservation is also important outside the laboratory.

acid and potassium dichromate added to modify the results. Mercuric chloride was chosen to give good cytoplasmic staining but it suffers from being a very harsh fixative causing excessive hardening and shrinkage if used alone. Although a good protein fixative, it is less good with nucleic acids and lipids. Acetic acid causes swelling, which counteracts the shrinkage; it gives a softer fixation, ameliorating the hard fixation of the mercuric chloride, and it fixes nucleic acids very well. Unfortunately it does not fix lipids at all. Potassium dichromate preserves some lipids, especially phospholipids of membranes. It improves cytoplasmic staining but it may dissolve nucleic acids (however, acetic acid counteracts this effect). The overall result is a good general fixation and Zenker's has become a widely accepted fixative.

In formulating a compound fixative, some provisos should be noted. The fixatives chosen may add their own disadvantages without counteracting the bad points of the other fixatives. This summation of bad points can result in worse fixation than if only one fixative was used.

Mixing fixatives with different penetrating powers may result in very uneven fixation with only the outer part of the tissue being fixed in the full mixture. The slowest penetrating fixative may lag so far behind the other fixatives that the inner parts are fixed only by the faster-diffusing components.

Problems can also result if the component chemicals react with each other. Aldehydes are reducing agents, whilst osmium tetroxide is an oxidizing agent, so any solution containing both will deteriorate rapidly.

Finally, the use of several component fixatives means that it becomes difficult to predict all of the chemical reactions occurring during fixation. Thus, compound fixatives are not usually the best fixatives for critical histochemistry.

Although compound fixatives can be an improvement on simple fixatives, they still cannot be ideal for every purpose and each is usually designed for different and specific purposes. **Micro-anatomical fixatives** (e.g. Zenker's) are excellent for preserving general tissue structure and fixing larger blocks evenly but will be less good for cytological detail. **Cytological fixatives** are often good at preserving fine cytological detail in small blocks but are less useful for giving even fixation if the blocks are larger. Within the cytological fixatives there is further specialization since nucleic acids and cytoplasm are very different materials. **Nuclear fixatives** (e.g. Carnoy's) will preserve nuclei very well, whilst **cytoplasmic fixatives** (e.g. Helly's) are preferred for cytoplasmic detail.

Sequential fixation

This is a similar concept to the use of compound fixatives with the benefits of one fixative being added to those of another, but the fixatives are used sequentially rather than as a single solution. The primary fixative is almost always an aldehyde but the secondary fixative varies, with post-chroming (potassium dichromate), post-subliming (mercuric chloride) and post-osmicating (osmium tetroxide) all having their place.

The importance of correct fixation

When choosing a fixative it is important to get it right. Properly fixed tissues are easier to prepare and the final results are better. Poor or inappropriate fixation makes later processing and staining more difficult and may make certain investigations impossible. Thus, before fixing tissues, and indeed before starting to remove them from the body, the final purpose of the sections must be considered and the fixative chosen to match the requirements of the technique. Trying to match a staining technique to an inappropriately fixed tissue always gives inferior results.

SUGGESTED FURTHER READING

Bignold, L.P. (2002) Hypothesis for the influence of fixatives on the chromatin patterns of interphase nuclei, based on shrinkage and retraction of nuclear and perinuclear structures. *British Journal of Biomedical Science* **59**, 105–113.

Hopwood, D. (2002) Fixation and fixatives. In *Theory and Practice of Histological Techniques*, 5th edn (eds J.D. Bancroft and M. Gamble). Edinburgh: Churchill Livingstone.

Kiernan, J.A. (2001) *Histological and Histochemical Methods*, 3rd edn. Oxford: Hodder Arnold.

SELF-ASSESSMENT QUESTIONS

1. In what ways will tissue removed from the body change with time?
2. How can post-mortem changes be prevented?
3. List the properties of a good fixative.
4. Dettol will kill bacteria including those that cause putrefaction. Will Dettol be a good fixative?
5. Schiff's reagent is used to detect naturally occurring aldehydes in tissues. It can be used easily on formaldehyde-fixed tissues but not on glutaraldehyde-fixed tissues. Why is there this difference?
6. Why should all fixatives be handled and treated carefully?

Processing and microtomy

Learning objectives
After studying this chapter you should confidently be able to:

■ **Describe why tissue needs support during sectioning.**
Tissues are soft and will flex and not cut cleanly. Tissues are most commonly embedded in paraffin wax for ease of sectioning.

■ **Describe how tissues can be impregnated with wax using intermediate reagents.**
Processing tissues involves dehydration to remove water, clearing in an organic solvent to remove the alcohol and finally impregnation in molten wax.

■ **Name some common and useful dehydrating and clearing agents.**
Ethanol is commonly used for dehydration but acetone, methanol and propylene oxide are alternatives. Clearing agents include xylene, chloroform and petrol hydrocarbons.

■ **Describe the preparation of mineralized tissues for sectioning.**
The mineral content can be removed by treatment with acids and the tissue can then be processed as usual. Alternatively, undecalcified sections can be prepared, for example by grinding the hard tissue to give a thin slice.

Even fixed human tissues are generally quite soft and need extra support to allow thin sections to be cut. Sections are usually cut between 3 and 6 μm thick and the easiest way to prepare sections of this thickness is to use a hard embedding medium such as paraffin wax to support the cells and to hold the tissue firmly. **Processing** is the method by which tissues are converted into a block for **microtomy**.

3.1 PARAFFIN WAX IMPREGNATION

The commonest embedding medium in routine histology is paraffin wax. Although called a wax, it is actually composed of long-chain paraffin hydrocarbons and is similar to the material used to make candles. Paraffin wax is molten above 60°C but is solid at room temperature and has a hardness similar to the tissues once they have been impregnated. However, the specimen cannot simply be immersed in the wax as wax and water are immiscible and putting the tissue in molten wax will result only in the tissue being coated in wax (see *Box 3.1*). The water in the tissue is instead replaced by

---

Box 3.1 Support needs to be deep into the tissue

Originally the support for tissues was much less intimate and did not penetrate into the tissue but simply surrounded it. Botanists still often support stems and leaves during cutting by wrapping them in elder pith to make a more rigid structure. This is less easy to do with animal tissues that are much more irregular in shape and are less intrinsically rigid than plant tissues. Histologists therefore used wax. The tissues were dipped in molten wax that moulded itself to the irregular shape of the tissue and helped support it. This was still not totally successful and it was not until the wax was permeated into the tissue as well as around it that effective sectioning was possible.

---

wax so that the support runs completely through the tissues and supports them internally as well as externally (wax impregnation). The replacement of the tissue water with wax involves several steps and is generally called processing. One or more intermediate processing reagents are needed to remove the water, replace it with a reagent miscible with wax and then finally impregnate with the wax.

Processing tissues to wax with a single reagent

Although there are some reagents that are miscible with water and wax, they are not popular in histology. For example, dioxane (diethylene dioxide) can be used as a single bath and will mix completely with water and paraffin wax. The tissue can simply be taken from the fixative (which is usually a water-based solution) and placed in dioxane. The dioxane will then replace the water, although a couple of changes of solution may be needed to completely remove all of the water from the tissue. Once all of the water has been removed, the tissue can be transferred into molten wax, which then replaces the dioxane. Again, more than one bath of reagent is needed to completely remove all of the dioxane. Unfortunately, dioxane has problems, In particular, it is quite toxic, it is relatively expensive and the final results are poorer than using other methods. For these reasons, it has never become a common or popular method despite its relative simplicity.

Replacement of tissue water with wax using two intermediate steps

Instead of using a single reagent, double-stage processing is usually used. The first stage removes water (**dehydration**) and the second stage replaces the dehydrating agent with a reagent that is miscible with wax (termed **clearing**). The tissues are then impregnated with wax, placed in a mould and the wax is solidified. Sections can be cut from the wax block and then stained. Calcified tissues such as bone are extremely brittle in their natural state but can be decalcified to leave only the soft tissue matrix of the bone (osteoid), which can then be processed normally. *Fig. 3.1* shows how the steps are arranged. Each of these steps will be considered in more detail but it is important to grasp the general scheme of processing tissues.

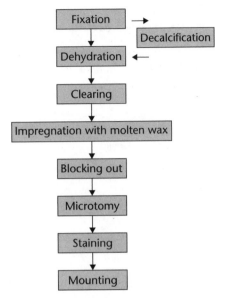

Figure 3.1
Flow of the specimen during processing. The fixed specimen is either transferred to
dehydrating agents directly or, if there is any mineralized bone present, it is decalcified
first before being dehydrated. The dehydration, clearing and impregnation with wax are
often done by a machine and can be considered as a single stage called **processing**

Choice of dehydration reagent

The first step in processing is dehydration of the tissue. In choosing a
reagent for dehydration, there are various properties that need to be considered. These are cost, safety, speed of action and its effect on tissues. The
speed of action is controlled by the viscosity of the solvent. Dehydration,
like most of the processing steps, is basically a diffusion process with the
solvent diffusing into the tissue and the water diffusing out. The rate of
diffusion into a relatively compact structure such as tissue is more dependent on the viscosity of the liquid than on simple molecular weight. Water
has a viscosity of 1 cP; higher numbers mean more viscous (thicker) fluids,
which will penetrate more slowly.

Safety considerations include both toxicity and flammability. Most of the
solvents used will burn but their flash points and fire risks vary. The properties of some dehydrating agents are listed in *Table 3.1*.

As with many steps in histological processing, the more rapid the removal
of water, the harsher the effect on the tissues. This applies equally to the
inherent speed of the reagent and to the graded series of strengths of the
reagent. Very gradual removal with a slow reagent may damage the tissues
less than rapid removal with a harsher reagent. It is always a trade-off
between speed and quality.

Table 3.1 Properties of dehydrating agents

Reagent	Viscosity	Toxicity	Fire hazard	Comments
Ethanol (IMS, 74OP)	1.2	?	+	Commonest reagent (see *Box 3.3*)
Methanol	0.6	++	+	Faster and harsher
Propanol	2.5	+	+	Slower
Acetone	0.4	++	++	Faster and harsh
Cellosolve (2-ethoxy ethanol)		+	+	Slower and gentler but destroys some elements
1-Epoxy propane (propylene oxide)		++ (carcinogen)	+++	Used in electron microscopy; inhibits some stains

Ethanol

Ethanol has long been used for removing water and is so ubiquitous in laboratories that if a method uses the term alcohol it will mean ethanol rather than any other alcohol. It is a fairly gentle reagent compared with many of the other agents that can be used. Its almost universal use is probably due to its low cost and low toxicity with little tissue damage. Ethanol will remove some materials from the tissue, but usually these same materials are removed by all dehydrating and clearing agents so this is not a problem unique to ethanol. Ethanol can be regarded as almost non-toxic in use (see *Box 3.2*) since the amounts liable to be ingested or inhaled, provided reasonable care is taken, are well below the levels known to cause damage.

During the process of dehydration it is usual to remove the water in a series of steps by using several baths of alcohol of gradually increasing strength (a 'graded series'). If the specimen is placed directly into concentrated alcohol, the tissue shrinks more and may become excessively hard. The actual concentrations of alcohol used in the graded series vary from laboratory to laboratory. Some processing schedules start with relatively weak mixtures (30% alcohol) and increase the strength very slowly, whilst others begin at 70% and move quickly to even higher concentrations. Most laboratories get good results, which suggests that any differences in the methods are small. It is usual to treat delicate tissues such as embryos with

Box 3.2 Safety of ethanol

Alcohol is unusual amongst laboratory chemicals in also being a foodstuff. It is included in the diets of many people. Alcohol is not seriously damaging to the skin and is the basis of many perfumes and aftershave lotions. Alcohol will slightly dry the skin by removing some of the natural oils and is also extremely painful if applied to cuts.

a more gradual removal as they are more easily damaged. Very tough tissues, however, may also benefit from a slower and gentler processing to prevent them becoming even tougher. Tough tissues can also be softened by adding other reagents to the dehydrating agents. The addition of phenol can have a beneficial effect on very tough materials.

Methanol

Methanol is important not only as a dehydrating agent in its own right but also because it is added to ethanol to give industrial methylated spirit (IMS), which is not drinkable (see *Box 3.3*) and so has a lower cost and is less strictly controlled than pure ethanol. Methanol is somewhat harsher than ethanol but is also faster and is sometimes used for rapid processing.

Higher alcohols such as propanol and butanol can be used as dehydrating agents but have no great advantages and are only occasionally used for specialized techniques where ethanol and methanol are unsuitable.

Box 3.3 Ethanol and excise regulations

Ethanol is cheap to produce but has the problem that the Customs and Excise people take a great deal of interest in, and duty from, anything alcoholic. Although laboratories can get the alcohol with reduced duty, they must keep accurate records to show that the alcohol is not being used illicitly. This explains the use of IMS instead of pure ethanol. Sometimes alcohol is referred to as 74OP spirit. This again is due to the Customs and Excise who used to test alcoholic spirits to 'prove' them. Originally, a spirit defined as 100° proof was the lowest strength of alcohol that, if poured on to gunpowder, would allow it to ignite. This was the original 'proof' of the spirit's strength. Anything stronger could be diluted and still pass the test so it was overproof (OP) spirit. Pure alcohol is equivalent to 174° proof, hence the term 74OP.

Acetone

Acetone, like methanol, is occasionally used as it will dehydrate a tissue more quickly than other reagents, but it does shrink and harden the tissue much more than ethanol. Acetone is also used more in electron microscopy (EM) than simple ethanol, as it is more readily miscible with the plastic resins used in EM. In EM, the hardening is less of a problem, as the resin gives stronger support than wax and shrinkage is usually less as the fixatives used harden the tissues more than the usual fixatives for wax processing. Acetone will dissolve more materials from the tissues than ethanol and is more of a danger as it has a low flash point and is more toxic than ethanol.

Propylene oxide

The use of this is almost entirely restricted to EM and even there some workers prefer to avoid it as it has a very high toxicity compared with other dehydrating agents. The miscibility of propylene oxide with resins is its only real advantage over other agents.

Cellosolve

Cellosolve has the reputation of being gentler than other reagents. Tissues may be left in cellosolve for long periods without becoming excessively hard and it has been recommended for embryos. Generally, it is not popular because of its cost. It readily absorbs water from the air so careful storage is essential.

Ensuring complete dehydration

Complete dehydration is essential, as the clearing reagents and waxes are usually intolerant of even small amounts of water. To ensure complete removal of all of the water it is important to have at least two baths of 100% alcohol (three or more are often used). The first 100% alcohol bath rapidly becomes contaminated with small amounts of water carried over from the previous lower concentration (e.g. 95% alcohol) bath. The second bath effectively removes all of the water. It is still essential to replace the reagents regularly as there will always be a gradual transfer of water from one bath to the next. It is possible to use anhydrous copper sulphate to test for water in the alcohol baths. When the alcohol is dry the copper sulphate remains white but when water gets into the alcohol it will turn blue and the reagent needs to be changed. To save on reagent costs, it is common simply to move these reagents one step lower down the chain when they become slightly contaminated. Thus, only the final 100% alcohol is replaced by fresh reagent. The old final bath becomes the penultimate bath and so on.

Safety is very important with dehydrating agents as they are used in such large quantities. Alcohol has a relatively low toxicity, whilst propylene oxide is very toxic. For this reason many people are turning away from propylene oxide, even for EM. Fire risks are also important since most laboratories now use electrically driven machines and these may produce sparks. I know of at least two laboratories that have caught fire and burnt down from fires that have started in the processing rooms.

Clearing

This is the next step and involves the removal of the dehydrating agent, usually alcohol, and its replacement with a solvent miscible with wax. It was originally named thus because many of the reagents had a similar refractive index to the tissues and so cleared them optically (as xylene does). Optical clearing means that the tissues become transparent once they have been completely permeated by the reagent. Although most modern reagents do not optically clear the tissues, they are still usually referred to as clearing agents (perhaps because they 'clear' the alcohol out of the tissues). Other names have been suggested (e.g. antemedia or dealcoholizing reagents) but the term clearing is still the most common. For hand processing of tissues, there is still an advantage in optical clearing, as it allows the person processing the tissue to see how clearing is progressing; when the tissue is completely transparent, clearing is complete.

Clearing agents

Many organic solvents can act as clearing agents. Many different agents have been used and they all have their own advantages and problems (see *Table 3.2*). Several properties are crucial in evaluating the usefulness of reagents:

1. Speed. Two factors are included: firstly, the speed of removal of alcohol from the tissues, and secondly, the speed of evaporation of the clearing agent from the wax bath. The speed of removal from wax is related to the boiling point of the clearing agent.
2. Harshness of their action and how much shrinkage or hardening they cause.
3. Flammability.
4. Toxicity.
5. Cost.

Table 3.2 Properties of clearing agents

Clearing agent	Boiling point (°C)	Refractive index	Toxicity	Flammability
Toluene	110.6	1.5	++	++
Xylene	138	1.5	+++	++
Chloroform	61.5	1.45	++	–
Cedarwood oil	Variable	1.5	0	Weak
Petroleum hydrocarbons	157	1.3–1.5	+	++
1,1,1-Trichloroethane	75	1.43	+	–

Whereas alcohol is universally used as a routine dehydrating agent, there is still variation in which clearing agent is used routinely in different laboratories. Clearing agents are generally much more toxic than alcohol and, being volatile, they need to be treated with caution (see *Box 3.4*). It is generally toxicity that forces the change from one solvent to another rather than poor section quality. For many years, benzene was the clearing agent of choice in many laboratories, but the increased risk of leukaemia in people exposed to the vapour made it less popular for use and today it is rarely used.

Toluene (methyl benzene) was used as a replacement for benzene but again suffers from the problem of toxicity. It is similar in many respects to xylene but not as popular.

Xylene. Many people still use xylene, which has a lower toxicity than benzene but is still quite toxic. Xylene is used less in preparing blocks, as its harsh action leaves tissues more brittle and harder than many of the other clearing agents. However, it is still very popular for clearing sections after staining where the hardness and brittleness are less of a disadvantage.

Box 3.4 Disposal of solvents

As well as being dangerous to use, clearing agents are also dangerous to dispose of. Many are combustible and can be burnt, but this requires very high temperatures and is not practicable for most laboratories. Passing the waste on to a specialist disposal firm is often the best alternative but does carry a high cost. This cost of disposal should be added to the purchase cost when considering which agent to use.

An alternative for large laboratories is recycling of the waste material. Specialist closed stills are available that will redistill solvents including alcohol and most clearing agents. The capital costs can be high, as they need a special room and careful monitoring to ensure safety. Providing the through-put is high enough, they can repay the costs in a couple of years. Recycling can be dangerous if picric acid is used, as it is explosive.

Not even very small amounts of clearing agents should be allowed to get into the normal waste disposal system, as they will not be effectively rinsed away and diluted. They are not miscible with water and will remain in the traps of sinks. Xylene tends to float, so a layer of xylene will remain floating in the trap and the fumes will be released. Constant exposure to small amounts of solvents will degrade the rubber and plastic components of the waste system and produce leaks.

Chlorinated solvents have also been used. Carbon tetrachloride (tetrachloromethane) was quite popular at one time, as it is almost non-flammable (it was used in fire extinguishers), but it has severe hepatotoxicity problems. Chloroform (trichloromethane) has a similar toxicity but is still used by some laboratories. 1,1,1-Trichloroethane (used as a dry-cleaning fluid) has a lower toxicity; however, its use is now restricted as it adversely affects the ozone layer.

Chlorinated hydrocarbons are usually denser and heavier than other clearing agents. This has two consequences. Firstly, and most obviously, they are heavier to lift and secondly, many tissues will float in them. This is worth remembering if a cassette holding tissues falls open in the processor, as you will need at look in the top of the reagent and not at the bottom as you might expect.

Petrol hydrocarbons/aliphatic hydrocarbons are now being promoted as a safer alternative to xylene. They appear to be suitable for tissue processing but have problems as clearing agents before coverslipping, as they are less miscible with common mounting media.

Cedarwood oil. This a slow-acting clearing agent, which has very little hardening effect on tissues. It is a very traditional clearing agent and was highly rated in the past, but is hardly ever used today because of its cost and slow speed of action. It has a distinctive odour that never seems to disappear completely from the wax, so the blocks have a faint but pleasant smell. Although it will burn, it does not readily catch fire and is not a real fire risk.

Many other reagents have been tried as clearing agents including simple petrol (inflammable but cheap), cooking oil (cheap and non-toxic) and essential oils such as lavender oil or sandalwood oil (very expensive but the laboratory smells lovely!).

Choice of clearing reagent

No one reagent has so far emerged as a clear winner. Each laboratory has different priorities. For some laboratories, price is more important than getting the very best quality, whereas others want perfection regardless of cost. Some laboratories use such small amounts of clearing agent that toxicity and flammability can be controlled and so this is less of a worry. Other laboratories use solvents on an industrial scale and need to consider safety in a different way.

The dehydrating agent must be removed completely from the tissue so three or more baths of clearing agent are needed to ensure complete replacement. Reagents need to be changed regularly as mentioned above for the alcohols. Again, the final bath can be reused as an earlier bath to save replacing all of the reagents at once.

Impregnation with molten wax

After clearing is complete, the tissues are passed through two to four baths of fresh molten wax. The wax is held at no more than 2–3°C above its melting point, rather than at much higher temperatures, as heat is very damaging to tissues.

Different waxes have different melting points. Usually a wax with a melting point in the in the range of 50–60°C is used. As a general rule, the higher the melting point of the wax, the harder the wax is at room temperature. Ideally, the hardness of the wax and the hardness of the tissue should be the same so that the texture of the wax and the block are even and when a section is cut, the knife moves smoothly through the block and does not 'jump' on encountering a different texture. In most laboratories a compromise is used, with one hardness being used for most specimens. The slight differences in texture between one tissue and the next are usually small enough to be ignored.

There are also specialist waxes that contain additives (such as plasticizers) or microcrystalline waxes to aid in the cutting. These are available ready prepared and are usually known by their commercial names. They often have excellent properties and have replaced not only simple paraffin wax but also some of the specialized embedding techniques (see Chapter 4).

Removal of clearing agents

The clearing agent needs to be completely removed from the final wax bath. If some persists in the block, it will later evaporate from the surface of the block. The block may initially cut quite well but after a few days or weeks the tissue will shrink, leaving the surface concave and below the surface of the wax.

The clearing agent is not just washed out of the tissue by the wax bath, it is also removed by evaporation. The wax bath is often at a high enough temperature to cause significant amounts of the clearing agent to 'boil off'. This evaporation is often the most sensitive way to tell when the final wax bath needs changing. If the final wax bath smells of clearing agent, then it needs changing.

Evaporation of the clearing agent and removal of air bubbles can be helped by using reduced pressure in the final wax bath(s). This is called 'vacuum embedding', although a true vacuum is not needed, simply a significantly reduced pressure (about 50–75 % of atmospheric pressure will suffice).

Blocking out of tissues

Once all of the clearing agent has been removed, the tissue is blocked out in a mould (see *Box 3.5*) containing fresh wax. It is oriented so that the correct surface will be cut during microtomy and the block is then cooled quickly. Rapid cooling prevents larger wax crystals forming and makes the block more homogeneous, improving the cutting quality of the block.

Once the tissue is embedded in the wax, it remains stable, so the next stages can be performed slowly, allowing careful preparation of fine sections. The block can also be stored for many years without deterioration. For unusual or important specimens, the blocks can be stored indefinitely and often prove a useful source of retrospective material for research. The use of archival tissue is subject to The Human Tissue Act (see Chapter 17).

Box 3.5 Moulds for blocking out

Blocking out originally used L-shaped brass blocks (Leuckhart's angles), which could be moved to make a variable-sized mould. The wax rapidly cools and solidifies so a fluid tight seal is not needed.

After cooling, the blocks were trimmed with a scalpel or small knife and then attached to a fibre or wood block by melting the lower surface and pressing it on to the surface. It was easy to get the labels mixed up with so many separate steps.

Next came disposable moulds and the integrated cassette and mould system, which is now commonly used. The blocks are directly mounted on the cassette they were processed in and the cassette fits into a special holder in the microtome. There is less scope for a mix up, the blocks are dealt with more rapidly and throughput is greater.

3.2 HAND VERSUS AUTOMATIC PROCESSING

It is possible to process the tissues manually or using an automated schedule on an automatic tissue processor.

Hand processing

Tissues can be processed by hand using a series of containers with the various reagents in sequence. This requires somebody to transfer the tissues. It is tedious and time-consuming but very flexible (each tissue can be treated differently). It is generally slower since there is not constant agitation of the reagent. If left without agitation, the reagent diffusing out of the specimen will form a static stagnant layer around the tissue and slow down the processing.

Hand processing is cheap to implement and is still used by laboratories with a very small throughput of blocks. Even large laboratories may occasionally use hand processing for unusual specimens where setting up an automatic processor for a single specimen would be impractical.

Automated processing

Automatic processing uses a machine to carry out all the changes and includes some method of programming so that the time in each reagent can be controlled. Typically about 12 changes of reagent are accommodated by a single machine and times in the baths can be varied from a few minutes up to several hours. The machines are intended to run unsupervised so that processing can be done overnight. The start can also be delayed so that the machine can run over a weekend without the specimens being left too long in the final reagent. The machines usually have facilities for thermostatically controlled wax baths and many can apply a partial vacuum to one or more steps. This allows the machine to carry out the complete processing schedule, taking the specimens from fixative right through to wax impregnation. Schedules can be changed quickly and easily and may be computer/microprocessor controlled. This makes processing very easy. Specimens are placed in the machine and can then be left unattended (see *Box 3.6*). Many laboratories have schedules arranged so that a specimen placed in the machine on an afternoon will have completed the processing schedule by the following morning and will be ready for blocking out into moulds when staff arrive. Paraffin processing often looks complex when written down, but is extremely easy with a machine to do the tedious work.

Many specimens (up to hundreds in large machines) are processed simultaneously. Each specimen is placed in a labelled cassette to keep it separate from all of the others and a batch of cassettes is placed in the machine. The actual structure and mechanism of the machines differ. In some, the reagents are in large beakers and the specimens are held in a basket, which

---

Box 3.6 Fire risks of processing

The use of flammable liquids such as alcohols and hydrocarbons in processing makes it a fire risk. This is especially true once the system becomes automated. Automatic processors are electric and have electrically heated wax baths. A spark from an electric motor or thermostat can easily result in a major fire. To prevent this, most modern machines are completely enclosed and the vapours are prevented from escaping by always using a partial vacuum so that the air flow is into the chamber. The reagents are pumped into and out of this evacuated chamber and stored in sealed containers when not in use. Older machines, which used relatively open baths of reagents, were always a fire risk. Some laboratories were destroyed by fire, which also meant the loss of irreplaceable diagnostic tissue samples.

is then moved from one beaker to the next. In other machines, there is only one bath into which the specimens are placed and the reagents are pumped into and out of the chamber. This allows a sealed system and a vacuum can be applied to the bath. Both types have similar applications; only the cost and number of specimens is different.

Automatic processing is generally faster, more reliable and can be done overnight. It is less flexible since all the specimens in one batch get the same times regardless of size, etc. Some newer machines are incorporating microwave treatment which speeds up the process, allowing blocks to be fully processed in a few hours. If the laboratory is large, then it may be able to justify several automatic processors set up with a variety of schedules so individual blocks can get more specialized treatment.

3.3 DECALCIFICATION

Tissues such as bone and teeth are strengthened and hardened by the addition of the mineral hydroxyapatite, a calcium phosphate salt, with smaller amounts of magnesium, potassium, chlorides and carbonates. The mineral content of the tissue is about 70% in bone, about 97% in dentine and over 99% in tooth enamel. Hydroxyapatite is hard and makes routine sectioning difficult. The tissue can be softened by removing the mineral; this process is usually called decalcification, although it also removes other materials in addition to calcium.

Box 3.7 Decalcification of teeth

The very high mineral content of enamel makes it almost impossible to decalcify teeth and still retain the enamel layer. The enamel has almost no organic content to hold it together, so once the mineral disappears the enamel layer becomes very fragile and falls apart. Enamel and dentine can also be decalcified *in situ* in the mouth by the acids produced by bacteria. Teeth are also attacked by highly acidic drinks such as lemon juice or cola. Cola drinks contain phosphoric acid and may have a pH of around 4. This is quite low enough to be used as a decalcifying solution.

Decalcification with acid solutions

Hydroxyapatite is soluble at low pH and can be removed by treating the tissues with acid:

$$Ca_{10}(PO_4)_6(OH)_2 = 10Ca^{2+} + 6PO_4^{3-} + 2OH^-$$

The mineral is usually in equilibrium with the body fluids, but if the pH is lowered, then the excess hydrogen ions combine with the hydroxyl ions to give water. This removal of the hydroxyl ions drives the reaction to the right, giving a net result of:

$$Ca_{10}(PO_4)_6(OH)_2 + 20H^+ \rightarrow 10Ca^{2+} + 6H_3PO_4 + 2H_2O$$

The calcium ions will form salts with whatever acid is being used (e.g. calcium chloride with hydrochloric acid).

Soft tissue damage caused by acid solutions

Mineral acids such as hydrochloric acid and nitric acid are generally faster than organic acids but cause more **maceration** of the tissues. Maceration involves swelling of tissues, loss of staining ability and generally poorer morphology. Maceration is result of the hydrogen ions causing hydrolysis of proteins and nucleic acids and is worse if the tissue is inadequately fixed. Although thorough fixation minimizes the effects of maceration, it cannot totally prevent some deterioration. Maceration is also increased by leaving tissues in acid for longer than necessary or by using higher temperatures to speed up decalcification. Decalcification is always a compromise between speed and quality of morphology.

Acid decalcifying solutions

Different acid decalcifying solutions give a choice between quality and speed. Acids that are used in practice include:

Nitric acid (e.g. Perenyi's fluid). This is very fast acting but causes severe maceration if used for more than a few hours. It is only suitable for very urgent cases. Old stocks of nitric acid often turn a yellowish colour and this exaggerates the disruption and also stains the tissue. The addition of urea is sometimes recommended to help prevent the disruption and discoloration.

Hydrochloric acid has been used and is often a part of commercial or proprietary decalcifying solutions. Although it works well, it does cause maceration, although not as much as nitric acid. It should not be mixed with formaldehyde as it can produce a carcinogen.

Formic acid is probably the most common decalcifying acid and is used at a concentration of between 5 and 30%. It is significantly slower than the mineral acids but causes less damage.

Acetic acid and peracetic acid can also be used but are even slower than formic acid. However, they do not adversely affect nuclear staining.

Some acids are unsuitable as decalcifying agents. Sulphuric acid, for example, forms insoluble calcium sulphate, which is extremely difficult to remove.

Chelating agents as non-acidic decalcifying solutions

An alternative to using acids is to use a chelating agent. These decalcify by continuously removing the small amount of free ionic calcium that is always present around the bone mineral. This removal acts in the same way as the removal of hydroxide ions drives the equilibrium to the right in the equation given above. However, chelating agents have a much slower action. The main chelating agent used is EDTA (ethylenediaminetetraacetic acid). Since this reaction can occur at neutral pH, there is no damage to fixed tissue and preservation is excellent, although decalcification is very slow (it may take months to completely decalcify larger pieces of bone or teeth).

Acceleration of decalcification

Many attempts have been made to speed up decalcification, but some methods also accelerate maceration. The most effective action is regular replacement of the decalcifying solution. This replenishes the acidity and speeds up decalcification. Simple agitation to prevent the layer of fluid around the specimen becoming saturated with calcium is also very effective. Constant agitation is not required; an occasional shake seems to work well, although any gentle automatic agitation will be beneficial.

Heating the solution certainly speeds up the reaction but also speeds up the maceration reactions, so gives no real benefit. The use of electrical currents (electrolysis) and ultrasonic treatment seem to speed up decalcification, but this seems to be mainly due to their heating effects rather than any more subtle effect. If the solutions are kept cool, then there is no real increase in speed.

By using an organic acid in a buffered state, it is possible to keep the hydrogen ion concentration more uniform. As the hydroxide ions neutralize the hydrogen ions in an unbuffered solution, the rate of decalcification falls as the pH rises. In a buffer, the hydrogen ions are replaced at the same rate as they are removed, so decalcification is more evenly paced.

The inclusion of an ion-exchange resin in the solution has been used to try and give the same replenishing effect. This seems to be rather more tedious to use than simply buffering the solution since the resin needs to be regenerated after use. Ion-exchange resins can only be used with organic acids and they prevent the use of the chemical end-point test (see below).

Buffering is advantageous, and one of the best decalcifying agents is a mixture of formic acid and trisodium citrate. The citrate acts as a buffer salt and also as a chelating agent. The pH is quite moderate and causes minimal maceration, but it is still quite a slow decalcifying solution.

Decalcification in fixatives

Acids must of course be avoided if the bone is to be examined as an undecalcified specimen (see *Box 3.8*). Sources of acid in processing include acetic and peracetic acids, picric acid and unbuffered formaldehyde solutions (these may contain formic acid). Acetic acid- and picric acid-containing fixatives will decalcify very small fragments of bone during fixation. This can be useful for bone marrow specimens where there may be a few tiny fragments of bone present but it is not worthwhile doing a full decalcifica-

> **Box 3.8 Undecalcified sections**
>
> Undecalcified sections are needed when the actual process of bone mineralization is being investigated. This occurs in bone diseases such as osteoporosis. There is no theoretical difference between undecalcified bone sections and soft tissue sectioning, but the practical problems and difficulties are much greater with the rigid and brittle mineralized tissues. They can also be prepared by the totally different method of ground sections. In this technique, rather than removing a section from a block by microtomy, the thin section is prepared by removing all of the unwanted block by grinding it away. One side of the specimen is ground flat and then attached to a slide. The exposed side of the block is then ground away until the required thinness is achieved. This is quite wasteful of tissue as only one section is prepared from each block. Machines to grind sections automatically are available as this is the standard way of making geological slides from rock samples. In fact, geologists consider bone to be very soft rather than hard. I suppose it is if you compare it with granite.

tion. Fixation in an acetic acid-containing fixative softens the tiny fragments allowing the tissue to cut without delaying the specimen.

Accurate determination of the end point of decalcification

The 'end point' of decalcification is the moment when the last calcium deposit is removed leaving only the soft tissues. The end point needs to be determined accurately so that the specimen is removed from the destructive acid bath as soon as possible. The end point can be determined by several methods.

X-rays

This is probably the most accurate method but is inconvenient for most laboratories. Tissues are placed on top of an X-ray film (held in a light-tight cassette) and exposed to sufficient X-rays to make the film very dark but not quite completely black. Any calcium deposits show as white areas on the developed X-ray film, whilst soft tissues appear as a faint grey background. This can be expensive as it requires X-ray films. It can be used to show how decalcification is proceeding, as well as indicating when it is complete.

Chemical testing

A sample of the decalcifying fluid is taken and neutralized with hydroxide solution. Adding ammonium oxalate to this neutralized solution will show whether calcium is present by producing a precipitate, which appears slightly hazy if viewed against a dark background. If calcium is detected, this means that decalcification is still proceeding and the decalcifying fluid should be changed and retested a few hours later. Once there is no faint precipitate, it can be assumed that decalcification is complete.

> **Box 3.9 Using a spare piece of bone to test for the end point**
>
> A slightly better method of manual testing by poking is to set up a decalcification using a test piece of bone the same size as the specimen and decalcify it in parallel with the specimen. This piece of bone can be bent, needled and even cut to see if it decalcified. When the test sample is decalcified the other piece is assumed to be complete. This method is not particularly accurate as the density of the bones may not be identical, but it is useful as a guide.

Manual testing

This includes testing by bending or poking with a needle (NOT recommended, but see *Box 3.9*). Although it is possible to detect calcified tissue by its rigidity, this method can cause damage to the tissue, especially if it is repeated many times.

Washing

Following decalcification the block should be washed free of acid in either a sodium sulphate solution or alcohol (simply washing in water causes further swelling) and the tissue can then be processed as for soft tissue.

3.4 MICROTOMY

The wax blocks can be cut using a microtome. This is a finely engineered machine capable of slicing sections regularly at 5 μm or less. There are many types of microtome from small hand-held ones to extremely large ones that can fill a small room. They all have certain characteristics in common:

1. A mechanism for holding the block firmly. The block is usually attached to a holder or chuck and this is clamped in a jaw mechanism.
2. A knife holder.
3. A mechanism to move the knife across the surface of the block to cut the section.
4. A feed mechanism to advance the block so that subsequent sections can be cut at the required thickness.

The engineering ingenuity that has gone into achieving these characteristics is quite remarkable and most microtomists have their own favourite type of microtome.

Some microtomes are better for particular purposes. The factors that make one microtome better than another, or at least better for one purpose, depend mainly on the specimen and what is required from it. Considerations include:

1. How big is the block? The bigger the block, the larger the microtome needed, but large microtomes can be inconvenient for small specimens.

2. How hard is the block? Very hard blocks of bone or tooth need a specialized microtome but such machines are usually somewhat tedious to use for soft specimens.
3. Are serial sections needed? Serial sections are where several adjacent sections are cut in order to follow structures, e.g. nerves, through the tissue or where exactly adjacent sections are used to apply more than one staining technique to the one specimen. A microtome that can produce ribbons is best for such work.
4. Cost.

Microtome types

Hand microtome

These are very simple with a small flat circular table around a central hollow pillar. The specimen is placed in the centre of the pillar and can be inched gradually up above the table. (It should be 'micrometred' up but that doesn't sound right in English.) By slicing across, using the table as a guide plate, thin sections can be cut. These are not suitable for serious histology and are mainly used for relatively thick sections of botanical specimens.

Rocking microtome

These are quite small microtomes with two rocking arms. One arm gives the cutting action, whilst the other acts as a feed mechanism. These small microtomes were once common but have largely disappeared from laboratory use. They are still used as 'student microtomes' as they are cheap and robust. They are limited to cutting small blocks and soft tissue since the actual cutting action is done by a spring. They were also very popular in cryostats (see Chapter 5) as they have no sliding parts (the only movement is a rocking movement), so they had no problems with lubrication at the low temperatures used in a cryostat (even thin oils become sticky at −20°C).

Rotary microtomes

These are more robust microtomes with a rotating handle. They are very popular in laboratories and come in a variety of sizes. They can produce nice ribbons of sections and are quite reliable if well maintained, but can be prone to wear if badly maintained, when they then become quite erratic in use. Once you are familiar with them, they can be quick and easy to use. They are not quite as good as a sliding microtome for very large or very hard blocks.

Sliding microtomes

These are usually much heavier and larger machines than the other types of microtome. The cutting action is by sliding a heavy 'sledge' under a knife. They can cut very large and hard blocks, but are heavier to use as a consequence. They are quite popular and in some laboratories are used to cut all specimens, even small soft ones.

Microtome knives

The knife used in a microtome is equally important. It must be very sharp and the edge must be free from blemishes. Knives can be solid and need sharpening or they can be disposable. Solid knives can be sharpened by hand, although this is no longer common, or sharpened by machines.

There is no great difficulty in understanding how knives are sharpened as it is fairly straightforward and logical. Sharpening involves removing metal from the edge of the knife to create a new sharp cutting edge. Large nicks are removed using a coarse abrasive (silicon carbide, also known as carborundum, or diamond powders) and then using finer abrasives to remove the scratches left by the coarse abrasives. Hand grinding usually uses hones or sharpening stones of different grades.

Sharpening machines can use powders (suspended in water or oil) and a hard glass or metal plate. These types of machine suffer from the fact that, as the plate wears away the metal of the knife to sharpen it, the knife also wears away the material of the plate and thus causes it to lose its original flat surface. The knives gradually become curved instead of having a straight edge.

The most popular sharpening machines now use a soft metal plate into which a diamond paste is rubbed. The plate becomes studded with very fine diamond particles and the knife is sharpened on a thin layer of diamond, which is regularly renewed; thus, the plate itself does not wear away. This requires the use of several plates, however, as each plate represents one grade of abrasive and you cannot mix coarse and fine abrasives on the same plate.

Whilst sharpening is occurring, the knife is wearing away. Since the knife is held at a constant angle this means that the knife develops a facet, which is the actual cutting edge. The facet grows larger with constant sharpening, so the knife becomes more difficult to sharpen and sections become more difficult to cut. Eventually the knife becomes unusable for fine sectioning and is either relegated to 'trimming' or is reground to give a new small facet but at a different angle.

Very acute angles of the facet are 'sharper' but lose their sharpness more

---

Box 3.10

There is nothing that brings out the argumentative side of histologists more than suggesting that the microtome or knife they are using is inferior. The relative benefits and shortcomings of these machines can be discussed at great length.

In reality, the only criterion is whether it produces a good section. Most microtomes in the hands of a good microtomist will cut good sections from most blocks. Only with the very hard or very large blocks does the choice of microtome become crucial.

Microtomy has improved greatly over the years and sections are now routinely cut much thinner than a few years ago. The advent of the disposable knife has been a major factor in this improvement.

There are a few unusual types of microtome in some specialist laboratories. The Tetrander and Jung K microtomes were produced for very large and very hard blocks, respectively, and would not look out of place in a heavy machine shop, as they are pretty substantial instruments.

Box 3.11 Knife profiles

Biconcave   Plano-concave   Wedge   D profile

Solid knives are available in a variety of cross-sectional shapes. The biconcave and plano-concave shapes are good for soft tissues and have a narrow leading edge that can produce an acutely angled and sharp facet. The wedge and D profile knives are more rigid and used for harder blocks. The wedge shape is usually preferred for frozen sections

---

quickly. Thin edges are less rigid and when used with hard blocks they may produce 'chattering'. Chatters are where the section thickness varies across the block as the knife edge moves slightly. The final section shows thick and thin stripes. Less acute facets last longer and are more rigid but cannot cut such fine sections (see *Box 3.11*).

Disposable knives are gradually replacing solid knives in routine histology. They involve less capital cost (for example, no knife-sharpening equipment is needed) and a fresh knife is always available. One of the horrors for a microtomist is when all of his knives are damaged at the same time and he is stuck until they are resharpened. Disposable knives possibly cost more in day-to-day running expenses, but the ease of use and the fact that it does not matter if the knife gets damaged usually outweigh this in a busy laboratory where urgency is paramount.

For very hard specimens, special knives may be required. These can be made of extra-hard materials, usually tungsten, and are not disposable. Also, very large specimens are not suitably catered for by the manufacturers of disposable knives, so non-disposable knives are needed for very large and very hard blocks.

Cutting the section

Cutting is not automatic it needs skill and sometimes can be difficult. It is a practical skill and is best learnt by actually doing it. Problems are usually caused by:

1. Poor impregnation. This means that the tissue is inadequately supported and will crumble or fold instead of cutting nicely. Poor support can also result from using wax of the wrong temperature (usually too soft) or if the room is too hot causing the wax to soften. Cooling the block with a block of ice may help.
2. A blunt knife. This is usually quite easy to spot in practice.
3. The wrong knife angle. This is probably one of the few things that can be tried quickly during cutting but once the angle is right it will not usually need changing between blocks.

Box 3.12 Use of Sellotape in cutting

To help cut difficult specimens, it is possible to give extra support by covering the surface of the block with a material such as Sellotape or specialized films that polymerize. The Sellotape is pressed firmly on to the face of the block and as the section is cut, the Sellotape and section are lifted off. The sections are then attached to slides using an adhesive but without being floated on to a water-bath. The Sellotape is usually removed using a solvent to dissolve the glue before the section is stained. This method is used for cutting undecalcified bone sections.

A solution of nitrocellulose in alcohol can also be used by painting it on to the block face. This leaves a thin layer of nitrocellulose on the block. This gives less support than Sellotape but is easier to remove.

---

4. Slackness in the microtome. This results in alternate thick and thin sections or in chattering, depending on how much slackness or unwanted movement there is.

There are many tricks and dodges, which are learnt with practice (e.g. see *Box 3.12*) and experience, and no amount of 'book learning' will ever replace simply sitting at a microtome and cutting.

Sections can be cut at different thickness. Thick sections are useful for low-power microscopy, for tracing long structures such as nerves as they travel through tissues and for some histochemical techniques. Thin sections are needed for fine intracellular detail and high-power microscopy (especially in photomicrography). For routine wax sections, a thickness of 3–6 µm is usual.

Floating and mounting

All microtomes have a chopping rather than a cutting action and this has a tendency to compress the section in the direction of cutting. This can result in wrinkles or folds in the section. To get rid of the wrinkles, the section is floated on to a bath of warm water. This does not melt the wax but softens it sufficiently for the tissues to recover their original shape and size. Gentle prodding with a soft brush can also help to flatten the section. For stubborn wrinkles, it is sometimes useful to float the section on to a few drops of alcohol on a slide first and then float it on to the warm water. The turbulence produced as the alcohol mixes with the warm water may sometimes gently ease out the wrinkles.

Sections can then be lifted on to a clean slide. The slide is held in the water-bath vertically and the section lifted on to it by withdrawing the slide still held vertically. This works much better than trying to slip the slide horizontally under the section and then trap it on the slide. Withdrawing the slide vertically also traps less water and is less likely to trap air bubbles under the section.

If a ribbon of sections has been cut, then either individual sections or a short length of the ribbon containing several sections can be cut from the ribbon either before floating out or on the surface of the waterbath and then picked up as for single sections. The slide should then be labelled. Some slides have ground glass areas that will accept a soft pencil writing on them but plain slides should be labelled by scratching with a diamond-tipped stylus. Ordinary felt-tip pens, paper labels and most forms of ink will not survive the staining and mounting process and the labelling will be lost.

Once picked up on to a slide, the sections are drained well and then dried on to the slide to achieve adhesion. This can be done at any temperature from 37°C to temperatures high enough to melt the wax. Lower temperatures cause less damage to the tissue. If the wax melts, then the tissue may disintegrate completely. However, at 37°C many hours may be needed for complete drying. If drying is incomplete, the sections will detach during staining. Drying can be done in an oven or on a hotplate. The oven method is somewhat slower than using the same temperature with a hotplate, but there is less contamination from dust settling on the slide if it is dried vertically in an oven rather than horizontally on a hotplate on an open bench.

If there are problems with sections adhering or if the staining method is particularly harsh and liable to remove the section, adhesion can be improved by coating the slides. Special slides coated with silane (3-amino-propyltriethoxysilane) are available; these have a surface charge, which helps the section cling to the slide. It is possible to coat ordinary slides with 2% silane in acetone and then drain and dry them, but this reagent is quite dangerous.

It is also possible to use chemical adhesives in the form of protein, such as egg albumen, serum, gelatine or poly-L-lysine, which are used to coat the slides prior to picking up the sections. Although these do help adhesion, they may stain with some techniques, causing background problems.

SUGGESTED FURTHER READING

Anderson, G. and Bancroft, J.D. (2002) Tissue processing and microtomy including frozen. In *Theory and Practice of Histological* Techniques, 5th edn (eds J.D. Bancroft and M. Gamble). Edinburgh: Churchill Livingstone.
Culling, C.F.A. (1975) *Handbook of Histopathological and Histochemical Techniques*. London: Butterworths.

SELF-ASSESSMENT QUESTIONS

1. Why are tissues commonly embedded in wax for section cutting?
2. Name, in order, the steps needed to prepare a paraffin wax block.
3. What is a 'graded series' of alcohol and what is its purpose? Name three alternatives to alcohol.
4. How did clearing agents get their name?
5. Name four clearing agents and compare their advantages and problems.
6. What is meant by vacuum embedding?
7. How can mineralized bone be softened for sectioning?
8. Outline how undecalcified bone sections can be prepared.

9. A piece of bone marrow is fixed in a mixture of methanol and acetic acid. Sections of the bone fragments show no sign of calcium. Does this indicate that the patient had osteomalacia (calcium deficiency)?

10. Outline the uses and advantages of tungsten knives, disposable knives and plano-concave knives in microtomy.

Other embedding techniques

Learning objectives
After studying this chapter you should confidently be able to:

■ **Name an alternative to wax embedding and outline the advantages of the medium.**
Plastics (resins) give firmer support and allow thinner sections to be cut.

■ **Briefly describe the preparation of plastic (resin)-embedded sections in light and electron microscopy.**
Processing tissues involves dehydration to remove water but clearing is not always needed. Tissues are impregnated in a fluid plastic monomer, which is then hardened by polymerization. The polymer is not always easy to remove and often remains there in the final section. Sections are commonly cut using glass or diamond knives.

■ **Compare the use of methacrylate and epoxy resins.**
Methacrylate resins can either be removed from tissues or are permeable to dyes and so stain similarly to wax sections. Methacrylates are therefore popular for light microscopy where very thin sections are needed or for very hard tissues. They are not stable in the electron microscope beam and are not used for electron microscopy. Epoxy resins are more stable and are the routine embedding materials for electron microscopy. They are more difficult to stain, so are less popular than methacrylates for light microscopy.

■ **Discuss alternative embedding materials.**
Ester, polyester and water-soluble waxes have been developed but cost and difficulty in use have restricted their popularity.

Although paraffin wax embedding is the commonest method of supporting tissues for sectioning, there is a variety of alternative embedding media that can be used. Some of these are of mainly historical interest, whilst others are more recent and are now routine. Even the 'historical' methods have a surprising durability, with most of them still being used for specialized purposes and they are still useful to overcome some modern research problems. They range from the use of very hard plastics and resins used to produce very thin sections, through wax-like materials with some quite different properties to paraffin wax, to the soft and pliable celloidin sections.

4.1 PLASTIC OR RESIN EMBEDDING

Plastics are very widely used as embedding media in histology. They are the main embedding method used in electron microscopy and have many applications in light microscopy. The terms plastic and resin tend to be used somewhat loosely in histology. To a chemist not all resins are plastics and not all plastics are resins but for most histologists the terms resin embedding and plastic embedding are simply alternatives.

These materials are usually very much harder than waxes and so give much better support to the tissues. This is better for hard materials such as undecalcified bone and allows much thinner sections to be prepared from soft tissues. Sections may be thinner than 100 nm (about one-fiftieth of the thickness of paraffin sections). This thinness is essential for electron microscopy and can be very useful for light microscopy as there is less confusion from overlapping cells and organelles. One slight problem is the loss of contrast in the sections due to their thinness. This means that staining must be more intense and so staining techniques must be changed for plastic sections. The traditional haematoxylin and eosin is often replaced with toluidine blue to stain the nucleus and a stronger cytoplasmic stain.

Plastics are quite unlike waxes in one major property. Waxes are converted from a solid to a liquid form by melting and will solidify again on cooling. Thus, tissues are impregnated in molten wax at about 60°C and converted to a solid block simply by cooling. The block can be gently remelted and reblocked without damaging the tissue. Plastics, however, are solidified by chemically converting them from a liquid monomer to a solid polymer by polymerization. This is irreversible, so reblocking is difficult or impossible.

The monomers of the plastics are often miscible with one or more dehydrating agents, particularly acetone and propylene oxide, so that clearing agents such as xylene often are not needed. Some monomers are even miscible with water and the tissue can be impregnated with the monomer directly from aqueous solutions without any need to dehydrate. The miscibility of the monomer and the solubility of the polymer are, however, totally different and once converted to a polymer they are often insoluble. Thus, for example, glycol methacrylate monomer is miscible with water but once polymerized to the solid polymer, the plastic is not only no longer soluble in water but is also insoluble in most other common solvents.

Methacrylates

These are related to Perspex and were the first plastic materials to be used for tissue embedding. They were introduced into histology during the early 1950s and have been used in various forms ever since (see *Box 4.1*). The early methacrylates were the butyl and methyl methacrylates and later glycol methacrylate was used (2-hydroxyethyl methacrylate), but since the 1980s, aromatic polyhydroxy dimethacrylate resins have been available.

$$CH_2=C\begin{array}{c}CH_3\\|\\|\\COOR\end{array}$$

$R = CH_3$	Methyl methacrylate
$R = (CH_2)_3CH_3$	Butyl methacrylate
$R = (CH_2)_2OH$	Glycol methacrylate

The tissue requires dehydration but not clearing since the monomers are miscible with alcohol and acetone. The dehydrating agent must be completely removed by several changes of monomer before attempting to polymerize the block. Acetone is more of a problem than alcohol for interfering with polymerization and so alcohol is recommended.

Box 4.1 Plastic embedding for museum specimens

Methacrylates can also be used for museum specimens since they can be produced in quite large blocks and are crystal-clear. The specimen is dehydrated and impregnated as usual, although with large specimens the impregnation time is extended. Polymerization must be slow. The block is then trimmed and polished. These embedded specimens are good for teaching as they are less easily damaged than the conventional glass jars filled with fluid. They can get scratched or slightly chipped but do not shatter if dropped. The occasional polish to remove scratches is all that is needed.

Methacrylates polymerize by chain elongation using an active radical. Adding a catalyst such as benzoyl peroxide produces active radicals. This molecule is highly unstable and is explosive but can be obtained as a more stable paste mixed with dibutyl phthalate. When the molecule is heated, it can split to provide two stable active radicals (see *Fig. 4.1*).

Figure 4.1
Splitting of benzoyl peroxide to give two phenyl radicals

The active radical then adds on to a monomer forming a new larger active radical, which in turn adds on to a monomer and hence the chain elongates (see *Fig. 4.2*). The chain elongation will continue until either there are no monomers to react or the free radical is inactivated by a free radical scavenger such as oxygen or acetone.

Polymerization of the resin is better if oxygen is removed by bubbling the monomer with nitrogen gas just before use. If the block is not polymerized in a sealed mould, then the upper part of the block may not

Figure 4.2
Polymerization of methacrylates

polymerize fully due to the oxygen. Some extra monomer should be used so that this upper soft layer can be removed without harming the embedded tissue.

Rapid high-temperature curing will result in more free radicals and the block will suffer, since the polymer chains will be shorter. A slower polymerization will give a better result. This is difficult since the reaction needs heat to start it off and once started it is exothermic and will get hotter and hotter. Thus, it is a delicate problem to heat the block enough to start the polymerization and then cool it to remove the heat and slow down the polymerization.

Problems with methyl and butyl methacrylates

Methacrylates have significant problems in use. First, they are often sold in an impure form with quinol materials to help to stabilize them. These can be removed by extracting the acrylic monomer with sodium hydroxide. The quinol dissolves in the sodium hydroxide solution, which can be discarded. The resin is then washed free of the hydroxide and finally dried with calcium chloride.

The monomer is strongly exothermic and will get very hot during polymerization. To minimize damage to the tissues, it is better to do some of the initial polymerization before impregnation. Thus, pre-polymerized monomer is made by starting the polymerization and then cooling the partially polymerized material to 0°C. An alternative is to use some low molecular weight beads dissolved in the monomer. If the heat is not controlled, then the heat may get so intense that the monomer may vaporize, causing cavities in the block.

Glycol methacrylate

Glycol methacrylate (2-hydroxyethyl methacrylate) is a useful addition to the resins since the monomer is hydrophilic and complete removal of water is not essential before impregnating in monomer. The tissue is often only dehydrated to 90% alcohol before being impregnated with the glycol methacrylate monomer. Once completely impregnated with monomer, which can take two or three changes, it can then be polymerized. Some forms of glycol methacrylate are contaminated with methacrylic acid, which can take up stains, and this can cause the problem of a heavy background colour. Low-acid monomers are preferable. Although the monomer is water-soluble, the cured resin is insoluble in most reagents and is not easily removed.

Aromatic polyhydroxy methacrylates

Aromatic polyhydroxy methacrylates have been available since the 1980s and have the hydrophilic characteristics of glycol methacrylate but are more stable in the electron microscope. These resins can also be cured by exposure to UV light and can be cured at very low temperature, allowing some enzyme histochemistry to be done.

Cutting and staining for methacrylates

Acrylic resins can be cut with ordinary steel or disposable knives but better results are usually obtained if they are sectioned using glass knives (see Chapter 16) for thin sections of soft tissue or tungsten knives for sections of hard, undecalcified tissues. Sections can be stained as free-floating sections without removing the plastic or they can be attached to slides using an adhesive and the methacrylate then softened or removed.

Methyl and butyl methacrylate can be dissolved using xylene and so can be stained using a wide variety of techniques similar to those used for paraffin sections. These methacrylates are no longer popular for electron microscopy because the resins disintegrate slowly in the electron beam, but they are still very useful for light microscopy and especially when working with hard tissues such as undecalcified bone and teeth. They are excellent for light microscopy as the resin is easily permeated by aqueous dyes and in the case of methyl methacrylate can even be removed by soaking in xylene. (The epoxy resins, which are preferred for electron microscopy, are more difficult to stain and impossible to remove.)

Glycol methacrylate is more difficult to remove and tissues are always stained with the resin still in place. The glycol resin is, however, still hydrophilic and allows penetration of many aqueous dyes, so staining is still fairly easy. It is this flexibility of staining with dyes that has meant that acrylic resins have retained their popularity for light microscopy, whilst electron microscopists have discarded them.

Epoxy resins

These are commercially produced resins and their exact chemical nature is often a commercial secret. They include Araldite, Epon and Spurr resins. They are generally much more viscous than the acrylic resins but have the advantage of causing very little shrinkage and do not produce damaging heat during polymerization.

The epoxy resins polymerize by a different mechanism involving the cross-linking of two different components and are more likely to produce cross-links between the extending polymer chains. Instead of using just a monomer and a small amount of catalyst, they need two major components that interact to form the polymer (see *Fig. 4.3*). Other materials can be added as accelerators and plasticizers such as dibutyl phthalate.

Figure 4.3
Epoxy resin polymerization. The epoxide group reacts with amines to form adducts. The adduct has an amine and a hydroxyl group, both of which can then further react with another epoxide group to give chain elongation and branching

The curing of these materials alters their characteristics. The higher the temperature, the harder the blocks will be, and they will also be more brittle. Curing for histology is usually done at 60°C for 12–24 h, which gives a tougher but less-hard block. At 120°C, the block will be cured in 1 h but will be hard and brittle.

Since the components of the resin can bond to amine groups, there is the possibility of the plastic bonding directly on to the proteins and nucleic acids in the tissues. The tissue becomes permanently attached to the resin and the degree of cross-linking means that, especially for small blocks, the whole block is essentially one large extended molecule including the tissues. The result of this is that staining is inhibited and antigens are blocked, so staining with dyes and immunohistochemical techniques are poor. It is almost impossible to remove the resin without destroying the tissue in the process. Some improvement can be obtained by breaking down some of the cross-links or etching the block with sodium hydroxide in alcohol. Staining is still reduced compared with other embedding techniques.

Epoxy resins can include some very toxic materials and should be treated with care. They are capable of linking on to the tissues in human skin and acting as a hapten group. This slightly alters the nature of the proteins in skin so that the immune system will treat them as foreign proteins and produce an immune reaction. This results in an allergic hypersensitivity to the resin materials. They should only be used inside a fume cupboard and gloves are needed when the monomers are being handled.

Cutting and staining for epoxy resins

As with the methacrylates, it is better to use tungsten or glass knives to cut these materials, although it is possible with steel knives. Sections are usually dried on to slides using an adhesive and stained as for paraffin wax sections. As mentioned above, a pretreatment with sodium hydroxide may help the dyes to penetrate a little further, but most staining will only occur at the surface rather than throughout the section.

Because they essentially form a single large molecule, epoxy resins are less liable to disintegrate in the electron beam. This means that they will remain intact for longer and will not contaminate the inside of the electron microscope.

4.2 ALTERNATIVE WAXES

These are materials that look and feel like wax but have quite different properties. They have lower melting points than standard paraffin wax but are still strong enough to act as a tissue support. These waxes often needed less processing and can accept tissues from dehydrating agents or even water. The result often is fewer artefacts and this can be a big advantage, but they have never become widely used for routine work because of the cost involved and even in research they are no longer used because the use of plastic embedding has made them redundant.

Water-soluble waxes

These are not really waxes at all but polyethylene glycols. They usually have a lower melting point than paraffin wax but are still similar in hardness to

---

Box 4.2 Preservation using water-soluble waxes

Water-soluble waxes are also used for impregnating many other things to protect and support them. They have the advantage of being easily removed if this becomes necessary and can be applied from either water or from alcoholic solutions. These waxes are being used to protect the 16th century warship *The Mary Rose*, which sank in the Solent in 1545 and was raised from the seabed in 1982. Because the timbers were waterlogged and liable to disintegrate if they were allowed to dry, they have been kept moist and then gradually impregnated with polyethylene glycols, which coat and support the wood.

A different medium, hydroxypropyl cellulose, was found to be the best way to solve a similar problem with books. The leather bindings of many old books have been restored in the famous old Long Room Library of Trinity College, Dublin, using this method. They did try using methacrylates to do the same supporting role for the drying and splintering covers but they tended to cause discoloration.

the common paraffin waxes used in histology. They are completely soluble in water, so tissues can be transferred into them without dehydration. The blocks are easy to cut and the tissue shrinks less since there are no dehydration and clearing steps and the impregnation is at a lower temperature. There are fewer artefacts than with the usual paraffin wax (for example, lipids can be retained in the section). The main reason that they are not commonly used is that after cutting they are very difficult to handle.

The sections cannot be conveniently floated on to a water bath for the tissue to relax and flatten after the rough action of being 'chopped' on a microtome. Tissues impregnated with water-soluble wax are difficult to store as either blocks or sections as they are hygroscopic and will gradually dissolve away in the moisture present in the air. For these reasons, they were never popular and are very rarely used today.

Ester and polyester wax

These were introduced by Steedman and consist of ethylene glycol esters. Polyester wax is sometimes referred to as Steedman's wax. They are based on glycol distearates.

Ester wax: *Polyester wax:*

Diethylene glycol distearate	60%		
Polyethylene distearate (300)	10%	Polyethylene distearate (400)	90%
Glyceryl monostearate	30%	Cetyl alcohol	10%

Ester wax melts at 45–47°C, whilst polyester wax melts at 38°C. Both are miscible with most dehydrating agents as well as clearing agents, so the amount of processing needed is reduced. These waxes are extremely hard, despite their low melting point, and ester wax will even allow sectioning of small pieces of undecalcified bone. These waxes are now rarely used.

Celloidin and low-viscosity nitrocellulose

This material is a derivative of cellulose (see *Box 4.3*) and although completely insoluble in water, it is soluble in a mixture of ethanol and diethyl ether. It is used in a different way to both wax and plastics by being used as a solution and then hardened by evaporating the solvent. This is a slow process and is very sensitive to the rate of evaporation.

The tissue is dehydrated in ethanol, treated with 1:1 ethanol and diethyl ether and then gradually infiltrated with a solution of celloidin in the same mixture. The tissue is then blocked out in a large mould and the solvent is evaporated slowly. The hardened block is then stored in alcohol. Storage in air results in the block becoming brittle as the remainder of the solvent evaporates.

Celloidin is good for tissues with widely differing textures. I have found it useful for whole eyes where there is a tough outer coat around a soft inner

---

Box 4.3 Celluloid

Celloidin or collodion is cellulose dinitrate and is a close relative of the explosive gun cotton. Although it is not explosive itself, it is highly flammable. It was widely used as a plastic when it was usually mixed with camphor to form celluloid. It was used to make the backing material for the early cinematic film. It is not stable when completely dry, so many of these old 'nitrate' films are now falling apart. The solution was also used as a wound dressing by painting an alcoholic solution over wounds to give a clear protective covering.

The decline in its commercial use has raised its price substantially and it is now a specialist chemical. It can be used for covering sections that are lifting, protecting microincinerated sections and coating crumbling blocks to enable sectioning. Although a valuable material for many tasks in histology it is unfortunately becoming too costly for routine use.

---

material (the humours) and it is the only method I have found that will reliably keep the retina attached.

Double embedding

In this technique the tissue is dehydrated and then impregnated with celloidin dissolved in methyl benzoate rather than the ether/alcohol used in the previous technique. The block is not allowed to dry in this method and instead is cleared in toluene and finally impregnated with molten paraffin wax. The tissue thus has a double support of celloidin and wax and this may help with some difficult tissues but without the cutting and storage problems of full celloidin embedding. Double embedding has largely become irrelevant as commercial histology waxes containing additives, which give similar support capabilities, have become widely available.

Thus, the support of tissues can be achieved in a number of ways. Each has its own particular advantages and problems. The choice of technique is often critical in obtaining good sections, so it is important to know that alternatives are available. In routine histology, they are not used as extensively as they might be because paraffin wax impregnation is readily available and used every day. Many routine histologists will often 'put up with' a paraffin block because it would be too much hassle to set up a processing schedule for one block.

SUGGESTED FURTHER READING

Anderson, G. and Bancroft, J.D. (2002) Tissue processing and microtomy including frozen. In *Theory and Practice of Histological Techniques*, 5th edn (eds J.D. Bancroft and M. Gamble). Edinburgh: Churchill Livingstone.
Culling, C.F.A. (1975) *Handbook of Histopathological and Histochemical Techniques*. London: Butterworths.

Hand, N.M. (2002) Plastic embedding media and techniques. In *Theory and Practice of Histological Techniques*, 5th edn (eds J.D. Bancroft and M. Gamble). Edinburgh: Churchill Livingstone.

SELF-ASSESSMENT QUESTIONS

1. What are the advantages of embedding in plastics?
2. Why are epoxy resins preferred for electron microscopy?
3. Why do epoxy resin sections not stain as well as wax or methacrylate sections?
4. Water-soluble waxes (polyethylene glycols) support tissues well during cutting but are difficult to flatten. Why?

Cryotechniques

Learning objectives
After studying this chapter you should confidently be able to:

■ **Outline the principles involved in the preparation of frozen sections.**
The water in tissues is frozen to form ice, which acts as a support for section cutting.

■ **Compare different methods of freezing tissues.**
Tissues must be frozen rapidly to avoid ice-crystal damage. Fast freezing can be achieved with liquid or solid CO_2 or liquid nitrogen. Slow freezing is only useful for macroscopic work and can be done using a deep-freeze cabinet.

■ **State the advantages of frozen sections compared with other embedding techniques.**
Frozen sections are quicker and allow rapid diagnosis. Frozen sections also retain more materials in the tissue and are good for histochemistry.

■ **Outline the process of freeze-drying.**
Freeze-drying involves rapid freezing followed by sublimation of the ice at low temperature and reduced pressure to remove water with minimal damage, loss of material or diffusion of cell components.

In the previous chapters on the main methods of preparing tissues, it has been emphasized that, in order to cut thin sections from soft human tissues such as liver or kidney, the tissue needs a rigid support. The previous methods involved removing the water from the tissues by treatment with dehydrating agents and replacing it with wax or other hard materials. However, there is an alternative to this chemical replacement of the water in the tissues with a firm wax and that is to physically convert the water itself into a solid (ice) by lowering the temperature.

5.1 CRYOTOMY

Cryotomy is the term used to describe the use of ice as a support for section cutting. Freezing is quicker than replacement (see *Box 5.1*) and does not

---

Box 5.1 Freezing techniques allow rapid diagnosis

The main use in hospitals for frozen sections is for the rapid diagnosis of tumours. Tumours can be benign (relatively innocuous) or malignant (the cancers) and the treatment of the two types can be very different. Benign tumours are removed with very little excess normal tissue but malignant tumours require a more extensive removal including local lymph nodes.

Clinical diagnosis is not always possible and a biopsy sample may be needed to confirm the diagnosis. With modern anaesthetics it is safer to keep a patient anaesthetized for an extra quarter of an hour than to sew them back up, send them back to the ward and give them a second operation 1 or 2 days later. The speed of the cryostat technique allows tissue to be frozen quickly, sectioned and stained ready for diagnosis within 15 min, so the surgeon can decide the extent of the removal once a microscopic diagnosis is made. This limits the patient to one trip to the operating theatre instead of two with a worrying wait whilst the tissue is processed.

---

involve treating the tissues with chemicals such as alcohol, which may remove important materials (such as lipids) from the tissues or may alter the chemical properties of tissue components (such as enzymes). Such techniques are usually called **frozen section techniques** and are an important way of preparing tissues for rapid diagnosis and for histochemistry.

There are several methods of cutting frozen sections, but the most important difference is whether the microtome is entirely enclosed in a deep-freeze cabinet (usually at −15 to −30°C) or on a laboratory bench at room temperature with only the block being kept cold. The first technique is the most popular and the instrument, which consists of a deep-freeze cabinet and the enclosed microtome, is called a **cryostat**.

Freezing and tissue damage

Freezing of tissues for frozen sections can damage the tissues and, although frozen sections involve less treatment of the tissue, artefacts are still produced and these depend on how the tissue is frozen.

Slow freezing and mechanical damage

The rate of freezing alters the size of the ice crystals. At slow freezing rates, the ice crystals will grow quite large and the crystals themselves expand as they freeze. This expansion results in mechanical damage to the tissue. Ice crystals may occur intracellularly and if they grow sufficiently large they can cause noticeable crevices in the tissue (ice-crystal artefact).

Water at atmospheric pressure is converted to ice at any temperature below 0°C, but it is in a dynamic state and will constantly be changing shape and interacting with adjacent ice crystals. Ice-crystal damage gets worse as blocks are stored, as the ice remodels and changes its shape and size. Only when the temperature of the ice drops very low, about −130°C for pure water, does it become stable and not recrystallize. The point at which recrystallization in tissues, which are filled with a salt solution, is inhibited is not known but it is probably somewhere below −90°C. Storage of blocks must

---

Box 5.2 Fast freezing kills cells

Although fast freezing is best for tissue structure, it is actually much more dangerous to living tissues that are not protected. Slow freezing causes less tissue damage than very rapid freezing. In slow freezing, most of the ice crystals form outside the cells and are made of pure ice. This increases the osmotic pressure of the fluid, as the same amount of salt is now in a smaller volume. The cells lose fluid to the extracellular spaces but there is no necrosis. Fast freezing freezes the cell cytoplasm as well as the extracellular tissues and this is intensely necrotizing

The freezing effect is not the cause of the necrosis seen in cold injuries such as frostbite and trench foot. These injuries are caused by the capillaries in the affected area constricting and reducing oxygenation of the tissues. Ischaemic damage results and this can cause the loss of fingers and toes.

---

be done in liquid nitrogen at −196°C to minimize this damage and cells should preferably be treated with a cryoprotectant solution such as 30% glycerol to reduce freezing damage.

Rapid freezing gives better tissue structure

Rapid freezing results in many smaller ice crystals that are less likely to cause visible alteration to the tissues. It follows that the higher the magnification that is going to be used on the tissue the smaller the ice crystals must be to avoid visible damage (see *Box 5.2*). Rapid freezing is needed for high magnifications. For low magnifications or macroscopic work (i.e. using the unaided human eye), the rate of freezing can be slower since the ice-crystal damage will not be seen. If the tissue is fixed before freezing, it will be able to resist damage more easily, so slower freezing of fixed tissue is less damaging than similar freezing of fresh tissue.

Slow freezing and osmotic damage

The fluids in tissues are not pure water but a solution of various salts, so when freezing occurs it is the effects on a salt solution that need to be considered, not simply the effects on water. Slow freezing of a salt solution results in the production of ice crystals that are pure water. It is only when the temperature gets below −21°C that the salt solution will freeze as a whole. Since water is being removed from the cellular fluid, the remaining solution becomes more concentrated. Water will be drawn out from the cells and they will shrink as a result.

Depression of freezing point

Salts dissolved in water lower the freezing point of the solution (depression of freezing point) and it requires a temperature of about −10°C before tissue fluid will freeze. The liquid left behind as the water crystallizes as pure ice may eventually become so concentrated that even at very low temperatures it may not freeze. The unfrozen areas will therefore remain liquid and the tissues in these regions will be unsupported. The result is that these areas will not section well and the sections may have distinctive

---

Box 5.3 Freezing ruptures cell membranes

The effects of freezing can be seen in frozen strawberries that retain their flavour but lose their texture. The firmness of strawberries is due to turgor pressure. This is a higher pressure inside the cell pressing against the cellulose cell wall like an inner tube and tyre. When frozen, the ice crystals rupture the cell membrane. The cell deflates like a punctured tyre and the strawberry loses its firm texture. Chemically it is unchanged but its physical integrity is lost. Freezing human tissue to keep it alive is not easy and requires replacement of the normal tissue fluid with cryopreservative and controlled freezing. The people who have paid thousands of pounds to have their bodies cryogenically stored are unlikely to be able to be restored, even with advancing technology, since all of their cells are likely to be damaged and repairing punctures in every cell in the body is totally impractical.

---

holes where the pools of unfrozen tissue occurred. The tissue appears to have holes in it and this can make it look like a waffle; this artefact has been called a **waffle artefact** (see *Colour plate 3*). The production of this artefact is dependent on the rate of cooling. If the rate of freezing is high enough, then the tissue freezes as one intact block without separating into water and salt solutions.

Rate of cooling and heat conduction

The rate at which tissues freeze depends on conduction from the warmer tissues to the coolant. The rate of conduction is dependent on the temperature difference between the coolant and the tissue, so the lower the temperature of the coolant, the faster the tissue freezes. Thus, even though the tissue may need to be cut at –20°C, it is usual to cool it with a cooling system that will be at a much lower temperature and then allow the block to warm up to the cutting temperature. This means the tissue reaches –20°C much quicker and so there is less deterioration.

Conduction depends on the area in contact with the coolant

The rate of freezing is also dependent on the area in contact with the coolant. With a solid coolant packed around the microtome chuck or a Peltier module, the only contact is with the base of the block. Cooling will spread through the tissues from the base and this can be seen as a white line moving up the block. Cooling will be slightly slower at the top of the block since the heat has to transfer through the block as well as through the chuck. Anything that slows down the transfer of heat will similarly slow down the rate of freezing. Microtome chucks should therefore be made of metal and putting thick layers of insulating materials such as cork on top of the chuck should be avoided.

With liquid coolants, the whole block can be immersed in the coolant and this increases the surface area for heat transfer and can speed up cooling. The disadvantage is that the fluid may itself damage the block. Liquid coolants can, of course, also be used simply to cool the chuck without totally immersing the specimen.

5.2 METHODS OF COOLING TISSUES FOR SECTIONING

Various techniques have been employed to reduce the temperature of the tissues below freezing.

Slow freezing methods

Slow freezing is taken here to mean a freezing technique in which it takes several minutes to freeze the tissue into a solid block and will produce larger crystals that may produce damage that is visible with high magnifications.

Freezing tissues in a deep-freeze cabinet

Simply putting the tissue into a deep-freeze cabinet at –20 to –30°C will eventually freeze the tissues. This is usually done histologically by putting the tissue into the chamber of a cryostat that is normally held at –20°C. Some cryostats have an extra-cold shelf or chamber that may be as low as –40°C that freezes the tissue more rapidly but this is still relatively slow. The use of a deep-freeze cabinet or a cryostat is a cheap and easy method of freezing tissues since it involves no special reagents or extra equipment. However, it is very slow and may take hours for anything other than very small blocks. This very slow freezing causes quite a lot of damage and is only suitable for macroscopic work such as whole-body autoradiography. Even quite low magnifications will reveal some damage from the frozen ice crystals.

Freezing tissues with a thermoelectric module

Peltier modules or thermoelectric modules are electrically activated heat pumps. When an electric current is passed through them, they absorb heat on one side and emit it on the other surface. By stacking several thermoelectric modules together, efficient heat removal can be achieved. The rate at which heat is extracted is controlled by the strength of the electric current. Increasing the current means a faster rate of freezing. Since the rate of heat pumping depends on the current, it means that the temperature of the block can easily be controlled by altering the current. Reversal of the current reverses the direction of the heat flow and is a convenient way to melt the lower surface of the block and allow it to be removed. These are not very popular as simple cooling devices but are used in some cryostats and other specialized instruments.

Rapid freezing methods

Rapid freezing techniques are now the most popular and the choice of method is often a matter of availability rather than strictly scientific choice. Most of these methods will give excellent results if carried out carefully.

Freezing using a fast-evaporating liquid

This method uses commercial spray cans containing fast-evaporating liquids (e.g. chlorofluorocarbons). As a liquid evaporates it will absorb latent heat of evaporation. This property applies to all liquids, but the faster they evaporate the faster they absorb heat. The liquids chosen for these sprays evaporate very quickly and therefore absorb heat very quickly. They tend to be expensive to use on a regular basis when compared with other methods of freezing and typically achieve a temperature of about −50°C.

They are very convenient since they can be transported easily and are therefore available to freeze tissues in places a long way from the laboratory. The sprays are a good reserve or emergency method of freezing since they can be stored without deteriorating. They can damage the outside of the block if sprayed directly on to the specimen since they are initially liquid and therefore act as solvents, but they do not penetrate beyond the very edge of the block so the inner regions are not affected.

Cooling with carbon dioxide

This method of cooling relies on the sudden expansion of high-pressure liquid CO_2 from a cylinder. The liquid CO_2 rapidly expands to a gas and absorbs heat in the expansion phase. The same effect is seen with CO_2 fire extinguishers, which produce a jet that appears white because of the production of cold CO_2 snow. Also like fire extinguishers, CO_2 cooling is very noisy. When the CO_2 is released, it expands rapidly, causing a very loud hissing noise.

CO_2 cylinders are reasonably convenient in the laboratory where they are only occasionally moved, but are more difficult to transport to distant sites. CO_2 cylinders are reasonably priced and readily available as they are also used for pumping (for example, beer in pubs). The cylinders must be used so that they run the liquid CO_2 out of the cylinder and not just the gas. This requires either a special siphoned cylinder, which can be used upright, or an ordinary one, which can be used inverted (with the outlet at the bottom). CO_2 blasts can reach temperatures as low as −70°C.

Cooling using solid carbon dioxide

Solid carbon dioxide is also known as 'cardice' or dry ice. It can be bought as large blocks and can also be prepared from liquid CO_2 by trapping the CO_2 snow produced when the liquid expands, as explained above. Solid CO_2 can be used as a dry material by packing it around the microtome chuck to cool it. Alternatively, solid CO_2 can be mixed with acetone to produce a freezing mixture in which chucks or tissues can be immersed. Both methods achieve a temperature of about −70°C. Buying blocks of CO_2 can be expensive and inconvenient as solid carbon dioxide must be delivered daily.

Cooling with liquid nitrogen

This liquefied gas is very cold (−196°C). Liquid nitrogen can be cheap if produced on site or bought in bulk. The very low temperature allows the possibility of very rapid freezing but there are some problems.

Liquid nitrogen has a tendency to boil when it comes in contact with warmer objects (see *Box 5.4*). The mechanical effects of boiling may damage some delicate tissues and the boiling slows down the rate of freezing. This

---

Box 5.4 Liquid nitrogen is safe if handled carefully

Although liquid nitrogen is very cold, it is still reasonably safe because of the boiling effect – liquid nitrogen will simply run off anything warm like skin with the drops of liquid nitrogen held aloft like a miniature hovercraft on a cushion of nitrogen gas. It is a party trick of some conjurors and exhibitionists to pour liquid nitrogen on their hands. This is not my idea of a safe trick and liquid nitrogen does become extremely dangerous if it becomes trapped and cannot roll away. So folds in skin or clothing become dangerous traps for the supercold liquid. If treated with caution it is safe, but mishandled it can be a disaster.

slowing is due to the boiling at the surface of the block producing a layer of nitrogen gas around the block that acts as a layer of insulation and inhibits the transfer of heat.

Various techniques are used to get around this problem. Some workers simply use liquid nitrogen to cool less volatile liquids such as isopentane, which do not boil, and then use the cooled isopentane to cool the actual block. The isopentane becomes quite viscous at these low temperatures and the viscosity is used as an indication of when the cooling has reached the correct temperature. Other workers use metal foil to enhance the rate of cooling. The speed of cooling can also be improved by using powdered starch ('glove powder') as a dusting on the surface of the block. The fine powder reduces the boiling effect in the same way as boiling beads do in a beaker of heated liquid.

Rather than cooling a liquid, liquid nitrogen can be used to cool large-blade metal forceps, which are then applied to the tissue. This technique can be used to freeze tissues whilst they are still in the body to eliminate the time between removal and freezing. This method only works well with very small pieces of tissue and special forceps that have extra-heavy jaws, which act as large heat sinks to draw the heat out of the tissue without themselves becoming warmed significantly.

Cutting sections using a freezing microtome

The freezing microtome technique uses a microtome with some convenient method of freezing the tissue on to the chuck (e.g. carbon dioxide blast or Peltier module) but only the specimen is kept cold. The rest of the microtome and the air around the microtome are at room temperature.

Tissue should be fixed first

The tissue usually needs to be fixed in formaldehyde to harden it and enable thin sections to be cut, as it is common for the sections to thaw out during the cutting process. Fixation in formaldehyde is best as it does not interfere with the freezing process and leaves the tissue fairly flexible. Mercury-, chromium- and osmium-based fixatives overharden the tissue, making thin sectioning difficult, and the salts can depress the freezing point of the tissue.

Alcohol-based fixatives will not freeze since the freezing point of alcohol is very low ($-112°C$). Unfixed sections can be cut using a freezing microtome, but they will often disintegrate during staining.

The tissue is frozen on to the chuck

Tissue can be attached to the microtome chuck simply using water or saline as an adhesive, although some workers prefer to use a gum syrup, which has a thicker consistency. A piece of filter paper soaked in water placed on top of the chuck is often useful as it makes it easier to remove the tissue cleanly after sectioning.

Tissue can be frozen solid by one of the methods discussed above; the thermoelectric module and CO_2 blasting are the most common. Once frozen, they are cut using a conventional microtome and knife, usually a non-disposable knife, since ice is somewhat harder than wax.

Collection of free-floating sections

If the sections are cut very quickly, they can be made to jump off the knife directly into a bath of fluid, although this is difficult to control. If the sections are cut more slowly, then they melt on the knife and can be removed using a brush moistened with water. Although it is possible to attach the sections on to a slide and then air-dry them to achieve adhesion, they are usually easily washed off, even when using an adhesive such as gelatine. More often the sections are left free-floating and transferred from one reagent to another by draping them over a bent glass rod ('glass hockey stick'). This is more difficult than using a section attached to a slide and the final stained section still needs to be attached to a slide before mounting under a coverslip.

Cold knife technique

The section can be prevented from melting by cooling the knife and this also helps to reduce crumpling. The knife can be cooled using solid CO_2 held on the knife or by repeatedly blasting the knife with CO_2, or even by clamping a Peltier module to the knife. The ideal situation is to keep the knife well below freezing at between -10 and $-20°C$. The sections still have a tendency to roll and must be teased out during cutting using a fine brush.

Box 5.5 Use of freezing microtomes in neurohistology

The freezing microtome has often been more popular with neurohistologists than with routine histologists. It is often quicker and simpler to cut large blocks of brain with a large freezing microtome than it is to process them through to other embedding media. The thicker sectioning associated with the freezing microtome is not a major problem. The sections needed for many neurological methods are often much thicker than for the rest of the body since the intention is to follow the nerve-cell processes. Free-floating sections are always more difficult to handle than ones attached to a slide, but have the advantage of two surfaces for dyes and reagents to penetrate.

In the full cold knife technique, the tissues are placed on to a slide and into fixative before thawing occurs. This is difficult in practice and most workers simply use a cooled knife to give better sections.

Although widely used at one time, most of the freezing microtome techniques are rarely used for most tissues, although they are still used in neurological histology.

Cryostats

The cryostat or cold microtome technique involves keeping all steps in the cutting method at low temperature, with the block, microtome knife and indeed the whole microtome as well as the final section being kept below freezing. The cryostat is therefore a specially designed deep-freeze cabinet into which a microtome fits and with connections to allow the common controls to be operated from outside the cabinet without the microtomist having to put his hands into the cold chamber. This not only keeps the operator's hands warm but also stops the cabinet temperature from rising too much. A light is usually fitted inside so that it is easy to see what is happening on the microtome. There is generally a transparent lid to allow viewing whilst still keeping the chamber cold. There is also usually an anti-misting system and an automatic defrost system.

Good quality sections from unfixed tissues

Sections produced in the cryostat are generally of a much better quality than those produced using a freezing microtome. In the cryostat, even unfixed tissue will section well. In fact, fresh tissue generally cuts better and is easier to handle than fixed tissue. It is much more usual to fix after cutting than before and since the section always remains frozen there is no need to thaw the sections, which can be fixed whilst still frozen. It is also very common not to fix the tissues until after staining. Unfixed tissues are widely used in histochemistry. Variations on this technique are the most common methods for preparing frozen sections.

Freezing is done outside the cryostat

Tissues are usually attached to the microtome chuck outside the cryostat and then quickly transferred into the cold chamber of the cryostat. The attachment to the microtome chuck is fairly straightforward. The metal microtome chuck has a piece of moist filter paper placed on top and the fresh tissue is placed on top of the filter paper and the chuck. The tissue is then frozen by one of the rapid freezing techniques.

Tissues can be supported

If it is difficult to keep the tissue in position, it can be surrounded and supported by a gum solution or one of the commercial products (OCT or Cryo-M-Bed) containing polyvinyl derivatives, which are inert, water soluble and colourless. These are thick viscous solutions that allow

---

Box 5.6 Improvements in anti-roll plates

Anti-roll plates have evolved over the years as various workers have tried to simplify the adjustments. The original technique was to wrap a piece of adhesive tape around each edge of the anti-roll plate as a rough indication of the gap needed. Adjustment screws were then added so the gap could be finely adjusted depending on the section thickness. The usual way of setting the thickness was to use a piece of newspaper as a 'feeler gauge'. The Times newspaper seemed to work best but I've no idea why! Teflon plates were then used to act as non-stick surfaces to ease the section down the knife more easily but were often opaque and so lost the visual feedback of how the section was cutting and seem to have vanished from use. Currently, anti-roll plates are made with a raised section at each end and this seems to work well – at least until the next innovation!

---

awkward-shaped pieces of tissue to be held temporarily in place whilst freezing occurs. Once they are frozen, these support media cut smoothly and evenly with a similar texture to soft tissues.

Cutting cryostat sections

The microtome fitted into the cryostat can be of any type, but sliding and complex rotary microtomes can be difficult to lubricate at such low temperatures, so modified rocking microtomes are often fitted instead. Sections cut at low temperature have a tendency to roll up, so most cryostats use an anti-roll plate to keep them flat (see *Box 5.6*). This is simply a transparent plate of Perspex arranged in such a way that it leaves a narrow gap between the plate and the knife. This gap is wide enough to allow the section to slide down but narrow enough to prevent rolling. The correct adjustment of the anti-roll plate is one of the most important factors in producing good sections. The anti-roll plate is also one of the reasons why even laboratories that regularly use disposable knives for their wax sectioning still use solid non-disposable knives in the cryostat. It is much more difficult to arrange the anti-roll plate with a disposable knife holder than with a solid knife.

Picking up sections on to a slide

Sections can be gently removed from the knife using a pair of forceps and, whilst still frozen, placed in a container of fixative or other reagent without being attached to slides. More commonly, however, sections are picked up on to warm (room temperature) slides or coverslips by gently placing the slide or coverslip on top of the cold section where it rests on the knife. With unfixed tissue the adhesion is good and some of the protein from the unfixed tissues seems to act as its own adhesive as it is coagulated by the sudden temperature change. Adhesion can be improved further by briefly air-drying the section or by brief fixation.

If the tissue has been fixed before cutting, adhesion is more difficult and the slides may need to have an adhesive applied before picking up the sections. Fixed tissues also cut less easily than unfixed tissues and the cutting can sometimes be improved by treating the section with a sucrose solution before freezing.

Individual component temperatures

The cabinet temperature, knife temperature and block temperature can all be varied, sometimes independently of each other. Most sectioning is done with all of these at the same temperature (isothermic cryotomy), but a colder knife is useful for thin sections. The temperature of the chamber in particular can have a large effect on the ease of cutting and the optimum temperature is not identical for all specimens. Materials such as liver and kidney often cut best at −10 to −15°C, whilst skin and prostate often cut better at −15 to −25°C. Undecalcified bone usually requires a very low temperature of −30 to −40°C.

Impregnation techniques

Some tissues are not able to fully support themselves as frozen sections and may require extra support; for example, the large air spaces in lung tissue offer no support during sectioning. Also, some specimens need a surrounding medium to keep them together and make a reasonable-sized block; this occurs, for example, with very small fragments of curettings or bone marrow fragments that are too small to be used individually as a block. These difficult specimens can first be impregnated with a water-soluble support and then frozen as a single block.

Impregnating media

Many media have been tried and all can be useful, but most have one or more disadvantages. Materials that have been tried include gelatine, which has a tendency to absorb many dyes, agar, which shows a strong metachromatic effect, methyl cellulose (used in Polycell wallpaper paste), which does not set well and is messy, and soaps and detergents.

Gelatine is probably the most popular medium. The gelatine is made up as a 10–20% solution and kept molten at 37°C. The tissue is immersed in this warm, molten solution. If impregnation is likely to be a long process, it is usually better to fix the tissue in formaldehyde before impregnation to prevent any post-mortem changes. However, the fixative needs to be thoroughly washed out or it will also fix the gelatine and spoil the impregnation. Once impregnated, the tissue is then blocked out in a mould and this is then placed in a refrigerator to harden the gelatine. A block is cut from the solid gelatine and can be frozen immediately or can be fixed in formaldehyde to harden the block further before being frozen.

Giant sections (Gough and Wentworth sections)

This impregnation technique forms the basis of the method for cutting giant sections of whole lung (see *Colour plate 4*). It is much easier to impregnate the lung with water-soluble gelatine than it is to process a whole lung through to paraffin wax. The fixed lung is impregnated with a weak solution of gelatine and then frozen in a deep-freeze cabinet. The small defects caused by slow freezing are less of a problem in this case, since the sections are not used with a microscope and are only used to give a cross-section for macroscopic viewing. The frozen lung is then sliced into sections, which are much thicker than is usual for microscopic sections (usually more than 300 μm thick) on a large microtome. The sections are then pressed and flattened on to absorbent paper, dried carefully and glazed with a layer of gelatine. The final section can be used to show the amount of macroscopic lung damage, for example, in coal miners. This technique has been modified for many other embedding media including Polycell wallpaper paste and Persil detergent. The original technique was described by Gough and Wentworth in 1948; hence the sections are often still called Gough and Wentworth sections, even when the technique has been heavily modified.

Freeze-drying

Another technique that uses freezing is the freeze-drying method. This uses freezing to temporarily preserve and stabilize the tissues as an alternative to fixing them. The water in the tissue is then removed by sublimation and the dry tissue can be impregnated directly with molten wax without the need for any intermediate reagents. The advantage of this technique is that the tissues are not disturbed by being treated with a solvent, so water-soluble materials are preserved. It has proved useful for many materials such as glycogen that are disturbed by other preparative methods, but the single most important use is to demonstrate the amine neurotransmitter materials. These amines (often called biogenic amines) include adrenaline, noradrenaline, dopamine and 5-hydroxytryptamine (serotonin). These amines can be made fluorescent by exposing them to aldehyde fixatives (often called formalin-induced fluorescence) once they are dry.

Box 5.7 Freeze-drying of food

Freeze-drying is applied in many other fields including the food industry. The ability to remove water from materials such as fresh coffee or peas without altering their chemical or physical nature is just as valuable in food preservation as it is in histology. It is also capable of preserving living cells, such as blood cells, and proteins, such as vaccines, without the need for refrigeration.

Sublimation rather than evaporation

The important characteristic of the freeze-drying technique is sublimation of the water. Sublimation is the conversion of solid ice directly into a vapour without passing through the liquid phase. Sublimation only occurs if the ice is put into a very high vacuum. Sublimation removes the water as vapour without damaging the tissue since it avoids the surface tension effects seen when a liquid evaporates.

Tissue is frozen and then warmed in a vacuum

The tissue is first very quickly frozen, usually referred to as **quenching** to distinguish it from slow freezing. This is best done using isopentane or a similar solvent with a high thermal conductivity cooled with liquid nitrogen. The frozen tissue is then put into a chamber with a Peltier module set to provide cooling and the tissue is kept at a low temperature to maintain it in a frozen state. The chamber is evacuated to a high vacuum (less than 1 torr or 133 mPa) to reduce the vapour pressure below that of ice and then it is slowly warmed up. Since a Peltier module is used for the cooling, the heat is applied simply by reversing the direction of the current and hence reversing the direction of heat flow, gently warming the tissue.

Sublimation keeps the tissue frozen

The ice sublimes as heat is applied. The tissue remains frozen, even though heat is being applied continuously. The reason for this is that as the ice undergoes sublimation it absorbs heat. The vapour pressure in the chamber is kept very low either by using a chemical desiccant (phosphorus pentoxide is the usual drying agent) or by having an even colder region in the chamber such as a metal tube filled with liquid nitrogen. Water vapour will condense on to the cold spot, even in the high vacuum, and this creates a vapour gradient between the tissue and the trap.

Impregnation with wax

The drying process is very slow and takes several hours to reach completion, even for very small pieces of tissue, as up to 80% of the tissue is water. When it is completely dried, the tissue is allowed to return to room temperature and can then be fixed using formaldehyde vapour or can be immediately impregnated with wax and made into a wax block for sectioning.

SUGGESTED FURTHER READING

Anderson, G. and Bancroft, J.D. (2002) Tissue processing and microtomy including frozen. In *Theory and Practice of Histological Techniques*, 5th edn (eds J.D. Bancroft and M. Gamble). Edinburgh: Churchill Livingstone.

Culling, C.F.A. (1975) *Handbook of Histopathological and Histochemical Techniques*. London: Butterworths.

SELF-ASSESSMENT QUESTIONS

1. Why does slow freezing damage tissues?
2. Name the reasons why frozen sections are used in (a) diagnosis of malignancy; (b) lipid staining; (c) enzyme techniques.
3. Outline the difference between a cryostat and a freezing microtome. Which is better?
4. What is the significance of liquid nitrogen boiling when it comes in contact with warm tissue?
5. Why do tissues still deteriorate even when stored at −20°C?

Staining theory

Learning objectives
After studying this chapter you should confidently be able to:

■ **Describe why sections need to be coloured with dyes.**
Staining is needed to give contrast between different components of the tissues and allow examination by light microscopy.

■ **Describe how dyes bind to tissues.**
Dyes bind by forming bonds with tissue components. Ionic and hydrogen bonding and van der Waals forces are probably all involved. Ionic staining is the most important and distinguishes between basophilic and acidophilic tissue components. Hydrogen bonding and van der Waals forces are less important but probably play a role in selectivity.

■ **Describe the use of mordants in staining.**
Mordants are metal salts that help bind some dyes to tissues. Haematoxylin is the most important mordanted dye.

■ **Define metachromasia and give examples of its use.**
Metachromasia produces a different colour in a tissue component to the colour of the dye solution. Toluidine blue is blue in solution but stains mast cell granules red.

■ **Describe the main properties of haematoxylin and staining using haematoxylin solutions.**
Haematoxylin is a natural dye that requires oxidation to haematein before use as a stain. Haematoxylin is a mordanted dye that can stain many different elements in tissue depending on the mordant used. Using different mordants it can be used to stain nuclei, connective tissue fibres, nerve cells, muscle striations and mitochondria. It is usually used regressively.

■ **Describe the use of silver as an impregnating metal.**
Silver solutions are easily reduced producing a dense black deposit and this reduction is autocatalytic. In argentaffin reactions, no extra reducing agent is needed, but argyrophil reactions require the addition of a reducing agent.

■ **Describe the reasons for mounting tissues and outline the types of mounting media.**
Mounting media and coverslips not only protect the specimen but also make it translucent, making examination easier. Mounting media may be resinous (organic-based) or water-based solvents.

If sections of human tissue are examined under the microscope immediately after sectioning, they appear very dull and uninteresting. The tissue lacks contrast because all of the fixed materials have a similar refractive index and a similar colour so that a dull grey colour is all that can be seen. To bring out the structure of the tissues, it is essential to stain the cells to see the different parts in contrasting colours.

Staining is not simply random colouring of the sections but depends on using differences in the chemistry of the tissue to show the various components in different colours. This is most commonly done using dyes that can bind to the tissue in a selective way. Thus, the colours that are seen reflect the nature of the tissue and are not just a pretty picture. By using two or more dyes, it is possible to bring out the different materials in several contrasting colours.

The commonest stain in use is the haematoxylin and eosin (H&E) stain, which colours the nuclei a dark blue or purple and stains the cytoplasm and connective tissue in shades of pink (see *Colour plate 5*).

6.1 STAINING MECHANISMS

The binding of dyes to tissues is no different to any other chemical bonding and the mechanisms rely on the same binding forces that occur in all other organic compounds. The dye must form some type of bond or link to the tissue or they will simply be rinsed out of the tissue when the section is washed in another reagent. The usual forms of bonding can be involved. Each type has its own characteristics and bond strengths.

Bond type	Strength (kcal mole^{-1})
Ionic bonds	40–110
Hydrogen bonds	2–7
Van der Waals forces	1-2
Covalent bonds	35–212
Hydrophobic interactions	4–8

Ionic bonding

Ionic bonding involves electrostatic attraction between oppositely charged ions. One ion is a fixed ion in the tissue section and the other is the dye ion. Anionic (negatively charged) dyes will bind to cations (positively charged) in the tissue, and cationic dyes will bind to tissue anions.

Ionic bonding is the single most important form of bonding in most histological staining. Almost all simple staining can be understood and controlled by understanding the ionic charges involved.

Negatively charged eosin ions will stain positively charged tissue ions

Eosin is an example of an anionic dye and is attracted to protein groups that are positively charged (cations) such as amino groups. First, the amino

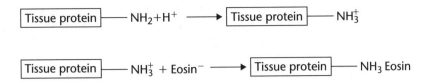

Figure 6.1
The ionization of tissue amines and subsequent binding of eosin

groups in the protein become ionized by binding to a hydrogen ion and this charged group then attracts the eosinic ion (see *Fig. 6.1*).

Eosin is usually sold as a salt such as sodium eosinate, which is readily soluble in water. Anionic dyes are also called acid dyes in histology because they are derived from coloured acids (in this case, eosinic acid) and not because of the pH of the solution. Anything that will stain with an acid dye is called **acidophilic**. In the case of materials staining with eosin, they could also be termed **eosinophilic**. Materials that are acidophilic include collagen, red blood cells and the cytoplasm of many cells.

Box 6.1 Controlling pH allows dyes to be removed

Sensitivity to pH is exploited in the removal of dyes. This is used in differentiation and is also important in getting dye splashes off skin and clothing. Basic dyes can be removed by using acids (usually acid alcohol), whilst acidic dyes are most easily removed with a solution of ammonia in alcohol. These should always be very dilute solutions and used with extreme care. The solutions are extremely painful if used on cuts or sensitive areas such as around the eyes. It is much better to avoid getting the dye on your skin in the first place.

Positively charged methylene blue ions will stain negatively charged tissue ions

Methylene blue is an example of a cationic dye and will bind to tissue anions such as carboxylic acid, sulphuric acid and phosphoric acid groups. These groups need to be ionized to bind the dyes (see *Fig. 6.2*).

Figure 6.2
The ionization of sulphate groups in mucins and their subsequent binding of methylene blue

Cationic dyes are commonly called basic dyes and so substances staining with such dyes are called **basophilic**. Substances that bind basic dyes include nucleic acids and acid mucins.

Binding of dyes depends on tissue ionization

Proteins normally contain both acidic and basic amino acids and so it might be expected that proteins would take up both dyes. In practice this does not occur because most staining is done at a neutral or slightly acid pH. At these acid pH levels, the carboxyl groups of most amino acids are not ionized. Dyes will only bind to tissue groups when they are ionized; if the groups are unionized they will not attract the dye ions and will remain unstained.

Acid pH levels favour staining with anionic dyes

Ionic bonding to dyes and therefore staining is pH sensitive since the ionization of tissue groups is affected by pH. At an acidic pH, the high concentration of hydrogen ions favours the ionization of amino groups and results in strong staining of proteins by eosin, as described above. However, the same acidic pH will have the opposite effect on staining by methylene blue since weak acids, such as the carboxylic acids found in proteins, will be inhibited from ionizing by the high concentrations of hydrogen ions. Stronger acids, such as the phosphate groups found in nucleic acids and sulphate groups found in mucins, are less easily inhibited and will still ionize at the pH levels generally used in staining. This means that in slightly acid solutions methylene blue will act as a differential stain, picking out the nuclei but leaving the proteins unstained. Altering the pH can inhibit dyes from ionizing, but total inhibition of ionization of the salt forms of dyes will only occur at extreme pH levels. The ionization of dyes can be assumed to be complete at normal staining pH levels.

Alkaline conditions favour staining with cationic dyes

Alkaline solutions will have the opposite effect. The lack of hydrogen ions will allow the weakly acidic groups in proteins to ionize and methylene blue will stain both the cytoplasm and the nucleus. To get maximal staining with methylene blue, it is best to use Löffler's formula, which uses potassium hydroxide to raise the pH. Methylene blue will then stain all of the proteins and the nucleic acids so the whole of the tissue will appear blue and there will no longer be any differential staining. Eosin staining is depressed at high pH since the amino groups are now unionized and no longer attract and bind the eosin.

By careful selection of the pH, it is possible to get highly selective staining of individual components. This is most apparent in the staining of mucins where pH is used to control the binding of alcian blue to the weak carboxylic acid-containing mucins and the strong sulphated mucins (see Chapter 7).

Ionic interactions are long-range forces and can attract dyes to tissues over relatively large distances. Since there are two different charges, they can repel as well as attract (see *Fig. 6.3*).

Figure 6.3
Effect of opposite charges. Although there is a negatively charged carboxyl group in the tissue that could bind the dye, the dye will not be attracted to it because of the two nearby positive charges. The net charge on the surface of the protein is positive, so the methylene blue ion is repelled

Salt concentrations affect dye staining

Ionic binding can be inhibited by high salt concentrations, although weak salt solutions can act to increase the staining. This paradoxical effect of both enhancing and inhibiting dyeing can be understood by the effects of the ions. In strong salt solutions, there will be competition between the dye and the salt ions so staining will be inhibited. In many ways this resembles the effect of acids on basic dyes where the hydrogen ion is competing for binding with the dye molecule. Salt will affect both acid and basic dyes. Low concentrations of salt will be less inhibitory since there will be more dye than salt and once a dye has bound, the binding of the dye will be stronger than the binding of the salt. The salt may enhance staining slightly since both ions will be interacting, so the dye may be able to bind to sites to which it was previously not attracted due to the salt ions masking a repelling charge (see *Fig. 6.4*).

Hydrogen bonding

Hydrogen bonding differs from other uses of the word 'bond' since it is a force of attraction between a hydrogen atom in one molecule and a small

Figure 6.4
Effect of 'salting on'. Compare this with *Fig. 6.3*. The methylene blue is now able to bind to the carboxyl group, since the repelling charges on the amino groups are temporarily neutralized with chloride ions. The net charge on the surface of the protein is negative

atom of high electronegativity in another molecule. Thus, it is an inter-molecular force, not an intramolecular force as in the common use of the word bond. The hydrogen bond has a very limited range and will only form if the two interacting groups are brought sufficiently close together.

Hydrogen bonding is not affected by pH or salt concentration but is affected by strong hydrogen-bonding agents including urea and water. Hydrogen bonds are highly selective as they can occur only between certain groups (one must act as a donor and the other as a recipient). They proba-bly play a role in the selectivity of dyes, but are usually secondary to ionic bonds unless special conditions are arranged to inhibit ionic interactions. This inhibition of ionic bonds can be achieved by using a non-aqueous solvent (water inhibits hydrogen bonding and favours ionization), a high salt concentration (which competes with the dye for tissue ion-binding sites) and an extreme pH (which is chosen to inhibit the ionization of tissue groups).

One or two instances of staining involve hydrogen bonding rather than ionic bonding. In the staining of elastin fibres hydrogen bonds are probably more important than ionic forces. More controversially the staining of amyloid by Congo red has been considered to be dominated by hydrogen-bond staining.

Van der Waals forces

These are short-range forces and will only have an effect if the two atoms are between about 0.12 and 0.2 nm apart. If they are further apart, then there is no effective bonding force. Van der Waals forces can occur between any two atoms and are not specific for any atom or group. If the surface shape of the tissue protein and the shape of the dye match, then many van der Waals bonds can be formed. Thus, although they are individually very

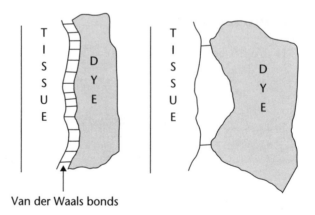

Van der Waals bonds

Figure 6.5
Van der Waals forces and dye binding. If the dye and tissue have similar shapes, more atoms can be brought close enough together to form van der Waals forces and this can add up to a significant binding force. If the dye and tissue shapes are not complementary, only a few atoms will be close enough to form van der Waals forces and the dye will be less strongly bound

---

> **Box 6.2 Van der Waals forces are important in section adhesion**
>
> Van der Waals forces are important in staining but in a quite different way to the binding of the dye. The adhesion of the section to the slide involves van der Waals interactions between the section and the glass. As the water evaporates from under the section, the lower surface of the section comes into contact with the flat smooth surface of the slide. Millions of van der Waals interactions are brought about and the section becomes firmly adherent.
>
> With the use of silane-treated slides, there is the addition of charge to the surface resulting in ionic bonding and the increased strength of adhesion may well reflect the difference in strength of the two bonds.

weak, they may add up to a significant binding force (see *Box 6.2*) if the dye and protein have complementary molecular surfaces (see *Fig. 6.5*).

Van der Waals forces are believed to have a role in selectivity but probably only play a minor role in actually binding of the dye to the tissue. The ability to form many van der Waals bonds is one explanation of the finding that larger dyes will bind more strongly than small dyes, even though they may have the same number of ionizable groups. Van der Waals bonds are unaffected by pH, ions and hydrogen-bonding agents.

Covalent bonds

These are very strong bonds and are not easily broken once formed. They do not seem to be important in most staining reactions. They are important in some histochemical techniques e.g. periodic acid–Schiff, and in the attachment of dyes to antibodies in immunofluorescence. The so-called **reactive dyes** use covalent bonds to bind but are not used much in histology.

Hydrophobic interactions

Although they are sometimes called hydrophobic bonds, the forces are not chemical bonds in the conventional sense since they hold dyes in tissues by the exclusion of water from the regions of hydrophobic groups. The exclusion of water stabilizes the two groups involved by entropy/enthalpy changes. Hydrophobic interactions again are short range and are unaffected by hydrogen-bonding agents or salts. Altering the pH may change a particular group from a hydrophilic to a hydrophobic form by altering its ionization and this will alter the staining with hydrophobic dyes. Hydrophobic interactions are important in selectivity and play a major role in the staining of lipids.

6.2 DYE STRUCTURE

Dyes are coloured organic compounds that can selectively bind to tissues. Most modern dyes are synthesized from simpler organic molecules, usually

---

Box 6.3 Synthetic dye discovery

Until the discovery of the first synthetic dye by W.H. Perkin in the 19th century, the only dyes available were natural ones. These tended to be somewhat drab and faded easily. The dye Tyrian purple was therefore a major discovery. Legend has it that this dye was discovered by the demigod Hercules. It is extracted from molluscs and by ancient standards was bright and did not fade quickly. It became a symbol of power and wealth in the ancient world and the dictionary still lists purple as meaning wealth and power.

The discovery of the first synthetic dye, Mauve, was entirely accidental. W.H. Perkin was a chemistry student trying to make the drug quinine from coal tar when he found some bright purple crystals. He borrowed some money and set up a factory to produce the dye and was rich enough to retire at 35.

---

benzene or one of its derivatives (see *Box 6.3*). The modification of these compounds into dyes is a huge industry and the chemistry of dye synthesis can be complex, but a simple example will show the general nature of dye structure.

Chromophores

Most simple organic compounds such as alkanes, benzene and alcohols are colourless to the human eye but will absorb light outside the visible spectrum. Benzene, for example, absorbs strongly in the UV region of the spectrum but appears water-white to the human eye. Benzene must be altered so that it will absorb visible light and so become a visible coloured compound that can be a useful as a dye. Any group that makes an organic compound coloured is called a **chromophore**. Benzene can be made to absorb visible light by adding a suitable chromophore. In the example below (see *Fig. 6.6*), the chromophore used is the nitro group. Adding a single nitro group gives nitrobenzene, which is a pale yellow colour; adding a second and third group intensifies the yellow colour and trinitrobenzene is a strong yellow colour.

Auxochromes

Trinitrobenzene, although coloured, is still not a dye, as it will not bind to tissues. Treating the section with trinitrobenzene will temporarily colour it yellow in the same way that a plastic sponge appears coloured when it is soaked in a coloured liquid but the colour will wash out as soon as the tissue is rinsed in a solvent. To turn a coloured compound into a dye requires the addition of an ionizable group that will allow binding to the tissues. Such binding groups are called **auxochromes**. The addition of an ionizable OH group turns trinitrobenzene into the dye trinitrophenol, which is more commonly called picric acid in histology. Picric acid is an acid dye (the OH group is phenolic and ionizes by losing a hydrogen ion) and is very useful

NO₂

₂ON   NO₂

Benzene
(colourless)

Trinitrobenzene
(yellow but not a dye)

Chromophore

NO₂

₂ON   NO₂

OH

Trinitrophenol
(picric acid,
a yellow dye)

Auxochrome

Figure 6.6
Conversion of benzene into a dye by the addition of a chromophore and an auxochrome

in histology (see *Box 6.4*); it is an essential part of the popular van Gieson counterstain.

The most important chromophoric group in dye structure is not the nitro group but the quininoid arrangement of the benzene ring (see *Fig. 6.7*). This has two double bonds at either end of the ring and two double bonds on either side. This arrangement strongly absorbs parts of the visible light spectrum.

Figure 6.7
Quininoid structure, an important chromophore

Box 6.4 Picric acid

Picric acid is a powerful explosive and needs to be kept moist. It was known as Lyddite after the explosive works at Lydd where it was manufactured. It was originally discovered by oxidizing indigo, a natural dye from an Asiatic plant. Picric acid is an unusual material in histological terms since it is a good fixative and forms the basis of the highly rated Bouin's fixative, and it is also a useful dye because it has a low molecular weight. It is used in histochemical tests to dissolve and thus identify the pigments found in malarial cells and following formalin fixation.

Changing substituent groups

The exact colour of a dye is highly dependent on many other features of the molecule including molecular size and other substituents on the ring. Most auxochromes alter the colour of the dye slightly (hence their name), as well as allowing the dye to bind to the tissue. Other groups or atoms are introduced solely to alter the colour and these are called modifier groups. Modifiers do not greatly alter the staining characteristics of the molecule, they simply alter the shade of colour.

Use of common dye names

Dyes are produced mainly for industrial uses such as textile dyeing, so a wide variety of different dyes have been synthesized to give a large range of colours. Dye manufacturers usually give the dyes they produce common names such as eosin or Congo red rather than their full chemical name and some of these names are copyrighted.

The dye structure shown in *Fig. 6.8* illustrates the complexity of many of these dyes. The full chemical name of this structure is 3,3'-((biphenyl)-4,4'-diylbis(azo))-bis(4-amino-1-naphthalenesulphonic acid) disodium salt, whilst its common name is Congo red. The common name is easier to remember and to say, so most histologists stick to using these.

Figure 6.8
Structure of Congo red

Different manufacturers may have different names for the same compound and this can be very confusing. If you ask for a dye by one name and get a bottle back with a different name on the label, you tend to think there has been a mistake. But if you order trypan blue you could get a bottle called chlorazol blue, which is the same dye by a different name. Eosin Y (yellowish eosin) has the following alternative names: acid red 87, bromoacid J, bromoacid S, bromoacid TS, bromoacid XL, bromoacid XX, bromofluorescein and bronze bromo.

Although a dye may have more than one name, it is usually easy to check with the supplier who will be able to put your mind at rest. More of a problem is the fact that different dyes can be sold by different manufacturers under the same name. For example, a dye called light green is usually considered an acid dye in histology and used for staining connective tissue, but the term light green is also used by some manufacturers for some basic dyes that will stain the nucleus and not the connective tissues. Buying the wrong dye can totally alter the results of a staining method.

The common dye names are derived from their industrial use rather than their histological use, e.g. fast green FCF (for **C**olouring **F**ood) and brown FK (for **K**ippers). In industrial terms, an acid dye is one that would be used from an acidic solution and not necessarily one that would be anionic. Sometimes the names coincide with histological properties, e.g. basic fuchsin is a basic dye, but they are sometimes misleading, e.g. neutral red is a basic dye in histological terminology.

The Colour Index

To overcome all of the confusion there is a standard list of all dyes, their synonyms and their structures. This is called the Colour Index (CI). This is a monumental work of reference produced by The Society of Dyers and Colourists and each dye is given an individual number and listed along with its name(s) and properties. Since each dye on the list has a unique number to identify it, this list is the most reliable way of identifying a dye. When naming a dye in the description of a techniques, the CI number should be given to avoid ambiguity, e.g. eosin Y (CI 45380).

CI numbers are arranged according to their structure, with the most important feature being their chromophoric group. For example, all nitroso dyes have numbers between 10000 and 10299, nitro dyes have numbers between 10300 and 10999, monoazo dyes have numbers between 11000 and 19999, and so on. There are 31 groups in all, with CI numbers up to 78000. Not all of these groups include important histological dyes; a few of the more important groups are listed below with examples of histological dyes from the group.

Nitro dyes. These have the nitro group -NO_2 as the chromophore, e.g. picric acid, martius yellow.

Azo dyes. These have the -N=N- group (azo) as the chromophore, e.g. orange G.

Triaryl methane dyes. These include the quininoid arrangement as the actual chromophore. The quininoid ring is shown as the one on the left in the diagram below, but since all three benzene rings are equivalent there can be rearrangement of the bonds and any of the benzene rings could take up this arrangement. There are a large number of dyes used in histology that fall into this category; a few examples are fuchsins, methyl violet, methyl blue and aniline blue.

Anthraquinone. Here the quininoid ring is seen as the middle of the three fused rings. Examples are alizarin and carmine.

Xanthene. Here the quininoid ring is the right hand one of the three fused rings and the ring is tilted compared with the previous example. Examples include eosin and xanthene.

Thiazine. This is very similar to the previous example in overall structure, but the middle ring now has S and N as constituent atoms. This group contains many important metachromatic dyes, such as toluidine blue, methylene blue and azure A.

Histological classification

In histology it is often more useful to classify dyes by their action on tissues and hence their uses in histology. Two dyes within the same chemical group may have quite different uses in histology. For example, the two anthraquinone dyes in the list above are used quite differently. Carmine is an important nuclear stain, whilst alizarin is most commonly used to detect calcium in tissues. Also, dyes that are from totally different groups may quite easily be exchanged in histological techniques. The histological classification is only a broad guide to how a dye will work in practice, since the actual binding relies on many properties and not just the simple ionic nature.

Basic dyes are cationic and will stain anionic or acidic materials such as carboxylates, sulphates (many complex carbohydrates are sulphated) and phosphates (particularly the phosphates in nucleic acids). Most are used as nuclear stains and staining of cytoplasmic carboxyl groups is deliberately suppressed by using a slightly acid pH. Acidic substances that stain with basic dyes are termed basophilic.

Acidic dyes are anionic and will stain cationic or basic groups in tissues such as amino groups. Most are used to stain proteins in the cytoplasm and connective tissues. Substances that stain with acid dyes are called acidophilic.

Neutral dyes are simply compounds of basic and acid dyes. In this case, both ions are coloured. Such dye complexes will stain both nucleus and cytoplasm from a single dye bath. Romanowsky stains are neutral dyes made from more complex mixtures. These are the commonest dyes used in haematology. They are less common in histology but still very useful and include Giemsa, Leishman and Wright's stains.

Amphoteric dyes also have both anionic and cationic groups, but these are on the same ion. Such dyes can stain either the nucleus or the cytoplasm if conditions are appropriate.

Natural dyes are simply dye substances extracted from natural sources. Although the main source of dyes for early microscopists, they have largely been replaced by synthetic dyes, which are usually more reliable, cheaper and can be supplied more readily. Natural dyes still in use include haematoxylin, carmine, orcein and litmus, although synthetic varieties are also available for some of these.

6.3 NON-DYE CONSTITUENTS OF STAINING SOLUTIONS

As well as dyes, most staining solutions contain other components to improve the staining.

Mordants

Mordanting is the use of a non-dyeing compound to improve the binding of the dye, with the mordant involved being able to mediate a dye–tissue interaction. Mordanting of dyes has a long history and was crucial in early textile dyeing to fix the stain to the fabric and make it into a fast dye. Fast in this sense does not mean rapid but resistant to washing out or fading, and both of these properties are critical in the dyeing of textiles. However, the term mordant was very vague in its original usage and covered a number

---

Box 6.5 Traditional mordants for textile dyes

The methods used to make dyes stable and resistant to washing were often quite elaborate. Alums were commonly used as mordants, so their transfer to histology is hardly surprising. Organic materials were also used including tannins from wood bark, gallic acids from tree galls and ammonia from urine. The dye woad was extracted from the leaves of *Isatis tinctoria* and is identical to indigo. The importation of indigo was strongly resisted by the dyers in Britain and the last woad mills closed only in the 1930s in Lincolnshire. This was despite woad processing having the reputation of being the smelliest of industrial processes.

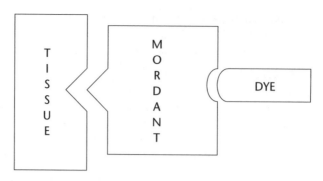

Figure 6.9

Mordanting. The dye can only bind strongly to the tissue when the mordant acts as a link between the two

of mechanisms of binding dyes. The term has been adopted for some histo-logical staining, but its use in histology is more restricted. It is usually only applied to conditions where the mordant acts as a link between the dye and the tissue and where the mordant is a metal salt (see *Fig. 6.9*).

The mechanism by which the mordant binds to the tissue is not certain but one likely mechanism is a dative covalency. The link to the dye would involve more than one such dative bond resulting in a chelate that was stable. The dye and mordant complex is sometimes called a **dye lake**. The groups on the dye forming the dative bonds are mainly oxygen-containing (e.g. in phenols, carboxyls and quinones) or nitrogen-containing (in amine, azo and nitro groups).

Since it is the mordant that binds to the tissue, the selectivity of the dye is controlled by selecting the mordant not the dye. The mordant gives greater stability to the stain and is not easily removed by water, alcohols or weak acids (i.e. it is a fast dye) and this makes it ideal when other stains are to be used afterwards, as the stain resists decolorization by the later reagents. Staining is commonly done with the dye and mordant present in the same solution, thus forming the dye lake in the stain before being applied to the tissue (e.g. Harris's haematoxylin and carmalum). The dye and mordant can also be used in two separate steps (e.g. Heidenhain's haematoxylin) and one or two techniques have used post-mordanting in which the dye is applied first and the mordant added afterwards.

Regressive use of mordanted dyes

It is also common to use mordanted dyes regressively (see *Box 6.6*). The differentiation is done by using strong acids (e.g. hydrochloric acid, often in alcoholic solution). Differentiation can also be done using excess mordant; for example, the iron alum in Heidenhain's haematoxylin can be used to slowly remove the excess haematoxylin. The excess mordant acts by displac-ing the dye lake and replacing it with a mordant with no attached dye. Theoretically it should be possible to devise a stain in which the balance of mordant to dye gives self-differentiation. A self-differentiating haematoxylin

---

Box 6.6 Progressive and regressive staining

The way in which dyes are used can differ. One distinction is between **progressive** and **regressive** staining. Progressive staining is the simplest, with the dye being applied to the section until the desired density of colour is reached. Regressive staining involves overstaining the tissue so it is darker than is needed and then removing the excess to bring the colour down to the required level. The removal of the excess dye is termed **differentiation**.

Regressive staining is often a better method of using stains. The reason is that dyes are rarely specific and will not only stain the structure being demonstrated but will also slightly colour the background, albeit less than the required structure. By removing some dye, the background can be cleared, since the background binding is usually weaker so the dye will be removed more readily. As long as the object being viewed has more dye than is required, differentiation will simply bring the colour down to the optimal level.

---

was described by Baker in 1962 but requires a constant and reliable dye, which is generally not available since most mordanting is done with natural dyes that vary in their composition from one year to the next.

Trapping agents

These differ from mordants in that they are always applied after the dye. They form large aggregates with the dye and result in the dye precipitating in the tissue. The large precipitate is more difficult to remove. The best-known example is the use of iodine to trap the violet dye inside the relatively impermeable wall of Gram-positive bacteria, whilst it can be removed from the more permeable Gram-negative organisms.

Accentuators and accelerators

Accentuators and accelerators are materials added to staining solutions to improve the staining reaction. Accentuators are generally simply used to control pH, e.g. potassium hydroxide in Löffler's methylene blue and phenol in carbol fuchsin. Accelerators are found in neurological techniques and are often hypnotic drugs such as barbiturates or chloral hydrate; their mechanism of enhancement is not known.

6.4 METACHROMATIC DYES AND METACHROMASIA

The term metachromasia is used when a dye stains a tissue component a different colour to the dye solution. For example, toluidine blue is a strong basic blue dye that stains nuclei a deep blue colour; however, it will also stain mast cell granules a pink colour. This colour shift that occurs with mast cells is called **metachromasia**, whilst the usual blue staining is called orthochromasia. Many dyes can show metachromasia but the thiazine group dyes are especially good for this type of staining.

Table 6.1 **Metachromasia and the spacing of acidic groups**

Target	Distance apart of acidic groups (nm)	Staining
Hyaluronic acid	1.03	Blue (orthochromatic)
Pectic acid	0.5	Blue/purple (weakly metachromatic)
Mast cell granules	<0.4	Red (strongly metachromatic)

Metachromasia is important as it is highly selective and only certain tissue structures can stain metachromatically. Substances that can be stained in this metachromatic way are called **chromotropes** and they include mucins, especially the sulphated mucins.

Mechanism of colour shift in metachromasia

The colour shift is always from a blue or violet dye to yellow or red staining. This means that the colour absorption shifts to shorter wavelengths, leaving only the longer wavelengths to be seen. This is believed to represent polymerization of the dye. The greater the degree of polymerization, the stronger the metachromasia. For example, toluidine blue will stain hyaluronic acid a blue colour, pectic acid (found in plants) a purple colour and mast cell granules a definite red colour. The difference is in the spacing of the acid groups, as shown in *Table 6.1* and *Fig. 6.10*.

Metachromasia requires water between the dye molecules to form the polymers and does not usually survive dehydration and clearing.

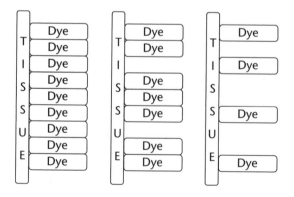

Figure 6.10
Metachromasia. The tissue on the left would be metachromatic as the dye has formed a polymeric form; the middle tissue would be weakly metachromatic as the polymeric forms are only a few molecules in size. The right-hand tissue would be orthochromatic as the dye molecules are widely spaced

6.5 EXAMPLES OF IMPORTANT DYES AND THEIR USES IN HISTOLOGY STAINS

Nuclear stains

Nuclear stains are very important in histology as the structure of the nucleus is often altered in disease. It is also easier to recognize tissue structure when only the nuclei are stained rather than when other structures are stained but the nucleus is unstained. Nuclear stains are important not only for looking at nuclear structure but also as counterstains for many staining techniques, since it is easier to recognize the location of the material in the tissue if a nuclear stain is used. For simple nuclear structure, a blue haematoxylin stain is ideal. However, for counterstaining this may not be the best stain to use, since a counterstain should be a different colour to the main technique so that it does not confuse identification. The blue/purple colours of haematoxylin often overlap with the colour of the main technique, so other nuclear counterstains are needed.

Haematoxylin

Haematoxylin is a natural product extracted from the heartwood of the tree *Haematoxylum campechianum*, which was named after the Campeche state in Mexico where it was originally found. It is now cultivated in the West Indies. The logwood of the tree is first extracted with hot water and the dye is then purified by precipitation with urea. The dry powder is usually quite pure (about 95%) but is not actually a dye. Haematoxylin is soluble in both water and alcohol but dissolves faster in alcohol, so stock solutions are often made by first dissolving the powder in alcohol and then diluting the alcoholic solution.

The formula of haematoxylin is shown below and it can be seen that there is no obvious chromophore and a solution of haematoxylin is not highly coloured.

Thus, haematoxylin itself is not a dye and for staining it must first be oxidized to haematein. Haematein has two fewer hydrogen atoms and the rearrangement of bonds introduces the quininoid ring structure and hence colour, as can be seen from the formula below:

Haematein is less soluble in water and alcohol than haematoxylin, but is soluble in ethylene glycol and glycerol. Haematein is only a weak acid dye, imparting a yellowish colour to the tissues, but when combined with a suitable mordant, haematein becomes probably the most widely used nuclear dye.

Haematein itself can be oxidized further to oxyhaematein, which is a weak acid dye but has no mordant dye capability:

Most working solutions do not completely oxidize the haematoxylin and the unoxidized part gradually oxidizes to haematein at the same time as some of the haematein oxidizes to oxyhaematein. This replenishes the working solution and greatly lengthens the life of the reagent. However, eventually all solutions will lose their strength and become useless. Oxidation is slower in acid conditions, so many solutions are deliberately kept acidic. During the natural oxidation, many haematoxylin solutions produce precipitates that must be removed by filtration before using the solution.

The oxidation of haematoxylin to haematein can occur in atmospheric oxygen, a process called ripening. This is a slow process and can take months, especially in cold and dark conditions, so that ripening is slower in the cold dark winter months than in the bright warm summer sunshine. This ripening is considered to give a longer shelf life but it is inconvenient if supplies run out, since it may take months to prepare a new batch.

Oxidation can also be carried out using oxidizing agents such as sodium iodate (200 mg per gram of haematoxylin), potassium permanganate

---

Box 6.7 Brazilin

Brazilin, extracted from trees of the genus *Caesalpinia*, is very similar to haematoxylin (only one OH different) and can be oxidized to brazilein. It can be used in the same way as haematoxylin but has never become as popular in histology. It is from this dye that the country of Brazil took its name.

Brazilin

Brazilein

(177 mg per gram of haematoxylin) or mercuric oxide (500 mg per gram of haematoxylin, although using smaller amounts than these traditional quantities will prolong the shelf life as explained above.

Mordants for haematoxylin

Haematoxylin is a very versatile stain and can be used to demonstrate many different tissue components in a highly selective way. The type of mordant used alters the specificity and colour of the stain.

Aluminium salts: haemalum. These are the commonest haematoxylin solutions and there are many different formulae but they all have similar results. Typical formulations include Harris's, Mayer's, Ehrlich's and Gill's haematoxylins. The mordant is usually either aluminium potassium sulphate (potash alum) or aluminium ammonium sulphate (ammonium alum). Because of their use of alum salts as mordants, these staining solutions are referred to as **haemalum** solutions. In acid solutions, the alum dye lakes are quite soluble and have a strong red colour. In alkaline conditions, the dye lakes are less soluble and have a strong blue colour. The dyeing bath is usually acidified and once staining is complete the section is rinsed in an alkaline solution. In hard water areas, the tap water is alkaline and simply rinsing in tap water will 'blue' the section. If the water is soft, then an alkaline solution can be prepared, e.g. lithium carbonate or tap-water substitutes. The haemalums are used regressively with a controlled differentiation in acid alcohol (1% HCl in 70% alcohol) followed by reblueing in water.

Ferric salts: iron haematoxylin. The ferric salts used are either ferric chloride or ferric ammonium sulphate (iron alum). The resulting stain is blacker and more intense, and will resist acidic counterstains such as van Gieson's better than haemalum. The ferric salts are oxidizing agents and will accelerate oxidation of the haematoxylin to haematein, which may result in overoxidation and loss of staining. The mordant is therefore either used separately (Heidenhain's) or the mordant and haematoxylin are mixed just before use (e.g. Weigert's). Differentiation is often done with excess mordant and requires microscopic control. There is no need to 'blue' the sections in an alkaline solution since the mordant produces an intense black colour regardless of the pH. The use of iron haematoxylins has declined following the introduction of the celestin blue–haemalum sequence, which also resists acid decoloration.

Other mordants that can be used to selectively stain specific tissue components are shown in *Table 6.2*.

Carmine and carminic acid

Carmine is a natural dye extracted from the red pigment cochineal, which is used in cooking. Cochineal itself is extracted from the bodies of the scale insect *Dactylopius coccus*. Carmine is actually a complex of aluminium and carminic acid rather than just the dye molecule. Commercial carmine powder is quite variable in its composition and in addition to the dye–aluminium complex also contains protein, calcium and other ions.

Table 6.2 Other mordants that can be used with haematoxylin

Tissue element demonstrated	Mordant
Nuclei	Al or Fe
Myelin	Cr or Cu
Elastic fibres	Fe
Collagen	Mo
Neuroglia	W
Axis cylinders	Pb
Mucin	Al
Fibrin	W
Mitochondria	Fe
Heavy metals (Pb, Cu) and Ca	None (the metal in the tissue acts as the mordant and binds the dye)

Carminic acid is a glycoside with a glucose derivative joined to an anthraquinone structure (see below).

Carminic acid is the pure dye and is only slightly soluble in water but dissolves much better in solutions of an aluminium salt, when it forms the carmine complex. Solutions of the complex are not stable and significant deterioration occurs after only a few weeks of storage. For precise staining, it is better if the carmine solution is prepared from purified carminic acid.

For many years carmine was a major stain with its main advantage being its permanence when compared with other dyes. The problem with many other stains was that when they were mounted in Canada balsam, the acidity of the mountant caused significant fading in just a few months. At the height of its popularity, carmine was used for many different techniques and a great many methods were devised using carmine. The unreliability of the dye supply and the rising cost of the natural product have led to it becoming much less popular. The loss of popularity occurred at the same time as laboratories switched to the use of modern synthetic mounting media, which cause much less fading of other dyes so there was less need for a stable nuclear stain.

A good carmine stain is easy for inexperienced workers to use, as overstaining is difficult. Any excess dye can easily be removed with 1% HCl.

The most popular stains were the carmalum techniques (e.g. Mayer's, Grenacher's) and acetocarmine.

Neutral red and safranine

These are popular red nuclear stains mainly used as counterstains to blue staining methods such as Perl's iron staining method. Both dyes are easily soluble in water and alcohol.

Neutral red can also be used as a vital stain when used at a very dilute (10^{-5}) concentration. Neutral red can act as an indicator, changing colour at pH 6.8–7.0 (turning yellowish in alkali). Neutral red stains nuclei red and cytoplasm pale yellow.

Methylene blue

This is a very widely used simple blue stain that does not require a mordant. It gives a quick and simple nuclear counterstain for red primary stains. It is readily soluble in water and alcohol.

Methylene blue was a major component of Romanowsky stains used in the staining of blood smears and bone marrow specimens. In the preparation of the Romanowsky dyes, it was used as 'polychrome methylene blue' (see *Box 6.8*). The polychroming produces a range of dyes from the original methylene blue of which azure B is probably the most important. Modern Romanowsky stains generally use mixtures of pure dyes rather than the empirical polychromed methylene blue.

Box 6.8 Polychrome methylene blue

One of the methods used to produce polychromed methylene blue was to allow fungi to grow in a solution of it. The metabolic actions of the fungi converted some of the dye to other compounds. The relationship between dyes and micro-organisms can be quite interesting. Many dyes will allow micro-organisms to grow in them and this changes their staining characteristics. Other dyes have been used as antibacterial agents and the selectivity of dyes led many people to believe that dyes might prove to be the 'magic bullets' that would kill selected bacteria and save humanity from infection.

Methyl green

This blue/green nuclear stain is a useful nuclear counterstain and is also an important part of many techniques that differentiate between DNA and RNA in tissues. It is often contaminated with methyl violet, but this can be removed by washing with chloroform.

Cytoplasmic stains

Cytoplasmic stains are often used as counterstains but can also be important to identify tissue components. Most techniques are also used to distinguish connective tissue fibres and other protein materials. The cytoplasmic stains should produce several different shades of colour so that the tissues can easily be distinguished. Most of the stains are acidic (anionic) dyes but can be used in mixtures to improve the contrast between different components.

Eosin

This is not a single dye but a variety of related dyes. All are derived from fluorescein, which is a useful fluorescent dye widely used to label antibodies but is useless for ordinary light microscopy. By substituting halogens or nitro groups for some hydrogens, a variety of shades of red can be produced from yellowish to bluish e.g. eosin Y (yellowish) changes to eosin B (bluish) if the bromine groups on positions 2′ and 7′ are changed to nitro groups.

The dyes are also fluorescent but are solely used as red dyes, although the parent dye fluorescein is widely used as a labelling compound in immuno-fluorescence. The sodium salts of the dyes are all freely soluble in water and fairly soluble in alcohol but will precipitate as eosinic acid if the pH is very low. However, adding dilute acids will improve eosin staining but may overdifferentiate the nuclear stain.

Eosin is a very good cytoplasmic stain as it gives several shades to the tissue. The range of shades can be extended even further if more than one dye is used in the solution. Some workers claim that up to seven different shades can be distinguished, although I have always found it difficult to distinguish more than about four.

Eosin solutions keep reasonably well unless they become contaminated by fungi, when they will develop significant growth. This growth can be inhibited by adding a small amount of thymol to the solution and this acidic material also enhances the staining.

Ethyl eosin is an ester rather than the more usual sodium salt and is only slightly soluble in water. It is used when eosin staining is needed from alcoholic solution. It must be differentiated in alcohol.

Eosin is also an important component of Romanowsky stains, which are all eosinates of azure dyes. Its pre-eminent role in staining is shown by the fact that many structures are referred to as eosinophilic when they will stain equally well with other acid dyes.

Eosin gives a good red cytoplasmic counterstain but if other colours are required then other dyes must be used.

Methyl blue and aniline blue

These are widely used blue anionic dyes with similar staining properties. Both are water soluble but insoluble in alcohol. They are often confused as both are also known as soluble blue and water blue. Both are quite large dye structures and are frequently used to stain connective tissue fibres.

Fast green FCF and light green SF

These are green anionic dyes similar to the blue dyes above and are frequently used as counterstains to red dyes. Fast green FCF is less prone to fading than light green SF.

Orange G, picric acid (trinitrophenol), metanil yellow and martius yellow

These are very pale-coloured dyes ideal for faint background staining or in conjunction with other acid dyes. Orange G is soluble in water but less so in alcohol and is a major component of the Papanicolaou stain used in cervical cytology.

Picric acid is a valuable stain in multiple acid dye techniques because of its small size.

Connective tissue methods

Connective tissue consists mainly of collagen fibres, elastic fibres, glycosaminoglycans and cells. The main way of distinguishing the fibres and cells is by using a combination of acid dyes to stain different structures in differing colours. There is still uncertainty about the exact mechanisms of these techniques but they seem to depend on differences in dye size and differing permeabilities of tissues.

Acid dye combinations

The differing molecular weights and sizes of dyes affect their diffusion rate and their ability to permeate into small spaces in the tissue. The larger dyes will also be able to form more van der Waals forces. Thus, when two acid dyes compete for binding to tissue, the larger dye will generally tend to displace the smaller dye. In addition, the smaller dyes tend to be paler colours (yellowish), whilst the larger dyes are dense colours. These effects combine so that smaller paler dyes are overwhelmed by larger denser dyes when they compete directly.

Tissue permeability is related to the amount of protein that is present and the amount of water between the proteins. Loose collagenous (areolar) tissue has many minute fluid spaces and is very permeable, whilst erythrocytes are packed full of haemoglobin and are much denser. Most other cells types, including muscle, lie between these two. The concept of the differential acid dyeing technique is that only the small dye will penetrate into the dense red cells. The red blood cells should thus be stained with the smallest dye. In the less-dense collagenous tissue, the large and small dyes will be in competition. The larger dye will dominate and the collagen will appear stained only with the largest dye.

Van Gieson's stain

This stain uses two acid dyes (acid fuschin and picric acid) to distinguish between acidophilic materials. Each dye, if used alone, would stain all cytoplasm and connective tissue. By combining them in a single solution, the tissue differences can be exploited. The open texture of the collagen, allowing free and rapid access to both dyes, stains red, whilst muscle and erythrocytes, which restrict access of larger dyes, stain yellow. Both dyes are mixed into a single solution along with hydrochloric acid to give a pH of 1–2.

Permeability and dye size considerations would suggests that the small dye will rapidly penetrate both the dense red blood cells and the looser connective tissues. The larger fuchsin molecules will penetrate into the connective tissues quite readily but will penetrate the denser red blood cells only slowly. Where both dyes are present, the fuchsin will displace or mask the paler picric acid with the result that the connective tissue will stain red but in the red blood cells the picric acid will not be displaced or masked and the red cells will stain yellow (see *Colour plate 6*).

Trichrome stains

These take the differential staining a stage further and use three different-sized dyes to selectively stain the three tissue densities. For example, picric acid (formula weight (FW) 229), acid fuchsin (FW 578) and methyl blue (FW 800) can be used as a trichrome mixture. The red blood cells are the densest tissue and stain with the smallest dye, the intermediate cytoplasm and muscle cells are stained red by the intermediate-sized dye and the collagenous tissue stains with the largest dye. In each case, only the largest dye of the competing dyes does the staining

Heteropolyacids aid trichrome staining

Trichromes differ from van Gieson's stain in that an extra reagent is used in the form of one of the heteropolyacids. The heteropolyacids are either phosphomolybdic (sometimes called molybdophosphoric) acid or phosphotungstic (tungstophosphoric) acid. These improve the staining but whether they simply act as colourless dyes or have a more active role in some form of mordanting is still unresolved. Trichromes also differ in that the three dyes are usually used separately and sequentially, rather than in a single mixed reagent as in van Gieson's stain.

Trichromes can to some extent be 'tuned' to differentiate between tissue fibres by selecting dyes of appropriate sizes and by controlling the size of tissue spaces. Alcoholic solutions seem to affect penetration by allowing dyes to permeate more freely, possibly by increasing the size of tissue spaces. This makes the molecules act as if they were a slightly smaller size.

Molecular size and permeability: not the full story

Although the explanation given here accounts nicely for much of the staining with multiple acid dyes (trichromes and van Gieson's), there are anomalies and the exact mechanisms are still very much undetermined. In particular, if the dyes are used alone they will readily stain all of the tissue. Thus, the fuchsin dye in van Gieson's stain will stain red blood cells, showing that it is able to penetrate these structures.

There is the possibility that the timing is crucial and that by using a limited time the red dye would not have long enough to penetrate into the cells. Even on theoretical grounds this seems unlikely; a red blood cell is less than 8 μm across at its widest point and less than 3 μm thick. For diffusion across such small distances to take more than 2 min (which is a typical staining time for van Gieson's stain) would suggest an extremely dense material.

If van Gieson's staining is extended to 30 min or more, there is no real major difference in the result.

Similar anomalies can also be seen when different combinations of dyes are used. It is always the smallest dye that stains the red blood cells and the largest that stains the collagen, but the same dye can stain both under different conditions. If acid fuchsin is used in combination with other dyes, it will stain erythrocytes if the other dye is larger, but will stain collagen and not erythrocytes if the other dye is smaller. The situation is more complex than the simple dye size and permeability would suggest, yet the concept does seem to hold in most practical applications and several good trichrome methods have been produced on the basis of this theory.

Dyes and quality control

As mentioned earlier most dyes are not produced for histologists but for textile dyers. The important property for textiles is a reliable final colour rather than chemical purity. Dye manufacturers therefore adjust their products to give consistent dyeing of fabrics rather than histological reliability. This means that dyes, unlike most biochemical reagents, are often impure substances and may contain significant amounts of other materials such as salts, dextrans and even other dyes. The actual content of the named dye rarely exceeds 95% and may be as little as 25% of the total weight. Different batches of dye will differ in their dye and contaminant content, which makes quality control in the histological laboratory difficult.

The non-dye constituents are often very important and may grossly affect the staining. To try to combat this problem, some laboratory suppliers offer **certified dyes** that have been tested biologically for their stated uses. Such dyes are more expensive but should match their stated uses reliably.

It is also worth repeating that some dyes have many names and it should always be made clear which dye is needed by using CI numbers; otherwise the dye may be completely different. When a staining method suddenly stops staining as expected, it is worth checking that you have not got a different batch of dye to the usual one.

There is a growing tendency for laboratories to buy in many reagents in a ready-prepared form rather than making up stains from the original

---

Box 6.8 Contaminated dyes

Dyes have always been impure so it became important to have a good source of dyes. Dyestuffs are quite expensive to manufacture, so it was not unknown for dyes to be 'cut' with less expensive materials to make them more profitable. Some older samples of dye certainly seemed to have an insoluble residue left after preparing the staining solution. One manufacturer, however, became famous for the quality of his stains and if you read the old textbooks you will find his dyes being recommended time after time in techniques as being the best available. Nobody thought his dyes were purer, just better. It was said that 'not only does Herr Grübler have the best dyes, he also has the best impurities'. Grübler dyes lost their leading role following the Second World War when importing of dyes from Germany became impossible and laboratories had to find other sources.

ingredients. This leads to more consistency in the laboratory as the scale of industrial production can be controlled more carefully than small irregularly prepared batches in the laboratory.

Checking dyes in a histology laboratory

Quality control of dyes within the laboratory is difficult, as many of the techniques used in quality control require complex equipment to analyse the dye samples (e.g. infrared spectroscopy, high-performance liquid chromatography), but some simple tests can usually be performed.

1. Chromatography. This will detect coloured contaminants of dyes and can be a sensitive way of comparing two dye batches. Simple paper chromatography using filter paper is often enough to pick out impure dye samples.
2. Measurement of absorption (including a full spectrum if a suitable spectrophotometer is available) can be used to determine the amount of dye in a sample and may also show contaminants.
3. Testing with standard dyeing techniques to determine whether the dye is suitable or needs altered staining times/conditions. Some dye batches may be suitable for one stain but not for others; for example, fuchsin samples may be good for use in Ziehl–Neelsen staining for mycobacterium but not for preparing Schiff's reagent.

Once the dye has been made up into a solution it may not be permanently stable. Dyes can alter due to oxidation by the air, bleaching by light, contamination by micro-organisms growing in the solution or chemical reactions between constituents of the dye solutions. Reagent bottles should be clearly labelled with the date of preparation and renewed at regular intervals or sooner if the staining seems to be suffering. If light accelerates the deterioration, then storage of the reagent in brown bottles to prevent light reaching the dye may help, although the dark glass will also mask any contamination and precipitation, so care must still be taken. Most techniques using reagents that need special storage (e.g. refrigeration) will usually give details.

6.6 SILVER IMPREGNATION

Metallic impregnation is an alternative way of increasing the contrast in tissues. The commonest metal to use in light microscopy is silver, which produces a dense, black, fine deposit of silver and silver oxide where the silver ions have been reduced. Silver impregnation is also called silver staining, but the mechanism is quite different to the effects of dyes and the structures are actually plated with the silver rather than the silver being reversibly bound to the section.

Advantages

Silver impregnation has a number of advantages compared with dyeing techniques and has a number of very common applications. The main advantages of silver techniques are:

1. They are stable and do not fade. The end product is metallic silver, which if properly fixed and washed is effectively permanent. The silver deposit in black and white photographs is similar to the material produced by silver impregnation and photographs from 150 years ago are still in excellent condition. Dyed sections rarely last more than 10 years without some signs of fading.
2. The silver deposit is densely black, which gives good contrast and is excellent for taking photographs.
3. Silver techniques are very sensitive methods and will detect many materials that are difficult to demonstrate by dyeing. These materials include reticulin fibres (see *Colour plate 7*), which are difficult to observe with haematoxylin and eosin staining but can be readily demonstrated with silver impregnation. Metal impregnation methods are more common in neurological methods, e.g. for axons, motor end plates and astroglia (see *Colour plate 8*).
4. Slender objects are thickened because they become silver-plated. This can be useful for fine fibres such as reticulin or for slender bacteria such as spirochetes.

Disadvantages

1. The techniques can be unreliable and capricious. They will sometimes work well and other times will not work at all. This can extend to different workers. There sometimes seems to be one person in the laboratory who can get a technique to work perfectly, whilst everyone else struggles, even when using the same reagents. Staining times can vary tremendously from one day to the next when a fresh batch of silver solution is prepared.
2. The silver solutions are often very alkaline. Strong alkaline solutions have a tendency to strip sections off the glass slides so extra care and adhesives are needed.
3. Silver techniques are so sensitive that they can sometimes give non-specific background deposits ('dirty preparations').
4. The techniques have a tendency to stain everything they come into contact with (hands, laboratory coats, benches, glassware, etc.). Silver is very difficult to remove without using dangerous reagents, so clothing is often permanently stained. Silver solutions are easy to wash out if they are caught early enough, but as they look just like water it is not always obvious that there has been a spillage. Once reduced, the safest way to remove silver deposits is by using an iodine solution, which converts the silver to silver iodide, which is then soluble in sodium thiosulphate solutions.
5. Some silver solutions have a tendency to become explosive if stored for more than 24 h.
6. Silver is expensive.
7. Silver cannot be discarded into the drains as it is a heavy metal poison.

Use of silver

Silver is not the only metal that can be used for impregnations but is the most useful as it is easily reduced and any reduced silver acts as a catalyst for the reduction of more silver. This autocatalytic activity makes silver useful in many fields other than histology. The use of silver is widespread in photography and the chemistry of photography and the chemistry of silver impregnation are very closely related.

Silver solutions are reduced during the impregnation, so silver techniques are primarily methods for reducing materials. There are three different ways of producing silver deposits. These are the argentaffin reaction, the argyrophil reaction and ion-exchange reactions.

The argentaffin reaction

In the argentaffin reaction, the tissue contains reducing groups that are sufficiently strong and present in sufficient quantity to give a visible deposit without added reducing agents. These groups are often aldehyde groups and silver solutions can be used to replace the Schiff's reagent in the periodic acid–Schiff technique (see Chapter 7) to give periodic acid–silver. The argentaffin reaction occurs particularly with reducing pigments and is strongest with the pigment of enterochromaffin cells, which derives its alternative name (argentaffin pigment) from the reaction. The strong reaction in this case is due to phenolic components (5-hydroxytryptamine, or serotonin). The reaction only needs the addition of the silver solution, such as in the Masson–Fontana technique, but tends to be very slow and may take up to 24 h to give a deposit.

The argyrophil reaction

Many tissue groups are able to adsorb silver, possibly by ionic mechanisms as for dyeing. The silver is mainly adsorbed as silver ions but small amounts are reduced to silver atoms. These silver atoms are deposited at the site of reduction. The initial reduction reaction with silver only deposits submicroscopic atoms of silver at particularly reactive sites. Probably only a few, perhaps as few as two, atoms are deposited in this initial stage and these are too small to be visible, even with high-power microscopy. These silver atoms then act as catalytic sites where more silver can be deposited by the reducing action of a developer (see *Fig. 6.11*), e.g. formaldehyde or hydroquinone (quinol). In this case the developer does the main reduction and the tissue simply provides places where there are silver atoms to catalyse the reduction. This type of reaction where an external reducer or developer is added is called an argyrophilic reaction.

Ion-exchange reactions

Ion exchange can also deposit silver and this is used to detect mineralization of bone using the von Kossa technique. The section is treated with silver solution (silver nitrate) and the phosphates and carbonates in the mineralized bone form insoluble silver salts. The silver salts are then blackened by

Figure 6.11
Silver deposition and reduction in the argyrophil reaction

UV light or hydroquinone solutions (see *Colour plate 7*). Although often said to demonstrate calcification of bone, the method actually detects carbonates and phosphates.

$$CaCO_3 + 2AgNO_3 \rightarrow Ag_2CO_3 + Ca(NO_3)_2$$

$$Ag_2CO_3 \text{ (UV treated)} \rightarrow Ag_2O + CO_2$$

$$\text{Black}$$

Silver solutions

Ammoniacal silver solutions are used as they are easily reduced. Silver solutions always need careful preparation and some diamine silver solutions can become explosive if kept for more than 24 h. If they are being used in a glass container, then a simple safety precaution is to wrap them up with adhesive tape (Sellotape); if an explosion occurs the glass fragments will be held by the sticky tape. It is important always to use distilled water in any silver method, as tap water will react with the silver salt.

Several silver solutions can be used in silver techniques but they are not directly interchangeable as they differ in their sensitivity to reduction.

Silver nitrate

This is the commonest form of silver salt used in the preparation of silver solutions. Simple silver nitrate solutions are sometimes used, e.g. von Kossa's solution, or as sensitizer solutions, e.g. Beilschowsky's method for nerve fibres, but for most techniques a more readily reduced form is needed.

Silver diamine

Silver diamine solutions are prepared by precipitating the silver with a hydroxide solution and then redissolving in a minimum amount of ammonium hydroxide. These solutions are very alkaline and this makes sections more liable to detach during staining, so an adhesive is often advisable. The final solution can be explosive if it is stored for more than 24 h, but has the advantage of being very sensitive.

$$2Ag^+ + 2OH^- \rightarrow Ag_2O + H_2O \quad \text{Precipitation of silver oxide}$$

$$Ag_2O + 4NH_3 + H_2O \rightarrow 2[Ag(NH_3)_2]^+ + 2OH^- \quad \text{Dissolving to form silver diamine}$$

Silver carbonate

Silver carbonate solutions are prepared by precipitating the silver using either lithium or sodium carbonate solution. The precipitate is filtered and washed. This removal of the precipitating salt is different to the previous example of silver diamine where the hydroxide is left in the solution. The precipitate is then dissolved using strong ammonia as for the diamine solution. Silver carbonate solutions are claimed to be even more sensitive than diamine solutions.

Hexamine silver solutions

These use hexamine (methenamine or hexamethylenetetramine). When mixed with silver nitrate, this produces a white precipitate that immediately redissolves without the need to titrate with strong ammonia.

Background deposits

Silver techniques often produce a non-specific deposit due to contaminants. Very small deposits can often be reduced by **toning**. This involves using 'gold chloride' (sodium chloroaurate):

$$3Ag + (AuCl_4)^- \rightarrow Au + 3AgCl + Cl^-$$

Thus, three silver atoms are replaced by one gold atom. For very small deposits this will result in a great reduction in size (thus reducing the background staining) but the large deposits of the impregnated tissue will hardly be affected. Gold toning also alters the colour from an intense black to a warmer brown/black colour.

Following completion of the technique, the sections are usually treated with 'hypo' (sodium thiosulphate, previously called hyposulphate). This is a photographic fixer that dissolves excess silver ions and prevents them later depositing as background. It is probably not necessary in histological preparations, as all of the silver is usually completely reduced so there is little risk of further reduction, but it is always done 'just in case'.

Silver techniques

Reticulin can be demonstrated using silver impregnation and the following is a fairly typical silver staining technique based on the method proposed by Laidlaw in 1929.

First the reticulin is oxidized to give aldehyde groups:

$$\boxed{\text{Reticulin}}\begin{array}{l}\diagup\text{OH} \\ \diagdown\text{OH}\end{array} \xrightarrow[\text{Oxidation}]{\text{KMnO}_4} \boxed{\text{Reticulin}}\begin{array}{l}\diagup\text{CHO} \\ \diagdown\text{CHO}\end{array}$$

Then the silver solution oxidizes the aldehydes to acids and in the process is itself reduced to silver atoms that precipitate at the site of reduction:

$$\boxed{\text{Reticulin}}\begin{array}{l}\diagup\text{CHO} \\ \diagdown\text{CHO}\end{array} + 4[\text{Ag(NO}_3)_2]^+ + 3\text{H}_2\text{O} \longrightarrow$$

$$\longrightarrow \boxed{\text{Reticulin}}\begin{array}{l}\diagup\text{COOH} \\ \diagdown\text{COOH}\end{array} + 4\text{Ag}\downarrow + 8\text{NH}_4^+ + 4\text{OH}^-$$

Aldehydes are one of the commoner reducing groups in tissues and silver solutions can often be used to detect the presence of aldehydes.

Silver techniques vary quite widely in their conditions

There are many variations on silver techniques that seem to give good results. It is largely a matter of preference which technique works best in a particular laboratory. There are probably differences between the laboratories that are not particularly mentioned or even controlled that make one method more suitable for one laboratory than another. These variations include tissue fixation and processing, water quality (both tap and distilled or deionized water), ambient temperature and ambient light.

The actual concentrations of silver vary quite markedly from 1 g per 100 ml (Foot method) to 10 g per 100 ml (Laidlaw method). Times and temperatures also vary from 30 s (Gordon and Sweet method) to 60 min (Perdrau method) and temperatures from room temperature of 20°C up to temperatures of 70°C (Lillie method).

This wide variation might suggest that the technique is quite insensitive to conditions and would work reliably, regardless of any slight technical errors, but this is not the case. Silver techniques are more difficult to get exactly right than most staining methods and require care, patience and experience to get an even impregnation and lack of non-specific background. The wide variation is actually a reflection of this, since many people have tried, and largely failed, to get an automatic and reliable technique.

6.7 GENERAL TREATMENT OF SECTIONS DURING STAINING

After drying to achieve adhesion, paraffin wax sections are still not ready to be stained, as they are totally impregnated with wax, which forms a water-proof coating and prevents dye access to the proteins.

Section rehydration

For staining, the wax must be removed and the section rehydrated. This is conveniently done using stainless steel racks that hold a number of slides and flat staining dishes. The dry labelled slides are placed in the rack and the wax is removed. Xylene is still the most commonly used reagent for this process. Xylene is less commonly used for processing tissues because of its tendency to cause shrinkage and hardening, but there is no problem with shrinkage at this stage because the tissues are firmly attached to a rigid slide, and harden-ing is no longer a difficulty as there is no further sectioning to be done. Removal of the wax needs to be complete; if any wax remains it will result in uneven staining. Treatment with xylene for 5 min is usually sufficient.

The sections can then be transferred through a series of graded alcohols (typically 100%, 95%, 70%) and finally into distilled water. They do not need prolonged times in any of these baths since penetration is very rapid through the thin sections; 30 s with gentle agitation will usually be enough.

This process of returning a paraffin section to water is usually called either dewaxing, or 'taking the section to water' (see *Box 6.8*) or occasionally by the somewhat grander phrase of **deceration**. One of these phrases will be found

---

Box 6.8 Dewaxing or 'taking to water'

If the section is frozen then the phrase 'take the section to water' can be ignored as the section is already in water. Often students do not think and try to process the tissue as if it was a paraffin section, which can totally ruin the section. For this reason, personally I prefer the phrase 'take the section to water' to 'dewaxing', as it is less prescriptive and suggests that the histologist needs to get the section into water from the medium the section is currently embedded in.

Sections are best dewaxed immediately before being stained. Once rehydrated, they will slowly deteriorate, especially if kept in water. Deterioration is not rapid and sections can be kept in water, alcohol or xylene for quite long periods, although they do gradually lose adhesion. This is similar to the 'soaking' of pans with dried-on food residue. Since soaking will remove dried-on food, it is hardly surprising that it will also remove dried-on sections. It is also bad practice to allow sections to dry out at any stage in the staining, as this can introduce minute air bubbles into the protein mesh, which is the cellular structure. These air bubbles may remain and not be removed when the tissue is again placed into reagent and will end up in the final preparation. There are occasionally instances when sections need to be dried, but these are the exception.

at the beginning of most staining schedules and must always be done when paraffin sections are used.

Once fully rehydrated, the sections can be stained in aqueous reagents until they are ready to be mounted.

Automated staining

Automated processing of tissues is widely accepted and a similar automation is possible with staining. The same general principles apply to both situations. Automation frees staff from a routine task that is relatively straightforward and allows them to do more demanding tasks. The use of an absolutely regular procedure ensures that there is little variation in results, so that direct comparisons are valid from one batch of stained sections to the next. This accuracy and reproducibility are crucial in some applications such as diagnostic and exfoliative cytology (see Chapter 12) where the colour of the cytoplasm is an important diagnostic feature.

The disadvantage is that there is less flexibility. All of the sections will be given the same treatment, regardless of their requirements. It is also only feasible for techniques that are carried out for a large number of samples. Machines are fine for doing hundreds of haematoxylin and eosin stains, but it is not reasonable to use a machine for stains where the technique is only required for two or three slides each day. It also does not lend itself to situations where different results are needed; for example, when photographing at low magnifications, an overstained section will give better results than the usual staining intensity. An ordinary stain will give insufficient contrast for the film's recording capabilities but a more-intense stain will give stronger differences between the tissue components.

Automated staining also demands reproducible reagents. If there is a change in a reagent's staining properties, the machine will not recognize this and compensate for the change in the way that a person would. Most histologists can easily compensate for gradual changes in reagents as they age or for sudden alterations from a new batch of stain without too many problems. Machines only follow the program and cannot tell that there is any need to change. Any alterations result in machines needing to be reprogrammed, for example, if a different batch of reagent is prepared. This inflexibility may also result in reagents being discarded sooner than they would be for manual staining in order to maintain a standard program.

Automated staining machines are also less flexible in producing single stains, even when they are already programmed for that stain. Thus, producing a single slide may hold up some types of machine; these machines must go through the full cycle before another section can even begin since the steps are uneven. These machines are inefficient for staining single sections. An alternative strategy is to have all the steps the same length (e.g. 1 min) so that sections can be added at any time and will follow the same path. The difficulty here is that, if a longer time is needed, then several baths of the same reagent are required. These machines often cannot cope with large numbers of sections in a short space of time.

Automated staining machines are very useful for absolute regularity with large numbers of sections needing the same treatment at the same time. They have found a significant role in two main areas:

1. Haematoxylin and eosin staining in histology, Papanicolaou staining in cytology and blood-film staining in haematology. This is because the sheer numbers needing staining make it worthwhile.
2. Immunohistochemistry, nucleic acid hybridization and similar techniques. Here the actual numbers are smaller but the need for absolute consistency is greater, so these techniques have moved to more automation.

The use of automatic coverslipping machines is often linked to automated staining. The process of mounting sections is very mundane, so automation is possible. There is less requirement for variety in mounting, so provided they are working well these machines are a useful addition to the laboratory.

6.8 SECTION MOUNTING

Use of coverslips

Mounting of sections under a coverslip is essential to get the best and clearest view of the specimen. You only need to compare an unmounted wet section at the end of staining with a properly mounted section to see the difference. The microscope manufacturers usually assume that the specimen will be mounted in a medium with a high refractive index and covered with a thin glass coverslip and calculate all of their optical corrections on that basis. The difference can be seen in *Fig. 6.12* where the optical paths through a wet section and a mounted section are compared. The unmounted section has twice as many refracting surfaces and the opaque tissue will transmit much less light.

The coverslip should have a thickness of 0.17 mm (No. 1 coverslip) for the best results, as this is the thickness used in optical calculations. Thicker

Figure 6.12
Effect of a coverslip on viewing sections. On the left, a section mounted in a high refractive medium has only two refractions, whilst a section in water has up to four refracting surfaces

coverslips such as a No. 2 coverslip will interfere marginally with the clarity and very thick coverslips may even prevent the oil-immersion lens being used as they can have a greater thickness than the normal working distance of the oil-immersion lens.

Mounting media

The mounting medium should have a high refractive index (RI). Most tissues have an RI of between 1.5 and 1.55, so a mounting medium with an RI in this range will give maximum clarity. There is no single mounting medium that is suitable for all specimens and stains. There are two major types of mounting media used and the difference is in the solvent. The commonest types are the resinous mounting media, which are based on hydrophobic organic solvents, usually xylene, and which need the section to be dehydrated and cleared before mounting. Water-based mounting media will accept tissues straight from distilled water and are used when a xylene-based medium would not be appropriate, e.g. if the dye or histochemical reaction product is soluble in xylene.

The properties that need to be considered in a mounting medium are:

1. Refractive index. If the RI is much lower than 1.5, then tissues will not be completely transparent and diffraction will occur. This is usually a disadvantage as it reduces clarity but it can sometimes be an advantage as it will give some contrast to even unstained tissues.
2. Clarity under normal conditions of use. Some media can become opaque as they dry out and are not suitable for long-term preservation.
3. Effects on the stain itself. Some mounting media will cause fading. This is most common with acidic mounting materials, which will cause significant fading, especially in the light. Some media may also act as solvents for the dyes and as a consequence the dye diffuses or leaches out into the mountant. This will gradually obscure the tissues.
4. Fluorescence. This is really only critical for fluorescence microscopy but it is generally a useful characteristic for a general mounting medium since it eliminates the need to use a special mountant when fluorescence is being used.
5. Setting. The ability of a mountant to dry or set quickly and hold the coverslip in place is very useful. Many aqueous-based media fail to harden sufficiently and the coverslip will need 'ringing' to preserve the section.

Resinous mounting media

Canada balsam. This was the original resinous mounting medium used in histology. Canada balsam is derived from the *Abies balsamea* fir tree and is available as a dried, brittle, yellow solid. It will melt at high temperature and is soluble in xylene. Approximately 60 g in 100 ml of xylene gives a good working mountant, although it takes a few days to dissolve completely. The yellow colour of the mountant hardly seems to matter when viewed through the microscope. The mountant is usually significantly acid and will cause fading, especially of basic dyes. It is relatively expensive and is mainly of historical importance rather than being a common mountant.

DPX. This is a synthetic polystyrene resin that is dissolved in xylene and has some plasticizer added. The initials come from the components: Distrene 80 (a commercial polystyrene), plasticizer (e.g. dibutyl phthalate) and xylene. It is a water-white clear solution and is one of the more popular mountants in use. It has very little tendency to fade dyes and hardens in about 24 h. The specimens do not need ringing.

Other synthetic media are available such as Permount or Entellan, which are commercial brand names.

When a section comes to the end of normal staining and is ready for mounting in a resinous mounting medium, it needs to be dehydrated and cleared in xylene before finally being mounted. This is simply the reverse of the dewaxing, but it is better not to use the same reagents as they gradually become contaminated with the other reagents, e.g. dewaxing will leave wax in the xylene, which can interfere with the mounting medium.

Aqueous mounting media

There is no fully satisfactory aqueous medium and several different ones are used for different purposes. They differ in the way in which the RI of water (1.33) is raised sufficiently to give a clear image. Most are best considered as temporary mounts and need ringing to hold the coverslip in place and prevent drying out. Tissues do not need any treatment before mounting and can be mounted directly from water or buffer.

Glycerol. Glycerol is a trihydric alcohol with a high RI. It can be used alone or with the addition of a buffer to control the pH. It is a useful medium for fluorescent staining, for example, for immunofluorescent antibody techniques. The addition of p-phenylenediamine is said to retard the fading of fluorescence. It neither hardens nor dries out and is usually used as a very short-term mountant, although it can be ringed for slightly longer use.

Glycerol jelly. This uses the addition of gelatine (up to 12% in some formulations) to allow the medium to set. The usual formulation has a lower RI (1.42) than most mounting media, so the clarity is reduced and some unstained structures will be visible. It is solid at room temperature and needs to be melted in a waterbath before use. It is very easy to get air bubbles trapped in this medium, so it is convenient to melt it and get rid of any air bubbles by warming it in a vacuum-embedding oven. Glycerol jelly is quite a good growth medium for some bacteria and fungi, so there is usually an antibacterial additive (e.g. phenol), but it still does not keep well. Sections may also allow the growth of organisms in storage, so it is best thought of as a temporary mount.

Apathy's medium. This uses a gum (gum arabic or gum acacia) and sucrose to raise the RI. It has an RI of around 1.5, so it can give nicely transparent preparations. It has a tendency to crystallize in storage and can set by drying but this is quite slow. Again, it may need the addition of an antibacterial agent to help preserve it.

Polyvinyl alcohol or polyvinylpyrollidone media. These are synthetic and less liable to bacterial contamination than the organic-based mountants, although the addition of phenol is still advisable. They dissolve in water or buffer but need constant stirring. They solidify slowly by evaporation but specimens can be ringed to prevent this. These are more permanent than the other water-based mounting media, but are still not as good as a resinous medium.

Temporary mounts need ringing

Ringing is the term used for sealing the edges of a coverslip when the mounting medium does not set. Ringing was originally so called because the coverslips were round and so there was a ring of the sealant round the coverslip. Ringing was done on a turntable to give a nice neat finish. Originally it used a gold size followed by a black asphaltum varnish. This produced a very neat finish and some commercial suppliers of prepared slides still finish many of their preparations in a similar way as it looks good. Most laboratories have dropped this and ringing is now just a temporary expedient rather than an aesthetic requirement.

Good temporary ringing can be achieved in a number of ways. Ordinary nail varnish works quite well and comes in a bottle with its own brush, which makes it convenient and simple. The only drawback is that it is dissolved in acetone, which may affect some materials, although I have never found this to be a problem.

Many styrene-based cements can also be used and again are convenient as they come in tubes ready to squeeze out around the coverslip. Again the solvent is a theoretical problem but I have not had problems. These cements can often be semi-permanent. Paraffin wax can also be used. A piece of warmed metal (such as the flat end of a broad spatula) is used to apply a layer of molten wax, which immediately sets. Provided the slide is dry, this is quick and easy but is easily broken and will not store well.

Storage of slides

Mounted slides should always be carefully labelled and stored horizontally until fully dry and set when they can be stored on their edge or end. Stained slides should be stored away from light as the dyes will fade even in the best mountant.

SUGGESTED FURTHER READING

Gamble, M. and Wilson, I. (2002) The hematoxylins and eosin. In *Theory and Practice of Histological Techniques*, 5th edn (eds J.D. Bancroft and M. Gamble). Edinburgh: Churchill Livingstone.

Horobin, R.W. (2002) Theory of staining and its practical implications. In *Theory and Practice of Histological Techniques*, 5th edn (eds J.D. Bancroft and M. Gamble). Edinburgh: Churchill Livingstone.

Kiernan, J.A. (2001) *Histological and Histochemical Methods*, 3rd edn. Oxford: Hodder Arnold.

Lamar Jones, M. (2002) Connective tissues and stains. In *Theory and Practice of Histological Techniques*, 5th edn (eds J.D. Bancroft and M. Gamble). Edinburgh: Churchill Livingstone.

SELF-ASSESSMENT QUESTIONS

1. What is the role of chromophores and auxochromes in dye structure?
2. How do basic and acidic dyes bring out the structure of tissues? Name one acidic and one basic dye.
3. How do pH and salt concentration alter dye binding?
4. A small amount of mordant causes staining but an excess of mordant removes the staining. Explain this oddity.
5. Why does haematoxylin mordanted with aluminium salts stain nuclei but other mordants cause haematoxylin to stain connective tissues or nerve fibres?
6. Toluidine blue will stain mast cell granules red. What is the name of this phenomenon? Why does the colour change occur?
7. Name one red and one blue nuclear stain. When would you use a red nuclear stain and when would you use a blue one?
8. Why do some haematoxylin solutions initially improve with keeping and then deteriorate?
9. Outline why permeability and dye size might explain trichrome staining with three acid dyes.
10. Distinguish between argentaffin and argyrophil silver impregnation.
11. Why is silver the best metal for metallic impregnation techniques?
12. Why might a lipid-staining technique recommend mounting in glycerol jelly instead of DPX?
13. Why do most laboratories routinely use a resinous mounting medium?

Histochemistry: general considerations and the histochemistry of carbohydrates and lipids

Learning objectives
After studying this chapter you should confidently be able to:

■ **Outline the problems associated with identifying and localizing chemicals in tissue sections.**
Histochemistry is limited by the need to have an insoluble coloured product to localize the site of reaction. Tissue preparation must retain the materials in their original site. Careful controls are needed to ensure that methods are sufficiently sensitive and selective.

■ **Describe the periodic acid–Schiff (PAS) reaction and be able to outline the problems in interpreting the PAS reaction.**
The PAS reaction detects materials containing sugars, including polysaccharides, mucins and glycoproteins. In the PAS reaction, the periodic acid oxidizes the adjacent hydroxyl groups to aldehydes, which then react with the Schiff's reagent. Difficulties include non-specific staining due to pre-existing aldehydes in tissues and identifying the source of a positive reaction from a wide range of materials that are PAS-positive.

■ **Describe how to identify and localize mucins in cells and tissues.**
Mucins can be classified into major groups using PAS, alcian blue and aldehyde fuchsin in combination. Further identification can be achieved using enzymes and controlled electrolyte concentration to inhibit staining.

■ **Describe the histological classification of mucins.**
Mucins are classed into neutral mucins, which have no acidic groups on the carbohydrate, and acidic mucins, which have acidic groups that react with alcian blue. The acidic mucins are further subdivided depending on the type and number of acidic groups into carboxylated, strongly sulphated and weakly sulphated types.

■ **Describe how lipids can be demonstrated in tissues.**
Many lipids can be demonstrated by their hydrophobic nature and the ability to concentrate fat-soluble dyes from an aqueous solvent (lysochromy or sudanophilia). Some lipids require special treatment before showing sudanophilia. Special techniques can be applied to identify subgroups of lipids.

Histochemistry is a method of investigating tissue structure that, instead of using relatively crude dyeing of the tissues, uses reasonably specific chemical tests to identify and pinpoint the location of chemicals within the tissues. In this regard, histochemistry is a modified form of chemistry or biochemistry.

There are a number of fairly specialized subdisciplines within histochemistry, each of which has its own problems and solutions. These include the histochemical identification of: carbohydrates and lipids (discussed in this chapter), nucleic acids, proteins and enzymes (see Chapter 8), and pigments and minerals (see Chapter 9).

7.1 LIMITATIONS OF HISTOCHEMISTRY

Histochemistry may have a lot in common with biochemistry but it has certain extra problems as biochemists investigating tissues usually have some quite significant advantages over histochemists.

- Histochemistry must produce a coloured final result to make it visible under the microscope. Biochemists can certainly employ methods that produce coloured final reaction products, but they can also quite happily employ methods that use materials only 'coloured' in the UV region and such results are invisible to the human eye and useless for microscopy.
- Histochemistry must produce a material that is insoluble so that the position of the chemical reaction in the tissue can be located accurately. Slight solubility of the final material is a problem as it can allow the coloured material to move from its true site to a nearby location and give a false localization.
- Histochemistry must be highly sensitive as it must accurately detect the material present within a single cell and in some cases within a single organelle such as a mitochondrion. Biochemists can often use several kilograms of tissue to make a single preparation and concentrate the material they are investigating.
- Histochemistry must never allow the material being investigated to be separated from its environment, as pinpointing its position in the tissue is the rationale for using histochemistry. The biochemist can separate and purify the material using a range of techniques such as chromatography, electrophoresis and dialysis. Indeed, the speed of movement of the material in such separation techniques is often the best method of identifying closely related materials.

Histochemistry is therefore often more difficult to achieve in practice and is often less certain in its identification than the equivalent biochemical detection. It is also much more difficult to get an accurate quantification (see section on Measurement and Microscopy in Chapter 15). Thus, it is best to think of biochemistry and histochemistry as complementary techniques that supplement each other rather than competing with each other; they give different information and, when used together, give a more complete picture of the chemistry of the cell than either could alone. Biochemistry can determine the types and quantities of material present in a tissue, whilst histochemistry can identify the position and distribution of the materials. Histochemistry also relies on the knowledge gained from biochemistry to enable satisfactory histochemical techniques to be developed.

7.2 USE OF CONTROLS IN HISTOCHEMISTRY

Controls are important in histochemistry and should include a minimum of a **positive control** and a **negative control**. Without controls the methods are little more than demonstration techniques, which, although still useful, cannot be considered as rigorous chemical testing.

Positive controls

The purpose of a positive control is to check that the technique is working satisfactorily. For this purpose, you need a weakly reacting material. The reason for using a positive control is to ensure that any material in the test section will be detected. If a strongly reacting control is used, it is possible that the test is working for a strong reaction but is insensitive to a weak reaction. A strongly reacting control may also be included to give a good positive result for comparison, but it should be in addition to a weak control, not a replacement. Where a material may have several forms that react differently (such a case would be amyloid, which has a number of different types), it may be necessary to have more than one positive control material (see *Box 7.1*). Thus, for amyloid the controls may include both the common AA and AL amyloid types (see Chapter 14) and perhaps even some of the less-common types if they are likely to occur in one or more of the test sections.

Where a technique is being used quantitatively, the use of a range of controls is needed to cover the range of results expected and to act as a standard for the quantitation.

The positive control should be as close as possible to the material being looked for in the test section. For example, using the periodic acid–Schiff (PAS) technique, it would be possible to check that the technique is working by using glycogen, a mucin, reticulin fibres or several other materials. If you are looking for glycoproteins in the pituitary, the control should be glycoprotein in the pituitary and not glycogen in the liver. The use of a slightly different substance is not as good a control as it may react differently.

The positive controls should be carried out at the same time and in the same way as the test sections. It is not enough to control the technique once at the beginning of the day and then use the result for several different batches of tests run at different times. A single positive control may be sufficient for a batch of sections that are tested at the same time, provided the test sections are similar in type and in the reaction expected.

Box 7.1 Control blocks can include many tissues

If many different tissues are being examined together, then the number of control sections can become tedious. In some cases, it is possible to have a large number of control tissues yet only one control section. The method is to pack a large number of test tissues into one block. The tissues may be blocked out separately in one mould or small rods of tissues can be cut and assembled into a single checkerboard or composite block. For control purposes, you only need a very small sample of tissue to see if the technique is working as expected, so as little as 1 mm² of tissue will suffice. A single checkerboard may contain 64 separate tissue samples in a single section. This is an effective way of reducing the number of control slides without compromising the number of control tissues. The only disadvantage is the time and effort needed to make the composite blocks.

Rods of tissue are assembled into a solid block and when sectioned appear as a checkerboard of tissues.

Negative controls

Negative controls are used to test the specificity of the reaction and ensure there are no false-positive results. The tissue should again be as close as possible to the test section in type and in expected reaction. In many cases it is possible to use another slide of the test section as a control by destroying the reactivity of the material being tested (see section on Treated tissues below.) It may be necessary to have a negative control for each section if there is some background colour that might be confused with the positive result. Only by comparing the negative and test sections can you be sure that the result is a genuine positive result.

Control results

The controls should always be examined first. If the results are satisfactory, then the test slides can be examined and the results analysed.

If there is any sign of a positive result in the negative control, then the method may not be specific and some factor other than the test material may be reacting. If the positive control is negative, or unexpectedly weakly reacting, then the method may not have been sufficiently sensitive or may have been performed wrongly. In both cases, the tests will need to be repeated. The controls may need to be investigated first to ensure that the results can be relied on before repeating the tests.

A simple rerun of the controls is a useful starting point, taking extra care to ensure that all the steps are carried out correctly. This will detect whether the results were due to a simple error in technique. The rerun can be done using fresh reagents to ensure that it is not a reagent error and different control slides to ensure that it is not a control section error. If the rerun fails to give the expected results, then the whole technique needs to be reassessed. Each step may need to be controlled separately to detect which step is going awry. This may result in a large number of controls but is the only way to ensure reliable results.

Controls can be of various types

The source of controls is important and it is sometimes necessary to use different types of control tissues especially when investigating unexpected results.

Control tissues

Positive control. This involves having tissues that you know contain the material you are looking for. The material can be a sample from a previous test that came up positive. Most laboratories are constantly looking for good positive-control materials to use in subsequent tests. The use of stock controls assumes that the material is stable enough to be kept. Some control materials do deteriorate during storage and may need regular replacement.

If the material cannot be stored or if there is no stock control available, it may be necessary to use fresh animal tissue. This would be the case for enzyme techniques where it may not be possible to store tissues as the enzymes may rapidly deteriorate. In this case, it is essential to use a tissue that you are certain contains the material being detected.

Negative control. Here it is essential to choose a tissue that does not contain the material being demonstrated to check for non-specific reactions. Ideally, the negative-control tissue should be from the same organ and the same species as the test sections.

Treated tissues

These are an excellent negative control since the actual substance being tested is treated to remove or destroy its staining ability. This can be used not only to ensure that the method is specific but also when the method is known to be non-specific. For example, the PAS technique is useful but stains many different materials and is not specific for glycogen. It can be used to demonstrate glycogen specifically by using a control in which the glycogen is removed by enzyme digestion with amylase. Other PAS-positive materials such as mucins, glycoproteins and reticulin will be unaffected. Thus, a material that stains in both the test and treated tissue control is not glycogen. Any staining that is positive in the test but missing from the amylase-treated tissue is glycogen. These controls are not as easy to examine and interpret as the use of sections that are naturally negative, but this is a vital method in many histochemical investigations.

The reactivity of the material can be destroyed in a number of ways:

1. Enzyme digestion, e.g. amylase for glycogen, collagenase for collagen, ribonuclease for RNA.
2. Extraction with a solvent, e.g. chloroform/methanol will dissolve lipids.
3. Use of a specific inhibitor, e.g. oxaloacetic acid will specifically inhibit succinic dehydrogenase but not other enzymes.
4. Heating to destroy enzyme activity, e.g. acid phosphatase using Gomori's lead phosphate technique; any coloration will be non-specific binding of the lead salts.
5. Blocking of reactive groups. This may involve reacting the group with reagent, e.g. acetylation of hydroxyl groups (using acetic anhydride in pyridine). The term is also loosely applied to complete removal of the group, e.g. deamination with nitrous acid (see *Box 7.2* for further comments).

Box 7.2 Blocking controls

The blocking methods are also used to prevent background reactions by removing the reactive material before performing the test. Thus, preformed aldehydes in tissues can be blocked by reduction with borohydride. This is useful, for example, after glutaraldehyde fixation when there are many free aldehydes from the glutaraldehyde. The use of any method using Schiff's reagent on glutaraldehyde-fixed tissues is therefore difficult unless these abnormal aldehydes from fixation are first blocked.

The use of blocking is also important in immunoperoxidase methods to destroy endogenous peroxidases (see Chapter 10).

Altered technique

It is possible to ensure that there is no non-specific reaction simply by omitting an essential step in the technique. For example, an easy negative control for an enzyme is to omit the substrate from the incubating solution. The absence of substrate means that the enzyme cannot catalyse its normal reaction so any positive result is non-specific. Similarly, omitting the periodate oxidation in PAS acts as a good test for any preformed aldehydes.

These types of control are very useful for investigating unexpected positive results. By omitting different steps in the procedure it is often possible to identify the source of the unexpected reaction. This control of individual steps is used in immunological and related techniques where there may be six or seven steps that could be the source of the false-positive reaction.

7.3 USE OF HISTOCHEMICAL INVESTIGATIONS

Histochemical tests as simple staining methods

Many histochemical techniques are used in routine histology not so much for the chemical information they can provide as for the fact that they are often better at showing a particular structure than simple dyes could ever be. Examples include the use of acetyl cholinesterase techniques to demonstrate motor end plates, the PAS technique to visualize goblet cells, nucleic acid techniques to identify plasma cells and lipid techniques to show myelin degeneration. In these cases, the histochemical controls are often omitted since the technique is not being used in its most critical way. This should not be taken to mean that the controls are never necessary, just that they can be omitted for simple demonstration methods; they would still be needed for more rigorous histochemical testing.

Staining techniques in conjunction with histochemical investigations

It is also true that many staining techniques that are not strictly histochemical are often used in histochemical investigations where they may confirm the results of another test. Two or more non-specific tests may between them give results that are quite acceptable as histochemical identification, even though individually they are not specific. Thus, alcian blue will stain many forms of mucin and aldehyde fuchsin will stain many materials including sulphated mucins, elastic fibres and some cell inclusions. If a material stains with alcian blue and with aldehyde fuchsin (in separate sections, not in the same individual section), then it can safely be assumed that the material is a sulphated mucin. Individually the two techniques are not specific but their combined results are at the very least highly selective.

Whether and how to fix

In all histochemistry, as indeed in all histological investigations, the early treatment of the tissue is vitally important. Improper treatment of the tissue, such as inappropriate fixation, will result in the material under investigation being altered, moved or even completely lost. As histochemistry

---

Box 7.3 Histochemistry is not always difficult

Histochemistry is sometimes perceived as being difficult and obscure. This is not true. Histochemistry is not always difficult or complex. The Perls technique for iron is one of the most sensitive of the histochemical techniques. In this case, ordinary paraffin wax sections will suffice since the material being identified is protein linked and therefore retained in paraffin sections. The reagents are not complex or critical and I use the technique in first-year degree practical classes. It works reliably for the students and they can observe the iron present within the spleen cells. Individual macrophages can be distinguished easily in their preparations. Any technique that can be done first time every time by inexperienced workers and still detect the minute amounts of iron present inside a single macrophage can hardly be called difficult.

Not all histochemistry is this easy, but a surprising amount can be performed with little difficulty given reasonable care.

involves precise chemical investigation, it is often done on unfixed tissue. This means that the tissues are unstable and must be used quickly. Once the histochemical reaction has occurred and the final insoluble product is formed, it is often possible to post-fix the tissues to make them more permanent.

7.4 CARBOHYDRATES

The carbohydrates found in tissues are mainly sugars and their derivatives. Simple sugars such as glucose and fructose are extremely difficult to preserve in tissue sections as they are very soluble in water. Distinguishing between simple sugars by chemical tests is quite difficult and glucose is also almost ubiquitous in cells and tissues. The identification of free monosaccharides is rarely attempted in tissues since the sugars are likely to have been lost or moved from their original site and any positive reactions are likely to be the glucose that is found everywhere.

Sugars can, however, be bound to a number of other materials to give a range of sugar-containing materials that are of interest to histochemists. The presence of any sugar can usually be identified by the periodic acid–Schiff (PAS) technique. This is the single most important technique in carbohydrate identification as it identifies most neutral sugar- and sialic acid-containing materials. It does not, however, identify the type of sugar; it simply indicates that a saccharide is present.

The PAS reaction

The PAS reaction involves a two-step chemical reaction in which there is an oxidation step in periodic acid to generate aldehyde groups from the carbohydrate, followed by the addition of a reagent sensitive for aldehydes (Schiff's reagent), which stains the site of the sugars. The method is widely quoted in descriptions of cells indicating whether the cell is PAS-positive or PAS-negative (see *Box 7.4*).

Box 7.4 Negative results with the PAS technique can still be useful

The PAS reaction is such a useful indicator that it is one of the few stains where a negative result is often quoted and many cellular components will be described in books as PAS-negative. The negative result means that no sugars are present, so it acts as a method of distinguishing glycoprotein hormones from simple proteins, e.g. in the pituitary.

This use of the negative result is quite unusual and means that it is used in situations where you expect no reaction. This means that controls need to be more stringent than normal since a negative result is expected and poor technique will give a negative result.

Other techniques that have this distinction include Sudan staining and the Perls method. It is also the case with the Gram bacterial stain where Gram-negative indicates a great deal about the structure of the bacterium.

Periodate oxidation

The oxidation reaction acts on the glycol (hydroxyls on adjacent carbons) part of the sugar and produces two aldehydes and at the same time splits the bond between the two carbons:

$$
\begin{array}{c}
\text{H}-\text{C}-\text{OH} \\
| \\
\text{H}-\text{C}-\text{OH}
\end{array}
\;+\text{IO}_4^-\;\longrightarrow\;
\begin{array}{c}
\text{H}-\text{C}=\text{O} \\
\\
\text{H}-\text{C}=\text{O}
\end{array}
\;+\text{IO}_3^-+\text{H}_2\text{O}
$$

Reaction with Schiff's reagent

The aldehydes then react with Schiff's reagent to produce a product that is a strong red/purple colour. The reaction can also occur with some derivatives of sugars and glycols, e.g. amino and alkylamino sugars. Most materials that contain sugars, such as glycoproteins, will be PAS-positive. Strongly sulphated mucins in connective tissue and hyaluronic acid are negative with the standard PAS technique, despite containing large numbers of sugar groups, but other mucins are PAS-positive. v

Oxidation agents

Periodic acid (HIO_4) is the most commonly used oxidant. It is made up as a 0.5 or 1% aqueous solution (0.044 M) and oxidation is for 5–10 min at room temperature. A longer oxidation may be needed for some materials to become Schiff-reactive (e.g. sulphated mucopolysaccharides). Adding extra steps to the technique may also increase the range of materials that can be demonstrated (e.g. borohydride treatment). Alcoholic periodic acid can be used instead of the aqueous solution if there is the possibility of the material dissolving in water (e.g. R.D. Hotchkiss, in 1948, recommended alcoholic periodate oxidation for glycogen).

Other oxidants can be used to give the same reaction, but most will continue oxidizing after the production of aldehydes, and this further oxidation of the aldehydes to acids results in loss of staining. This further oxidation does not happen with periodic acid and it is this that makes periodic acid the most popular method. Other oxidants that can be used include chromic acid, potassium permanganate, lead tetra-acetate and sodium bismuthate. These oxidants need more precise timing to obtain maximal staining and it is this critical timing that makes them much less popular. However, they are occasionally included in other staining methods; for example, chromic acid oxidation is used in the Gridley technique for fungi.

Schiff's reagent

Schiff's reagent is a sensitive reagent for detecting aldehydes and stains them a pink/purple colour. It is quite specific for aldehydes. Even the related ketones do not react with the PAS method. Schiff's reagent consists of a solution of basic fuchsin (pararosaniline) that has been decolorized with sulphurous acid. The sulphurous acid adds an extra sulphurous group to the central carbon of the dye. This disrupts the chromophore group with consequent loss of colour.

Pararosaniline with
the quininoid chromophore
as the bottom ring

Schiff's reagent
has no quininoid ring
and is colourless

On reacting with the tissue, it seems likely that the alkylsulphonic derivative of the dye is formed. This entails a rearrangement of the sulphonic group and restores the chromophoric group, but this is not simple restoration of the original dye colour since the product is a significantly different colour to the original dye.

The quininoid ring chromophore is restored
when the Schiff's reagent reacts with an aldehyde

To prepare Schiff's reagent therefore requires a solution of basic fuchsin or pararosaniline. The fuchsin needs to be specifically for the preparation of Schiff's reagent as not all 'basic fuchsins' are suitable.

Varieties of Schiff's reagent

The sulphurous acid needed to decolorize the dye can be produced using the following methods:

- Sulphite or metabisulphite and HCl at 50°C (de Thomasi method). This is one of the most popular recipes.
- Metabisulphite and HCl at room temperature with prolonged shaking (Lillie method). This 'cold Schiff' is more acidic than the previous recipe.
- Thionyl chloride (Barger and Lamarter method).
- Bubbling sulphur dioxide through the solution (Itikawa and Oguru method).
- Sodium dithionite (Alexander method).

Sensitivity and shelf-life

Although these different methods all produce effective reagents, there are differences in their sensitivity and shelf-life. The amount of sulphurous acid seems to be the main difference affecting the Schiff's reagent. If there is an excess of sulphurous acid, the Schiff's reagent will have better storage qualities but may have reduced sensitivity. Schiff's reagent should be stored at 0–4°C when it may keep for months.

After the sulphurous decolorization, Schiff's reagent is often a yellowish colour and this can be removed by treating the solution with activated charcoal. A slight yellowish tinge does not seem to matter and Schiff's reagent will still work fine, but if a pink colour is produced, this indicates degradation of the reagent and it should be discarded. Because of the problems involved in preparing Schiff's reagent, many laboratories now prefer to buy it from a commercial supplier.

Washing out

In the original techniques, the Schiff's reagent was washed out of the tissues using sulphurous reagents as a rinsing solution. For most routine purposes, the use of sulphurous acid rinses after the Schiff's reagent has largely been dropped in favour of simply washing in running water for several minutes; however, sulphurous rinses may still be needed for critical applications. The water wash generally increases the intensity of the colour as any excess sulphurous acid is removed.

Alternative reagents

A PAS-stained section can be counterstained in many ways but the use of a nuclear stain such as haematoxylin is usually sufficient. The traditional Schiff's reagent prepared from fuchsin or pararosaniline can be replaced by reagents prepared with other dyes such as thionin. Instead of Schiff's reagent, the aldehydes can be detected with a silver reagent, usually methenamine (hexamine) silver. This technique is called the PA–silver method but is less popular.

Interpreting the results of a PAS reaction

Many materials are PAS-positive but if badly carried out the PAS technique can also give false-positive results, so controlling and interpreting the results are very important before relying on the PAS reaction as a method of identifying a material.

False-positive reactions. The first type of false-positive PAS reaction is given by an improper Schiff's reagent. If all of the dye has not been decolorized or if the Schiff's reagent is old, the section may develop a pink colour independent of the presence of aldehydes. This should not happen if the Schiff's reagent is prepared correctly, is reasonably fresh and has been stored correctly. Schiff's reagent should always be examined for signs of deterioration before it is used, but deterioration of the reagent is always a possible explanation if results seem unusual.

The second type of false-positive reaction occurs when there are preformed aldehydes within the tissue before the periodic acid oxidation. These aldehydes will react with the Schiff's reagent and give the same colour as if it was a PAS-positive substance. Preformed aldehydes can come from the use of an aldehyde fixative. Formaldehyde fixation is not normally a problem as the formaldehyde is effectively washed out of the tissue during processing, but other aldehydes, particularly glutaraldehyde, can cause difficulties.

Preformed aldehydes also occur naturally in small amounts in tissues, and particularly after mercuric chloride fixation they can appear as the so-called **plasmal** reaction. The plasmal reaction is mainly due to lipids ('plasmalogens') and so this is more likely in frozen sections, but it can occur sometimes in paraffin sections. Blocking of fixative-derived or preformed aldehydes is possible, e.g. using sodium borohydride, but is not a common procedure.

To ensure that non-specific reactions are not occurring, a second section can be carried through the technique but omitting the periodic acid oxidation. Any material or component stained in both sections is not PAS-positive but something else, usually a preformed aldehyde.

False-negative reactions. The cause of false-negative reactions may be a reagent that is not working effectively or inadequate treatment with one or more reagents. A positive-control section where you are sure that the material is present should be stained alongside the test section to ensure that the technique is working. The control should be a weak rather than a strong positive and should be as close in type and material to the test section as possible.

A negative result when a positive reaction was expected may also be due to poor technique; staining a slide upside down is one example. The test should be repeated ensuring that no errors occur.

The materials being detected may have been lost due to processing or delayed fixation. If this is the case, the only way to correct it is to get a new specimen.

PAS-positive materials

Some of the more commonly encountered materials that can be PAS-positive are shown below. This is not a comprehensive list but indicates the range of materials that need to be considered when a positive reaction is found.

Amyloid	Glycogen
Basement membranes	Hyaline membrane of neonatal lung
Cartilage	Lipochrome pigments
Cellulose	Pituitary basophil granules
Cerebroside lipids	Starch
Chitin	Thyroid colloid
Epithelial mucins	Zymogen granules in pancreas
Fungi (chitin)	

If PAS is being used for a specific confirmation, then the identity of the material will probably be obvious. The problem of identification can arise if there is an unexpected positive reaction or if the identification of a material needs to be confirmed beyond doubt.

There is no simple procedure to be certain of the identity of a PAS-positive material. Several techniques can be applied:

1. Simple appearance can often be useful. Some PAS-positive materials can be recognized simply by their shape (morphology), e.g. fungal hyphae are sufficiently distinctive for their morphological appearance to be enough for a positive identification.

2. Stain a second section with another technique that selectively stains the material that you believe is the source of the PAS reaction. For example, starch can be identified by treating it with iodine when it will develop a distinctive blue colour. Even if the other technique is not itself specific, the combination of PAS reactivity and staining with a second technique may be unique, e.g. lipochrome pigments also stain with the Ziehl–Neelson technique and Sudan black, so anything that stains positive with all three methods can be identified as lipofuscin.

3. Dissolving or destroying the material chemically, e.g. dissolving glycolipids in hydrophobic solvents shows that they are soluble in organic solvents and this is a strong indication of their lipid nature. This requires two sections to be stained together. One section is pretreated with a lipid solvent and after the extraction both sections are stained using the PAS technique. Materials that stain in both sections are not glycolipids since they are insoluble in the lipid solvent. Glycolipids will show positively in the section that was not extracted but will not stain in the treated section.

4. Enzyme digestion. Really this is the same as (3) but enzymes are such precise reagents that this can be used as a positive identification and is therefore worthy of separate consideration. This is useful for glycogen. Diastase (amylase) specifically digests glycogen and starch. Since starch is not a normal constituent of animal tissues, this makes it highly selective and starch can be eliminated by iodine staining. Predigesting one section with amylase and comparing it with an undigested section, both of which have been stained by PAS, allows identification of the

glycogen. It also, of course, eliminates glycogen as a possible material when both sections are positive.

Specific carbohydrates found in tissues

Polysaccharides: glycogen and starch

Glycogen is the major form of carbohydrate found in human tissues and acts as the main energy store in many cells such as muscle and liver (see *Box 7.5*). Glycogen is one of the commonest materials giving a PAS-positive reaction in tissues. Glycogen is a polymeric form of glucose (the glucose is mainly α-1,4 linked in straight chains but there are some α-1,6 links, which give branched chains). It is related to starch, which has the same general chemical composition but is generally found as larger polymeric molecules. Since only one material (glucose) makes up these materials, they are termed homoglycans. Two forms can be identified by electron microscopy:

- α-glycogen, which forms distinctive rosettes of β particles;
- β-glycogen, in which the individual components of the rosettes are free as individual 20–40 nm particles.

Glycogen is found in many cells, with large amounts in liver and muscle cells.

Glycogen relocation within the cell during fixation. Glycogen illustrates an important characteristic of histochemistry, namely the role of fixation in the successful demonstration of a tissue material. The preservation of glycogen is important. If it is not fixed properly, glycogen can be lost completely or its location within the tissue can be altered. Routine fixation with formaldehyde is not ideal as some of the glycogen is lost, so the amount left in the section is diminished. Glycogen is also relocated by 'streaming' in the cytoplasm and becomes polarized within the cell. In streaming, the glycogen is effectively washed to the far side of the cell by the fixative where it then becomes fixed. Using an alcohol-based fixative retains more glycogen and diminishes the streaming artefact (Gendre's fluid is recommended to

---

Box 7.5 The glycogen content of cells is variable

The amount of glycogen is quite variable in tissues as it is used continuously as an energy source by cells. The amount of glucose can alter quite markedly depending on diet and activity. Long-distance runners attempt to manipulate their glycogen stores by eating a high-protein/low-carbohydrate diet until shortly before a race. The lack of dietary carbohydrate depletes their liver and muscle cells of glycogen since protein cannot be converted easily into carbohydrate by the cell's metabolism. Then, for a few hours before the race, they eat a high-carbohydrate diet, which causes the cells to actively store as much glycogen as possible. This carbohydrate loading means that they can have maximum glycogen stores for the race. Glycogen is a much more readily available energy store, so the muscles will be that little bit more efficient than if they were running on lipids, the next available source of energy.

give the best results). However, the best preservation is achieved by avoiding fixation altogether and using freeze-drying to prepare the tissue.

Starch contamination. The presence of starch in animal tissues usually means contamination of the specimen, the commonest source being the glove powder used in many rubber gloves to make them easier to put on (see *Box 7.6*). Starch can be distinguished from glycogen by staining with iodine (starch stains blue, glycogen stains brown); also starch is usually in the form of grains that show Maltese-cross birefringence with a polarizing microscope.

Box 7.6 Contamination from rubber gloves

Starch was originally used to replace mineral talc as a glove powder. Lubrication is needed with latex gloves to allow them to slip on to the hands easily. Talc is a magnesium silicate and remained in the body, causing problems including 'talc granulomas'. Starch was used to perform the same task as it is more easily degraded in the body. Starch has now been found to have fewer although still significant problems and can delay wound healing. The Medical Devices Agency in the UK recommended that the use of powdered gloves should be discontinued. Gloves made of plastic, which is not as sticky as rubber latex, are now common in surgical practice. Non-surgical gloves may still use glove powder.

Cellulose

Cellulose is another homoglycan of glucose but is β-1,4 linked. It is usually found in plant materials but this can include cotton wool, gauze, filter paper and clothing, so cellulose fibres are one of the commonest contaminants of tissues. Cellulose fibres are usually easy to recognize: they are PAS-positive, birefringent, insoluble in all common reagents and resistant to enzyme digestion by amylase.

Chitin

Chitin is a homoglycan of *N*-acetylglucosamine and is β-1,4 linked. It is found in the exoskeleton of invertebrates. It is of only minor importance in mammalian histochemistry where it occurs as either a contaminant or as part of a complete invertebrate parasite.

Many PAS-positive substances are protein–sugar combinations

Many of the most important compounds containing sugars are mixtures of protein and sugars. These can be many and varied in form, structure and function. They are studied by many different disciplines and this has led to a variety of nomenclatures that do not always agree with each other. One simple distinction is between glycoproteins and proteoglycans. The major distinction here is between the dominant chemical in the combination:

Glycoproteins are proteins that have some sugar added as a post-translational modification but are predominantly protein. They are widespread as membrane proteins where the sugars act as 'stoppers' to prevent the proteins slipping back through the membrane. The sugars always occur on the outside of the cell and form the **glycocalyx** (the carbohydrate cell coat) where they act as antigens and cell-recognition structures. They also occur as serum proteins such as immunoglobulins, structural proteins such as collagen and as secretions, both exocrine and endocrine. Their histochemical properties are determined mainly by the protein but they do give a positive PAS reaction.

Proteoglycans are mainly carbohydrate in nature with a small protein core surrounded by large polysaccharide chains. It is this group that has confusing nomenclature. They are often known in histology by the imprecise terms of mucins or mucopolysaccharides. The histological classification of mucins that will be followed here is that of Cook (1974).

7.5   MUCINS

Mucins are a group of substances with certain physical, chemical and staining characteristics in common. They all contain large amounts of sugars attached to a small amount of protein and they all stain PAS-positive. Many mucins react with the dye alcian blue at acidic pH. Many also show metachromasia and this forms the basis of the histological classification.

Identification of mucin type can be important in some diseases (see *Box 7.7*).

Box 7.7 Diseases of mucin metabolism

Mucins are normally very useful substances, but if the body loses the ability to destroy mucins, they can accumulate and cause severe disruption. This happens in a number of rare diseases called mucopolysaccharidoses. These are inherited gene defects in which the affected individuals accumulate mucinous substances inside and between cells. The accumulations occur because of an enzyme defect in the lysosomes. The severity of the disease and the type of accumulated material depends on which enzymes are defective or missing.

Affected babies often appear normal at birth and may develop normally at first. It is often only when the child seems to develop frequent infections that the disease is diagnosed. The effects are progressive and vary widely in their severity. Patients often develop coarse facial features (hence the term 'gargoylism' for these diseases). Thick skin and unusual hair growth also disfigure these patients. Skeletal involvement often causes distortion of the body. Corneal abnormalities are not uncommon and can lead to impaired vision. Internal organs may enlarge, e.g. the liver (hepatomegaly) and spleen (splenomegaly). There will be mental retardation in severe cases. Their overall growth is usually stunted and their life expectancy is usually short.

There are several variants of the disease of which the best known are Hunter's disease and Hurler's disease.

Histological classification of mucins

The histological classification of mucins is based on staining properties. Two major groups of mucins can be identified:

Neutral mucins

Neutral mucins are PAS-positive but alcian blue-negative and display no metachromasia with thiazine dyes such as toluidine blue.

Acid mucins

Acid mucins are PAS-positive and also stain with alcian blue; they demonstrate some degree of metachromasia. Acid mucins can be further subdivided based on their staining behaviour with regard to pH due to the type and number of the ionizable acidic groups:

Strongly sulphated acid mucins stain with alcian blue and are metachromatic, even at very low pH (less than pH 1). They are mostly connective tissue mucins, e.g. cartilage, chondroitin sulphates, keratan sulphates.

Weakly sulphated mucins stain with alcian blue and are metachromatic only when the pH is greater than 1, e.g. epithelial mucins in colonic goblet cells.

Weakly acidic (carboxylated) mucins stain with alcian blue and are metachromatic only when the pH is greater than 2.5, e.g. epithelial mucins of the salivary gland and the connective tissue hyaluronic acid. These can be further subdivided by the type of acid group (either uronic acid or sialic acid), which can be identified by enzyme digestion with hyaluronidase or sialidase followed by alcian blue staining.

Identification of mucins

Identification of mucins is most conveniently done by using several staining techniques. The routine stains such as PAS and alcian blue give information that is useful, but they can be even more useful if more than one technique is applied to the same section in a sequence so that the techniques interfere with each other and effectively compete for the carbohydrate.

PAS reaction

This is positive for all groups of mucins. However, if the mucin is stained first with another technique (e.g. alcian blue), the dye will prevent or block the PAS reaction and the mucin will not then stain PAS-positive.

Alcian blue reaction

This is a cationic dye with an unusual structure (it is a copper phthalocyanine dye) and if the pH is kept acidic it will only stain acid mucins. It does not stain nuclei, probably due to the size and shape of the dye and the conformation of the DNA. Although other cationic dyes can be used to stain mucins, it is this lack of nuclear reactivity combined with a strong colour that resists fading that has made alcian blue so popular in staining mucins.

By varying the pH or salt concentration, alcian blue can identify the different types of mucin.

Aldehyde fuchsin reaction

This stains substances containing sulphur groups a strong purple colour. It will stain sulphated mucins very strongly. However, it will also stain many other tissue components purple (e.g. elastic fibres), even though they are not mucins. Thus, only components that stain with both alcian blue and aldehyde fuchsin can be classified as sulphated mucins. By staining with aldehyde fuchsin first, it is possible to inhibit or mask alcian blue staining. The mechanism for the affinity of aldehyde fuchsin for sulphated mucins is not known and the stain should be regarded as an empirical test (i.e. no rational reason); however, it seems to work reliably.

Critical electrolyte concentration

This technique uses differing concentrations of magnesium chloride (or different pH levels) to inhibit alcian blue staining in mucins. The dyes are made up in the appropriate concentration of the salt as shown below and then used to stain sections.

$MgCl_2$	pH	Type of mucin
<0.06 M	>2.5	All acid mucins are alcian blue-positive
0.2–0.3 M	1–2	All sulphated mucins are alcian blue-positive
>0.5 M	<1	Only strongly sulphated acid mucins are alcian blue-positive

If a group of sections is treated with the range of concentrations, then it follows that if a mucin is stained under all of the conditions, it is a strongly sulphated mucin. If a mucin stains in the first two solutions but not in the highest concentration, then it cannot be a strongly sulphated mucin and must be a weakly sulphated mucin. If it only stains alcian blue-positive in the weakest concentration of salt, then the mucin must be a carboxylated mucin.

Combining these techniques

By combining these techniques it is possible to identify the major groups of mucins.

Alcian blue/PAS. The alcian blue blocks the PAS reaction in acid mucins and so distinguishes between neutral and acid mucins. Acid mucins stain blue and neutral mucins stain purple from the PAS (see *Colour plate 9*).

Aldehyde fuchsin/alcian blue. The aldehyde fuchsin stains the sulphated mucins dark purple, whilst the carboxylated mucins take up the alcian blue.

Finer distinctions can be made by using enzymes to differentiate between the carboxylated mucins and by using the critical electrolyte concentration technique to distinguish between the strongly sulphated and weakly sulphated acid mucins (see *Fig. 7.1*).

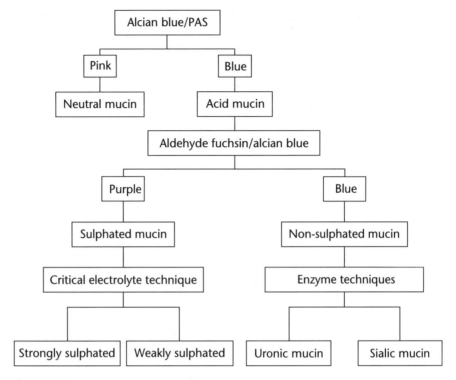

Figure 7.1
Scheme to identify the major mucin types by staining two sections with alcian blue/PAS and aldehyde fuchsin/alcian blue

The scheme in *Fig. 7.1* looks easier to do than it is in practice. The colours can sometimes be vague and inconclusive, some mucins react poorly in practice and there may be conflicting results in some cases. None the less, the scheme is useful for identifying mucins.

7.6 FATS AND LIPIDS

Lipids are usually defined by their solubility in fat solvents and their insolubility in water. Solubility is referred to by the terms:

- **hydrophobic**, which refers to materials that are insoluble in water but soluble in organic solvents;
- **hydrophilic**, which refers to materials that are soluble in water but not soluble in organic solvents; and
- **amphipathic**, which refers to materials that have parts of the molecule that are hydrophobic and parts that are hydrophilic.

All lipids are therefore at least partly hydrophobic but are otherwise often quite varied and they may have very little in common except their solubility.

For example, the differences in structure, distribution and function between a steroid hormone such as testosterone and the adipose fat found in the subcutaneous tissues is much greater than the similarities in their solubility. Nevertheless, in histological terms, the solubility of lipids has been of crucial importance. The identification and location of lipids is generally less well understood and less frequently investigated histologically because the traditional wax sectioning techniques remove the lipids (see *Box 7.8* for further comments). It is almost a truism to say that lipids are materials that cannot be investigated in paraffin wax sections. Because of this, historically most histologists have chosen to investigate other things.

Box 7.8 Problems with processing fatty tissues

Even though fats are soluble in the solvents used for clearing, they can still cause problems in the cutting of wax blocks. Lipids will act as a waterproofing layer and will prevent the complete dehydration of blocks that are rich in fats. The fat itself will be dissolved gradually by the clearing agent and the block will then be left incompletely dehydrated. The water content may be very small, but unless the clearing agent is water-tolerant and can complete the dehydration, the final block will have some water trapped within the tissues. During storage, this water can evaporate causing the tissue to shrink, leaving a depressed block.

If there is much fat, then it may not be completely dissolved by the clearing agent. The final block will be not be impregnated properly and will not section easily, if at all.

Types of fats and lipids

The classification and structure of lipids have been confused and different methods of grouping the various types have been used. Metabolically there are two types of lipid: these are the **steroids**, which have a complex ring structure as the hydrophobic part of the molecule, and **lipids**, in which the hydrophobic part of the molecule is an aliphatic fatty acid. In many biochemical textbooks, these two materials are dealt with quite separately since the metabolic pathways dealing with steroids are completely different to those dealing with fatty acids. Histology textbooks more commonly use a classification that is based on whether the lipid is conjugated or not. In many of the demonstration techniques used in histology, the critical difference is often whether the lipid is a hydrophobic lipid or an amphipathic lipid.

Conjugated and unconjugated lipids

The list below shows the different categories of conjugated (esters or amides) and unconjugated lipids.

Conjugated lipids:
1. Neutral fats
2. Waxes   ⎫ Hydrophobic lipids
3. Cholesterol esters
4. Phosphoglycerides
   Phosphatidyl choline
   Phosphatidyl ethanolamines
   Phosphatidyl serine   ⎬ Phospholipids
   Ether phosphatides
   Phosphatidyl inositol
   Diphosphatidyl glycerols
5. Sphingomyelins   Hydrophilic lipids
6. Ceramides
7. Glycolipids

Unconjugated lipids:
1. Fatty acids
2. Steroids
   Cholesterol   ⎬ Hydrophobic lipids
   Steroid hormones

Section preparation for lipids

The first thing that must be considered in investigating lipids is how they can be preserved and sectioned.

Fixation is difficult for lipids. Most fixatives used in histology are protein fixatives and do not fix lipids; at best they leave them unaffected (e.g. formaldehyde), at worst they may even destroy them (e.g. alcohol). Only two fixatives have any significant fixative action on lipids and neither is commonly used. The first is osmium tetroxide, which adds on to double bonds in tissues including those in unsaturated lipids.

This fixes the lipid but also blackens it. This makes osmium-fixed lipid unsuitable for most histochemistry. Osmium tetroxide is, however, very important in electron microscopy since the fixation and blackening preserves and stains membranes, which are a vital part of the ultrastructure of cells.

The second fixative that can preserve lipids is potassium dichromate, which can preserve some phospholipids, although it has little effect on triglycerides or steroids. This has been used in histochemistry in the Marchi technique and the Baker technique for phospholipids, but otherwise the prolonged dichromate fixation needed to fix the phospholipids is not common.

The majority of lipid histochemistry is therefore done on unfixed lipid because, even if the sections have been fixed to preserve protein, the fixatives usually have no effect on the lipid. The sections are usually cut frozen. This means that the best fixative is formaldehyde, which allows good frozen sections and does not alter lipids. The addition of 10% calcium chloride is believed to help preserve phospholipids but should be kept short (<2 days) to prevent the formation of soaps with free fatty acids. Fixation is often delayed until after sectioning (or even after staining) when fixation times can be considerably reduced.

Sections are almost always prepared by a frozen section technique, with cryostat sections generally being preferred and fixation being done after cutting.

Neutral lipids

Simple neutral lipids can be localized very easily using **lysochrome** methods, which rely on the hydrophobic nature of the lipid. Lysochrome staining relies on using a dye that is very soluble in lipids but relatively insoluble in aqueous solvents.

If the dye is made up in an aqueous solvent, then when it is applied to the tissues the hydrophobic dye will become concentrated in the tissue lipids, even when used at only at a low concentration in the watery phase. Such a solution of hydrophobic dye will rapidly colour the lipid by a simple solution mechanism, leaving the hydrophilic proteins and nucleic acids uncoloured, as it is much more soluble in the hydrophobic lipid than in the aqueous solvent (see *Fig. 7.2* and *Colour plate 10*).

The first techniques used in this way relied on Sudan dyes (Sudan I, II, III and IV) and this type of reaction is still often called **sudanophilia**. Only Sudan III and IV were ever popular in histology and these have now been replaced by an even more highly coloured and hydrophobic dye, oil red O. In either case the hydrophobic dye must be dissolved at high concentration

---

Box 7.9 Lipids in accidents

The staining of lipids is one method of determining whether a person died instantaneously in an accident, even if they are not examined until many hours or days later. In an accident in which bones are broken, the fatty material in the bone marrow will be released into the bloodstream. The fatty material does not dissolve but remains as a solid fat embolism. The embolisms are carried around in the bloodstream until they reach a capillary where they lodge. The first capillary bed that the droplets encounter is usually in the lung. Thus, in a fatal accident, if a fresh section of lung is taken and stained by a lysochromy technique, then the finding of lipid droplets from the marrow shows that the heart went on beating after the bones were broken so the person did not die instantaneously.

Apply dye solution to tissue

Lipid absorbs dye but protein does not

Figure 7.2
Process for neutral lipid staining

in an aqueous solvent in which it is not very soluble. This contradiction means that it is not usually a simple solution.

One of the earliest reliable techniques was that of Herxheimer who used acetone and alcohol. This has significant solvent ability for the dye but unfortunately it will also dissolve some lipids. It gives excellent demonstration of major fat deposits such as adipose tissue but may dissolve very small droplets of lipid such as might be found inside non-adipose cells. Since then, the lipid-dissolving ability of the solvent has been reduced in a variety of ways (see, for example, *Box 7.10*).

Lillie and Ashburne introduced isopropanol as a solvent. The stock solution of the dye is a saturated solution in 100% isopropanol, but for use the stock solution is diluted immediately before being used to give a final concentration of 60% isopropanol. This weaker alcoholic solution has much less solvent action on the lipid, but in diluting the stock a supersaturated solution is produced, which gives a high concentration of dye. The supersaturated solution is unstable and must be used immediately.

Box 7.10 Avoiding the use of solvents

The dangers of dissolving the lipid by using an organic solvent as the dye carrier led to an attempt to avoid using a solvent. The gelatine method developed by Govan used gelatine as a carrier instead. In this method, the dye was first dissolved in acetone and this was mixed with a hot solution of gelatine. The acetone evaporated, leaving the dye trapped within the colloidal suspension of the gelatine. The method does work but the slight theoretical advantage of not having any solvent present did not compensate for a complex and messy technique and this method has not stood the test of time. A good theoretical idea does not always translate into a useful and workable method.

Chiffelle and Putt used propylene glycol and Gomori used triethyl phosphate, both of which are claimed not to dissolve lipid although they will dissolve the dyes.

Most laboratories use one of these three techniques, depending mainly on personal preference.

Since all of the solvents use the dye at close to saturation, it is important to filter the dye solutions to remove any precipitate and to prevent evaporation during staining, which would cause deposits to occur. Removal of excess dye solution is usually done with the same solvent that was used for the dye and this is then followed by washing in water. This rinse in solvent helps to prevent any precipitation of the dye and keeps the background clear. The most commonly used dyes are red and are usually counterstained with haematoxylin.

Temperature alters lysochrome dye solubility

Staining at room temperature will demonstrate neutral lipids but not most phospholipids, cholesterol or their derivatives, which are crystalline at room temperature. These can be rendered sudanophilic by heating to above their melting point during staining. Protein-bound lipid also may not be demonstrated by the simple technique as the protein restricts the entry of the hydrophobic dye. These protein-bound lipids are sometimes called masked lipids; they can still be demonstrated provided the lipid can be detached from the dye, e.g. by hydrolysis with acid.

Free fatty acids and phosphoglycerides, being more amphipathic, have a greater tendency to be extracted by the solvents used but their solubility can be reduced by bromination, which also converts any cholesterol to a compound that is liquid at room temperature and so will also stain.

Sudan black

One further Sudan dye used is Sudan black. This is a mixture of two main hydrophobic dyes plus several hydrophilic components. It is a more aggressive dye mixture and will often stain lipids that are partly hydrophilic (amphipathic), which would be left unstained by oil red O. Unfortunately, it will sometimes stain other tissue components as well as lipids, making interpretation more difficult. This unwanted staining increases as the dye solution ages and is less pronounced with fresh dye solutions.

A negative control for lysochrome techniques can be performed by using a section extracted with a 2:1 chloroform:methanol mixture for 1 h. The solvent will extract all of the lipids and so destroy any true sudanophilia. Any coloration after the extraction will be non-specific and not lipid.

Phospholipids

These are lipids that contain a phosphate group. They are mainly phosphoglycerides and are principally associated with membranes, including the myelin sheaths of nerves. The presence of the phosphate group renders them more hydrophilic (i.e. they are amphipathic) than the neutral fats, so they stain less readily with lysochrome techniques and are more rapidly and easily extracted than other lipids unless they are bound to protein.

Baker's acid haematein staining

This involves the reaction of phospholipids, especially choline-containing phospholipids, with potassium dichromate. The dichromate adds on to the lipids:

The chromium can then act as a mordant for the haematein dye and the phospholipids stain blue. Any lipid unaffected by the dichromate will be lost during dehydration and clearing, so the reaction is reasonably selective. It is usually controlled by using a second sample, which is treated with a simple solvent extraction before treatment with dichromate. The control differentiates phospholipids from tissue ions that may act as mordants. This technique, as well as being a histochemical technique, is also a good way of demonstrating mitochondria.

The original technique was a block-staining method and involved prolonged exposure to all of the reagents (a total of 3–5 days), but this can be reduced by using cryostat sections instead of blocks of tissue, which also makes controls more realistic as adjacent sections can be used for the test and the control.

Marchi techniques for myelin

This relies on the following properties:

1. Osmium tetroxide is soluble in both hydrophobic and amphipathic lipids.
2. Osmium tetroxide is an oxidizing agent that oxidizes and blackens lipids.
3. Hydrophilic oxidizing agents such as potassium dichromate or potassium chlorate are only able to penetrate amphipathic lipids.
4. The oxidizing and blackening effect of osmium tetroxide is inhibited by other oxidizing agents.

Thus, if a mixed reagent of osmium tetroxide and potassium dichromate (a hydrophilic oxidizing agent) is applied to tissues, the amphipathic lipids will absorb both the osmium tetroxide and the potassium dichromate. Since the dichromate will inhibit the blackening effect of the osmium tetroxide, the amphipathic lipids will not become blackened. The hydrophobic lipids will absorb the osmium tetroxide but not the potassium dichromate, so they will become blackened. The total effect, therefore, is that hydrophobic lipids will be blackened but more hydrophilic or amphipathic lipids will not.

This is one way of identifying degenerating myelin. Normal myelin consists of hydrophilic phospholipid, whilst degenerating myelin is converted to hydrophobic neutral lipid. With Marchi-type techniques, normal myelin is unstained and degenerate myelin is black. The original Marchi method used potassium dichromate, but the Swank–Davenport method of using potassium chlorate is now generally preferred.

Osmium tetroxide α-naphthylamine (OTAN)

This is similar to the Marchi-type techniques, but the osmium that is bound by phospholipids but not blackened is visualized using α-naphthylamine, which gives an orange/red or orange/brown complex with the osmium. The OTAN technique has lost popularity because its specificity has been questioned, and because hydrophobic lipids and some proteins may also be stained. In addition, α-naphthylamine can be carcinogenic, especially if contaminated with β-naphthylamine.

Steroids: cholesterol

Cholesterol is the only steroid that is present in large enough quantities to be detectable in tissue sections. Large amounts of cholesterol may form crystals within the tissues and when they dissolve out during processing, their presence is indicated by angular gaps in the tissues referred to as cholesterol clefts. Cholesterol is also associated with disease (see *Box 7.11*).

Cholesterol is not normally sudanophilic

Cholesterol will not be stained by the normal lysochrome technique as it has a high melting point and is crystalline at room temperature. By staining at a temperature above its melting point (150°C), it will become

---

Box 7.11 Cholesterol in disease

Large amounts of cholesterol are found mainly in degenerating tissues, such as in necrosis. The cholesterol is a normal constituent of cell membranes but is difficult for the body to remove. As tissues degenerate, cholesterol accumulates. This occurs, for example, in atherosclerosis. The wall of an artery becomes damaged and as cells disintegrate cholesterol accumulates, partly from the degenerating cells and partly from **low-density lipoprotein** (LDL), which carries cholesterol in the blood and also gets trapped in the vessel wall. The lipid is ingested by macrophages, which develop a foamy-looking cytoplasm ('foam cells'). Repair mechanisms are activated and result in a fibrotic plaque. The lesion gets worse with time and can lead to narrowing of the arterial lumen and even complete blockage. The degeneration is slow and may even reverse if the cholesterol can be removed by **high-density lipoprotein** (HDL). The exact mechanism of this degeneration is still unresolved but high levels of LDL cholesterol are bad for the arteries and high levels of HDL are good for avoiding cardiovascular disease.

sudanophilic, but staining at this high temperature is inconvenient. It can also be rendered sudanophilic by treatment with bromine water (2.5% aqueous bromine), when it is converted into an oily liquid that will stain with Sudan black.

The PAN method

The best specific staining method for cholesterol is the perchloric acid/naphthaquinone reaction (PAN). The perchloric acid converts the cholesterol to a diene, which then reacts with 1,2-naphthaquinone to give a blue product. In practice, the cholesterol first needs to be oxidized, which can be done using ferric chloride. The reagent also includes ethanol and formaldehyde, but their exact roles are not completely clear. The reaction is usually done on a hotplate at 70°C and the reagent is constantly brushed on to the section to prevent drying.

Cholesterol esters can be distinguished from free cholesterol by treating a second section with digitonin. This precipitates free cholesterol as a digitonide, which is insoluble in acetone. The section is then treated with acetone. The acetone dissolves the cholesterol esters but leaves the cholesterol digitonide. The PAN technique is then applied to the extracted section. Material reacting in both sections is free cholesterol, whilst any material reacting in the straight PAN but absent from the digitonin-treated slide is a cholesterol ester.

Free fatty acids

Free fatty acids are unusual in normal tissues but can occur in acute pancreatitis when the release of lipases results in the fats being enzymically hydrolysed. Free fatty acids can be demonstrated by treating the section with copper salts. Any fatty acid will form insoluble copper soaps with the copper ions. The copper soaps can then be demonstrated with copper-detecting reagents such as rubeanic acid (dithio-oxamide).

In many cases, the free fatty acids will already have formed calcium soaps if they have been in contact with solutions containing calcium ions. This may occur in the body or if the tissues have been fixed in formal calcium. These calcium soaps need to be hydrolysed with hydrochloric acid before being treated with the copper ions.

Phosphatidyl ethanolamine-based lipids (plasmalogens)

Plasmalogens can be detected by the plasmal reaction (from which they get their name). This involves treatment with mercuric chloride, which reacts with the vinyl ether linkage found in plasmalogens. This releases an aldehyde, which can be detected using Schiff's reagent. The reaction may even occur without pretreatment of the tissues with mercuric chloride if the Schiff's reagent is highly acid and the treatment with Schiff's is prolonged, as the acidity can have a similar bond-splitting effect.

Unsaturated lipids

The double bonds in lipids can be detected in a number of ways. As mentioned above, osmium tetroxide adds across double bonds and blackens the lipid in the process. Double bonds can also be oxidized to aldehydes, which can then be detected using Schiff's reagent. The oxidation can be achieved by using a powerful oxidizing agent such as performic acid (performic acid–Schiff, PAAS), but will occur slowly, even with atmospheric oxygen. This slow oxidation will result in aldehydes occurring in the section without any pretreatment and is called a pseudoplasmal reaction. This is a nuisance when using Schiff's reagent as it can give a non-specific background colour to the sections. The oxidation by air can be speeded up by irradiating the section with UV light and the UV Schiff technique is an alternative to using the PAAS and avoids the use of the highly corrosive performic acid.

Glycolipids

These will give a positive reaction with the PAS technique but require controls to distinguish them from mucins and other carbohydrates. The simplest is an extraction with chloroform/methanol. There can also be confusion with plasmalogens, which can give a positive reaction with Schiff's reagent and pseudoplasmal reactions.

Extraction techniques as controls and for identification

Lipids can be identified by their solubility. Extraction is a standard technique in lipid biochemistry and the difference in solubility of the different lipids forms the basis of chromatography, which is the best way of identifying individual lipids. In histology, the solubility of a lipid is determined by lipid staining of two equivalent sections, one of which has been extracted with a particular solvent. By using different solvents, it is possible to selectively remove different lipids. The example given in *Table 7.1* shows the method of Keilig.

Box 7.12 Diseases of lipid metabolism

As with the mucopolysaccharidoses, if there is a defect in the destruction of lipids it can lead to a disease in which lipids build up. Tay–Sachs disease is a genetic disease in which the hexosaminidase enzyme of lysosomes is defective. This prevents the destruction of one type of glycolipid (gangliosides), which accumulates in the lysosomes. The childhood form of this disease is particularly associated with Jewish populations originating in Eastern Europe (Ashkenazi Jews). The Ashkenazi Jews have a much higher incidence of the gene in the population, with perhaps as many as 1 in 25 people being a carrier of the gene compared with 1 in 500 in the general population. Affected children are therefore much commoner in these Jewish populations. The disease causes swelling of neurones, which can lead to seizures, poor development and blindness. The disease begins to affect the child from about the age of 3 months and leads to death at around 4–5 years old.

Table 7.1 **Selective removal of lipids by the Keilig method**

Solvent	Lipids dissolved
Cold acetone	Glycerides, cholesterol and its esters and other steroids
Hot acetone	Cerebroside lipids
Hot ether	Lecithin and cephalins
Hot chloroform and methanol	All lipids

The table gives a false impression of the ease and accuracy of the method. For example, it is usually necessary to use a Soxhlet apparatus and continuous refluxing for long periods to ensure removal of the lipid. The problems with extraction are:

1. The lipid may relocalize rather than dissolve. This may be unrelated to the solvent since heating itself alters the lipid and it may move significantly during the treatment, giving the impression that it has dissolved whilst it has only flowed to a different area of the tissue.
2. The solubility is determined on pure lipids, but in tissues the lipids are often mixtures and this can affect their solubility in solvents.
3. Lipids in tissues are often intimately bound to proteins, which may alter their solubility.
4. Lipids in sections have often been exposed to fixatives, which may affect their solubility.

In practice, extraction techniques are rarely used as a major way of identifying individual lipids but they can be very useful control methods.

SUGGESTED FURTHER READING

Bancroft, J.D. and Cook, H.C. (1994) *Manual of Histological Techniques and their Diagnostic Application.* Edinburgh: Churchill Livingstone.
Kiernan, J.A. (2001) *Histological and Histochemical Methods*, 3rd edn. Oxford: Hodder Arnold.
Lamar Jones, M. (2002) Lipids. In *Theory and Practice of Histological Techniques*, 5th edn (eds J.D. Bancroft and M. Gamble). Edinburgh: Churchill Livingstone.
Sheehan. D.C. and Hrapchak, B. (1980) *Theory and Practice of Histotechnology.* St Louis: Mosby.
Totty, B.A. (2002) Mucins. In *Theory and Practice of Histological Techniques*, 5th edn (eds J.D. Bancroft and M. Gamble). Edinburgh: Churchill Livingstone.

SELF-ASSESSMENT QUESTIONS

1. What are the extra difficulties involved in identifying chemicals in sections compared with in solution?

2. What types of material stain with the PAS technique?
3. Why is periodic acid preferred as the oxidizing agent compared with chromic acid or potassium permanganate?
4. List the main types of mucin.
5. Outline the principle of the critical electrolyte concentration technique of using alcian blue.
6. How could you distinguish between hyaluronic acid and sialic acid, both of which stain with alcian blue?
7. Why are lipid techniques unpopular with many histologists?
8. What is the principle of staining lipids with Sudan-type dyes?
9. Which, if any, fixatives can fix lipids?
10. Why does normal myelin react differently with lipid-staining techniques compared with degenerating myelin?

CHAPTER 8

Histochemistry of nucleic acids, proteins and enzymes

Learning objectives
After studying this chapter you should confidently be able to:

■ **Describe the methods of staining nucleic acids in sections.**
RNA and DNA can be stained using basic dyes or more selective techniques. DNA can be specifically demonstrated using the Feulgen technique or using fluorescent dyes such as ethidium bromide. To distinguish DNA from RNA, it is possible to use selective methods such as methyl green–pyronin or acridine orange or by selective destruction using enzymes.

■ **Describe the main methods for identifying proteins in sections.**
Proteins can be stained with simple stains like eosin or by using more selective methods for particular proteins, e.g. acid orcein for elastin and martius/scarlet/blue for fibrin. Individual proteins are best identified by immunotechniques. Proteins with enzyme activity can be demonstrated by their action on a substrate to produce an insoluble coloured product.

■ **Discuss the difficulties of retaining enzyme activity in sections.**
Enzymes are easily inactivated by fixation, processing or other handling of tissues or by simple exposure to room temperature. Even if they remain active, many enzymes will become delocalized or even completely lost from the tissue.

■ **Outline the problems involved in quantifying enzyme activity in sections.**
Enzymes may be inactivated or may diffuse out of the tissues before quantitation can be done. The kinetics of enzymes in sections may not follow Beer–Lambert kinetics because of diffusion limitation.

8.1 NUCLEIC ACIDS

The general structure of the nucleic acids is a backbone of alternating pentose sugar and phosphate groups. Each sugar has a nitrogenous base attached to it. The base can be either a purine or a pyrimidine. The backbone can interact with similar nucleic acid strands to form double strands by hydrogen bonding between the purine and pyrimidine bases. There are four different bases that can occur in any nucleic acid and the sequence of these bases is the basis of the genetic code. Nucleic acids include several quite different forms of material that differ in their chemical composition and structural forms.

DNA and RNA

Ribonucleic nucleic acid (RNA) has a simple ribose sugar in the main backbone of the molecule, whilst deoxyribonucleic acid (DNA) has the deoxyribose form of the sugar in its backbone. They differ slightly in their bases such that DNA includes the base thymine, whilst RNA uses uracil in the same position; in both forms the other three bases are the same (adenine, guanine and cytosine).

DNA is found almost exclusively in the nucleus (very small amounts are found in the mitochondria). Whilst all of the RNA is actually produced inside the nucleus, it is usually quickly transported into the cytoplasm, so that most of the RNA in a cell is found in the cytoplasm or in the nucleolus, which produces the ribosomal RNA.

Probably the most important differences in the properties of the nucleic acids, from a histochemical point of view, are the size of the molecule, the shape of the molecule and whether there is any attached protein.

DNA double helix

DNA forms a double helix and is strongly associated with histone proteins. This combination forms nucleoprotein and is the material usually referred to by histologists as chromatin. The DNA is wrapped around the histones and each structure forms a characteristic unit called a nucleosome. The DNA in a cell usually forms very large molecules with each chromosome being a single DNA molecule. Thus, an average human chromosome consists of around 1×10^8 nucleotides and the DNA helix would measure about 5 cm if straightened out completely. The wrapping around the histones reduces this to around 1 mm total length and more coiling and folding reduce it even further. Thus, the DNA within the cell is always highly coiled.

Active and inert DNA

Depending on how tightly packed, or condensed, it is, the DNA is described as being heterochromatic (darkly staining and very tightly packed) or euchromatic (lighter staining and less densely packed). Heterochromatin is inactive and not transcribed, whilst euchromatin is being actively used by the cell. The DNA may also be modified by being methylated. In methylation, some of the cytosine bases are changed to 5-methyl cytosine. This conversion is catalysed by enzymes. Methylation is believed to be a method of controlling gene activity as inactive genes tend to be more heavily methylated.

Different forms of RNA

RNA occurs in several different forms within the cell:

Ribosomal RNA (rRNA) does not form a double helix and is always associated with protein. This RNA forms part of the small structures called ribosomes. Although too small to be adequately resolved as individual structures by the light microscope, ribosomes can form larger aggregates (polyribosomes), which can be visible in the cytoplasm.

Transfer RNA (tRNA) does not form a double helix but forms a series of hairpin loops of RNA. Transfer RNA is not bound to protein.

Messenger RNA (mRNA) does not form a double helix but occurs as a single-stranded RNA and is not firmly bound to protein.

The differences in function of the three forms of RNA are of only minor importance in most histological investigations since all three forms of RNA are associated in different ways with the production of protein. Thus, for most histological purposes, they are all indicators of active protein synthesis and provided any one of them is retained, the loss of the other forms is less critical. It is only when mRNA is needed in hybridization studies (see Chapter 13) that it is essential to retain a particular kind of RNA.

Fixation affects either the physical or chemical structure of nucleic acids

In paraffin sections, only nucleic acid that is firmly attached to protein will be consistently retained since most fixatives act on proteins and not on nucleic acids. This means that only DNA and rRNA are retained by all fixatives and can always be demonstrated in tissues. Some fixatives, whilst not truly fixing the nucleic acid, may still alter it either chemically or physically.

Additive fixatives usually combine with and alter the reactive groups of nucleic acids, whilst non-additive fixatives alter the double helix regions of DNA and so disturb its physical form. There is no fixative that retains both the chemical and physical form of nucleic acids. Some methods rely on chemical reactivity, whilst others use physical form to trap the dyes. Whenever nucleic acids are to be investigated, it is essential to use a fixative that retains the particular characteristic of the nucleic acid that is used in the demonstration method.

Generally, fixatives containing acetic acid give better preservation and are preferred for DNA studies, but formaldehyde is satisfactory for DNA and rRNA.

Staining techniques

The commonest staining methods for nucleic acid are the basic dyes. Nucleic acids are strongly basophilic and will stain with almost any basic dye. This is good for morphological purposes but basophilia is not limited to nucleic acids and needs controlling with enzymes in order to get specific identification.

Feulgen technique

The Feulgen technique is specific for DNA and will not stain RNA or any other components of cells. The technique uses Schiff's reagent, which reacts with aldehydes (see Chapter 7). The DNA in tissues does not contain any free aldehydes, but aldehydes can be produced by acid hydrolysis. The hydrolysis removes the bases from the DNA leaving pentose sugars that contain aldehyde groups and therefore stain pink with Schiff's reagent.

Hydrolysis of DNA is usually done with 1 M HCl at 60°C. Care must be taken to get the timing of the hydrolysis correct or the DNA will be completely hydrolysed to soluble fragments of nucleic acid and these will wash out of the section and the staining will be reduced. Any RNA is completely hydrolysed by the usual hydrolysis conditions and does not stain.

The Feulgen technique is quantitative when performed correctly, and the amount of DNA in each cell can be measured by microdensitometry. The amount of DNA in an individual cell is usually constant in most human cells except when:

- The cell is actively dividing. Before division can occur, the cell must duplicate the DNA so that when the cell splits into two, both daughter cells will get a complete set of chromosomes.
- The cell has an unusual chromosome number.

Both of these can be associated with malignant cells, so investigations are currently underway to determine whether an automatic technique can be developed that will reliably identify malignant cells by measuring their DNA content.

The Feulgen hydrolysis step is dependent on the fixative used. Picric acid performs the same hydrolysis as HCl, so material fixed with picric acid is not suitable for the Feulgen technique nor is tissue decalcified in acid solutions.

The following are the optimum times for some fixatives and show the effects of fixation on the nucleic acid: formaldehyde, 8 min; Carnoy's, 8 min; Helly's, 5 min; Susa's, 18 min. If there is as little as 30 s error in the timing, the results will be less than optimal and will be non-quantitative.

Fluorescent stains

There are a number of very valuable fluorescent dyes that can be used to demonstrate nucleic acids. These include quinacrine, Hoechst 33258, ethidium bromide, acridine orange and methyl green–pyronin.

Intercalating dyes. Quinacrine, Hoechst 33258 and ethidium bromide act by intercalating into the double helix. Intercalation is where the dye slides between the stacks of bases and is dependent on the double helix structure. These dyes are only used to stain DNA and can be used as vital stains to show DNA in living cells. Quinacrine has been used to identify chromosome bands (so-called Q-banding) used in identifying chromosomal structure and diagnosing chromosome disorders. This is because it produces bright fluorescence in adenine/thymine-rich regions and less fluorescence in guanine/cytosine-rich regions. When quinacrine is used on the condensed chromosomes found in mitosis, it gives a banding pattern of bright and dim transverse bands. The non-fluorescent dark bands represent regions rich in guanine and cytosine, whilst the brighter fluorescent bands represent regions rich in adenine and thymine.

Acridine orange. Acridine orange is different to the previous dyes in that it can be used for both DNA and RNA. With acridine orange staining, double-stranded DNA fluoresces green, whilst single-stranded RNA fluoresces red. As staining depends on the conformation of the strands to distinguish the two types of nucleic acid, it follows that any treatment that alters the structure will destroy this differentiation. Formaldehyde-fixed and paraffin-processed materials do not work reliably with this technique but it has been used successfully on alcohol-fixed smears.

Methyl green–pyronin

The methyl green–pyronin technique uses two different basic dyes to differentiate between DNA and RNA. In some ways it is the equivalent of the van Gieson or trichrome method of using acid dyes. The dyes used are methyl green, a triaryl methane dye, and pyronin Y, a xanthene dye. The dyes differ in molecular weight, molecular size and molecular shape. When used at pH 4.6, they compete for binding to the nucleic acids and differentially stain the DNA a green colour and the RNA a red colour (see *Box 8.1*).

The mechanism of this differential staining is disputed. It seems likely that the larger methyl green stains by binding to the outside of the DNA helix and is bound by the phosphate groups and possibly by linking non-ionically to the protein and sugars. Pyronin, being a smaller, more planar molecule, can probably intercalate between the bases and stain nucleic acids in this way. The differences in staining probably reflect the differences in structure, with intercalation being more easily achieved with the more open structure of RNA than with the compact double helix of DNA.

This technique has many variants; this is probably because it is sometimes fickle and erratic in the results it gives. It is sensitive to pH and needs to be buffered at pH 4–5 (there is some dispute as to the best pH, with most methods using pH 4.8 but others recommending a pH as low as 4). The pyronin is rapidly extracted by ethanol dehydration, so the section is usually dehydrated in butanol instead. Dye purity seems to be a problem, with the methyl green usually being heavily contaminated, and repeated extraction with chloroform is recommended to remove the methyl violet. The method is also sensitive to dye strength. All these factors make it difficult to get uniform results in every laboratory on every occasion it is used.

Box 8.1 Pyroninophilia

The identification of RNA by this technique is referred to as **pyroninophilia**. The term is applied to cells such as lymphoblasts and plasma cells that are active in the production of antibodies. Although the presence of nucleic acids in the cytoplasm can be indicated by cytoplasmic basophilia, the term pyroninophilia is more limited and only refers to nucleic acids, whereas basophilia refers to any acidic material in the cytoplasm.

Using specific enzymes and chemical extraction as controls

There is always doubt as to the nature of a stained material when using dyes for histochemical identification so it is important to control these methods using an extraction technique. This is done by selectively destroying one or both nucleic acids and comparing the digested section with an undigested one. Both sections are stained by the technique being used and only if the stain disappears from the digested section can it be reliably assumed that the material is the nucleic acid. If the colour is present in both sections, it is a non-specific reaction, probably due to the dye binding to a protein. This digestion is usually sufficiently specific that it can be used with a relatively non-selective basic stain such as methylene blue as a simple method of locating a specific nucleic acid.

Enzymatic digestion. This is highly specific if done correctly but needs careful control as enzymes are sensitive to fixation, pH and the presence of ions and the enzyme must be pure. The enzymes are readily available commercially and, providing pure forms of the enzymes are used rather than impure extracts, they are highly specific. Impure forms of enzymes prepared from materials such as pancreas can be contaminated with proteases. **Deoxyribonuclease** is usually prepared from pancreatic tissue and used as a dilute solution (0.05 mg ml^{-1}) in buffer at pH 7.6. Deoxyribonuclease requires magnesium ions to work effectively, so it is usually better to add magnesium chloride or sulphate to the buffer to ensure optimum activity. **Ribonuclease** is usually used as a simple solution in distilled water but at a higher concentration (0.5 mg ml^{-1}). Extraction is done by incubating at 37°C and then washing in water to remove the digestion products.

In situ hybridization

In addition to the general staining techniques, mRNA and DNA can be identified by hybridization with labelled probes. This method identifies specific sequences of DNA and will be covered in more detail in Chapter 13.

8.2 PROTEINS

Proteins are the most important structural component in most sections as they are better fixed and more easily retained than most other tissue materials. However, individual proteins are difficult to identify as all proteins are very similar chemically and differ mainly in size and shape and neither of these properties is easy to identify in tissue sections.

Several different approaches are available for the staining of proteins.

General protein stains

Proteins are usually acidophilic and will stain with a wide range of dyes. These include acid dyes such as eosin, ponceau red and Coomassie blue. Although these dyes are useful to indicate the total quantity of protein present within the tissues, they are not selective for particular proteins. These dyes are used as general counterstains to give general colour to tissues and are also widely used in electrophoresis to show the protein bands. If used correctly, they can bind to tissues stoichiometrically and can be used to measure the total amount of protein present accurately. The use of dyes as a quantitative measure is more commonly done in electrophoresis than in histology. The density of staining is used by most microscopists as a guide to the total amount of material present, but this is just used as a subjective guide and is not accurately measured.

Digestion techniques

These use specific enzymes to remove and thus identify proteins. By comparing two sections stained with a general protein stain, it should be possible to see whether a particular protein has disappeared. Collagen, for example, can be identified by collagenase. This resembles the use of deoxyribonuclease in identifying DNA but is less specific. Although the names of the enzymes, such as collagenase, often suggest a high degree of specificity, they are usually much less specific than might be expected and the name of the protease indicates only a differential rate, not an absolute specificity. Thus, collagenase will act more quickly on collagen than on other proteins, but will still have some proteolytic activity towards other proteins. Despite this, they are still useful as controls in other techniques.

Selective protein techniques

A few techniques are available that are claimed to be selective for specific proteins. Although these techniques can sometimes be highly selective and very useful for histological purposes, they are often not fully specific and other proteins or tissue components will also take up the stain, albeit to a lesser extent.

Elastic fibres and elastin stains

Elastic fibres may be changed by disease (see *Box 8.2*) and are different to most proteins in having relatively few polar amino acids and many hydrophobic side chains. This unusual amino acid structure means that they

---

Box 8.2 Elastosis

The term elastosis refers to a deterioration in the connective tissues of the skin. There is a general loss of connective tissue fibres, not just elastic fibres, and the fibres that remain are abnormal. The changes gradually occur with wear and tear on the skin of normal living but are accelerated by exposure to sunlight. This change can be seen by examining different areas of skin from the same person. Skin that is regularly exposed to sunlight is more affected than skin only a short distance away that is not subjected to the same amount of light (e.g. behind the ears). In elastosis the skin loses its elasticity, develops wrinkles and is more easily damaged.

stain rather poorly with the usual ionic dyeing techniques such as haematoxylin and eosin, van Gieson's and trichromes and instead need more specialized techniques (see *Colour plate 11*). These possibly rely more on van der Waals bonds or hydrogen bonds than ionic bonding and many use an extreme pH that limits the staining of other fibres and proteins.

Relatively selective techniques include: Gomori's aldehyde fuchsin technique, Weigert's resorcinol fuchsin, Verhoeff's haematoxylin technique and the Taenzer–Unna orcein technique.

Oxytalan fibres

These stain rather poorly by most techniques but after oxidation (e.g. with peracetic acid) they stain as for elastic fibres. They are found in tendons, periodontal membranes and ligaments.

Fibrin

Fibrin is produced from the precursor fibrinogen by the coagulation of blood and is also present in some inflammatory exudates (see *Colour plate 12*). Fibrin is not stable in the body and gradually alters with ages. Fibrin can be demonstrated by different techniques as these changes occur and as it is gradually replaced during healing (see *Fig. 8.1*). Fibrin that is less than 24 h old is difficult to stain specifically by any technique and this also means that fibrinogen in plasma will not stain by these selective methods.

The Gram staining technique is useful mainly because it is also used in staining bacteria. The use of the Gram stain in an inflammatory condition will therefore show fibrin at the same time as the bacteria causing the inflammation. The phosphotungstic acid–haematoxylin (PTAH) technique is excellent for many structures and will show fibrin as a dark blue fibre. PTAH is not specific for fibrin but is a useful confirmatory stain. The martius/scarlet/blue (MSB) and Masson 4/44 methods are both trichrome techniques that were specially designed to be selective for fibrin, but again they are not specific and both need careful control and differentiation to achieve the desired result.

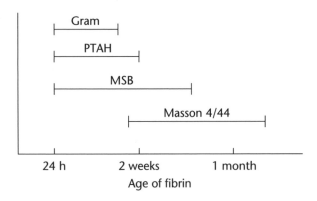

Figure 8.1
Staining techniques for fibrin as it ages

Fibrinoid

Fibrinoid is an amorphous material that stains similarly to fibrin but is associated with necrosis and disease rather than simple bleeding. It consists of fibrin (possibly aged or degrading), other plasma proteins and perhaps some mucopolysaccharide.

Amyloid

Amyloid is a pathological protein. Amyloid is formed in several diseases from a variety of precursor proteins. It stains selectively with congo red and thioflavine dyes. Amyloid is considered in more detail in Chapter 14.

Specific amino acid techniques

There are a range of biochemically based spot tests that will detect individual amino acids (e.g. Millon's for tyrosine) or specific groups associated with several amino acids (e.g. ninhydrin–Schiff for amino groups). The amino acid techniques demonstrate only protein-bound amino acids since free amino acids are readily lost into solvents including water.

In most cases, all proteins will react since all proteins contain a wide range of amino acids. This makes them somewhat pointless for general use as it is easier simply to use a general stain such as eosin (but see *Box 8.3*). A few examples of spot tests are given in *Table 8.1*.

Control of spot tests for amino acids is achieved either by selective removal, e.g. amino groups with nitrous acid:

$$R\text{-}NH_2 + HNO_2 \rightarrow R\text{-}OH + N_2 + H_2O$$

or by blocking, e.g. acetylation of amine groups with acetic anhydride:

$$R\text{-}NH_2 + CH_3COOCOCH_3 \rightarrow R\text{-}NHCOCH_3 + CH_3COOH$$

Single amino acids are rarely demonstrated in diagnosis but may sometimes be demonstrated in research. When performing these techniques, it must be remembered that the fixation and other treatments that are used in tissue preparation are likely to alter the reactivity of the proteins. Glutaraldehyde and to a lesser extent formaldehyde will bind to amino

Table 8.1 Examples of spot tests for single amino acids

Group	Amino acid(s)	Technique
Amine	E.g. lysine	Ninhydrin–Schiff
Phenyl	Tyrosine	Millon
Disulphide/sulphydryl	E.g. cysteine	Performic acid–alcian blue
Indole	Tryptophan	DMAB–nitrite (see *Box 8.3*)
Guanidyl	Arginine	Sakaguchi

Box 8.3 Tryptophan and amyloid

The *p*-dimethylaminobenzaldehyde (DMAB) method for tryptophan has been used as a method of demonstrating the pathological protein amyloid. This will work well with certain types of amyloid that have high levels of tryptophan in their polypeptides but is not a generally reliable method of identifying all amyloids. The low levels of tryptophan in most proteins make this method more useful than most of the other single amino acid techniques. Most proteins will barely react. It is only in cells such as Paneth cells and zymogen granules in the pancreas that significant reaction will be seen.

---

groups, mercury-containing fixatives will affect sulphur-containing groups and picric acid will form picrates with proteins. The best fixatives for the histochemistry of amino acids in proteins are the non-additive fixatives such as alcohol or Carnoy's.

Immunological techniques

These are the most specific and accurate but will only detect a particular protein. Immunological techniques are probably the best method of localizing individual proteins and have become very important in identifying cells, diseases and metabolic changes in cells. They are so important that they will be dealt with as a separate chapter (Chapter 10).

Specific action of the protein

Receptors and other binding proteins can be detected by using labelled ligands. These techniques usually resemble the immunotechniques in their methodology. The most important of this group of techniques are the enzyme techniques where the enzyme is located by its action on a substrate. These are less specific than immunological techniques; for example, acid phosphatase is a broad title for many enzymes. However, they are often useful as they indicate function rather than single protein species (see *Box 8.4*).

Box 8.4 Isoenzymes

Many enzymes have more than one type present within the body. These are isoenzymes or isozymes and often can be separated by electrophoresis. This technique is of little use in sections where localization of the enzyme is critical. However, many isoenzymes can also be identified by differences in their sensitivity to inhibitors or pH.

Acid phosphatase is found in many cells but one form is resistant to inhibition by tartrate ions. Tartrate-resistant acid phosphatase (TRAP) is limited to the osteoclasts that resorb bone, so osteoclasts can be identified by using a TRAP technique.

Similar inhibition methods are available for a range of enzymes and can identify subtypes of enzyme reasonably well.

8.3 ENZYMES

Enzyme histochemistry is the localization of enzymes in tissues by their specific action on a substrate.

Tissue preparation for enzyme techniques

Enzyme activity is an extremely labile phenomenon and most enzymes are rapidly inactivated by most tissue preparative methods. For this reason, paraffin wax- and plastic-embedded sections are almost entirely useless for demonstrating enzyme activity and cryostat sections are the more usual way of preparing the sections.

Fixation can sometimes be useful to help stop enzymes diffusing and this can be done either on the block before sectioning or immediately after cutting when the section can be rapidly fixed. Fixing the section rather than the block is often better as the length of fixation can be kept brief since penetration into a thin section is rapid compared with a large block of tissue.

For electron microscopy (EM), where the block needs to be embedded in plastic to obtain thin enough sections, the staining is done on the fresh tissue before processing ('block staining'). This means that only one method can be performed on each block of tissue and a separate block is needed for each enzyme being investigated. This is not necessarily as drastic as it sounds since EM blocks can be very small; indeed, a cryostat section for light microscopy can be used as an EM block. However, it does mean that each block has to be processed and sectioned separately. Once the enzyme technique is finished, the block can then be fixed as usual since there is no longer any difficulty if the enzyme is inactivated. The tissue is then processed and cut as for any other EM block.

Enzyme demonstration techniques

For histology it is usually more important to get accurate localization than precise quantitation and so the techniques are often quite different from biochemical techniques. In particular they must produce a visible (i.e. coloured) insoluble product. Various methods of localization have been tried with differing degrees of success.

Immunotechniques

Antibodies against the enzyme can be used to localize the enzyme by any of the usual immunotechniques. However, immunotechniques do not show enzyme activity, simply the presence of an antigenic protein. Thus, some inborn errors of metabolism may show high levels of enzyme even though there is no active enzyme present. In these cases, the cell may be producing an aberrant protein but the mutated enzyme has no catalytic activity.

Substrate film techniques

Substrate film techniques can detect digestion but are inaccurate and non-specific. The enzyme is detected by allowing it to diffuse out of the section into a thin film of substrate layered on to the slide (see *Fig. 8.2*). This can be done for proteases with a layer of protein or for nucleases with a film of DNA. The enzyme digests the film leaving a hole in the film. The film and section are then stained and any holes in the stained film indicate where the enzyme activity is located. This technique is not popular and has very limited application. It is only applicable to a few enzymes that break down a substrate that can be made into a suitable film. It gives relatively poor specificity and poor localization.

Figure 8.2
Substrate film technique. The upper diagram shows a layer of substrate before digestion and the lower diagram shows holes where the enzyme has digested the film

Dissolved substrate techniques

These are the most common techniques and provide the most useful way of detecting enzyme activity. They use dissolved reagents and by careful choice of reagents it is arranged so that one of the final products of the reaction is coloured and insoluble.

Variations on the technique include the following:

■ The natural reaction product is coloured and insoluble, e.g. DOPA oxidase.
■ The reaction produces a product that, although not itself insoluble, can be precipitated as a coloured product. This is a very useful way of detecting many enzyme reactions, e.g. the azo dye technique for phosphatase.
■ The reaction produces a product that, although not itself insoluble, can be precipitated. However, the precipitate is not coloured and must be treated further to produce the colour, e.g. the Gomori phosphatase technique.

Hydrolytic enzymes

Only two major types of enzyme can be easily and reliably identified in sections. These are **hydrolytic enzymes**, in which the substrate is split using water, and **oxidoreductase enzymes**, in which there is a change in redox potential. A few other individual enzymes can be demonstrated but these are the exception.

Hydrolytic enzymes were the first enzymes to be localized in tissue sections and the relevant techniques were introduced by Gomori. The basic idea of the technique has remained but the method has been modified to give more reliable results. The enzymes that were demonstrated by these initial techniques were phosphatases. Phosphatases split organic phosphate molecules releasing inorganic phosphate ions that are then precipitated by ions in the substrate solution and the precipitate is then visualized.

Gomori's acid phosphatase

The method uses β-glycerophosphate as the substrate and incorporates lead ions into the substrate solution to trap the phosphate ions. Lead phosphate is insoluble in acid solutions and so is precipitated at the site of enzyme activity. The lead phosphate is then visualized using a sulphide treatment to convert it to a black precipitate (see *Colour plate 13*).

This method is easily adapted to other substrates that contain phosphates, e.g. ATP (for ATPases). It suffers from the disadvantage that lead ions can bind non-specifically to tissues (especially nuclei) and so requires careful technique and good controls to ensure that the sites of enzyme activity are correctly located. Lead is also an unnatural ion in cells and can act as an enzyme poison.

When these methods were first used to localize phosphatase enzymes, there was initially some doubt about their specificity and reliability. The lead ions, for example, could easily be absorbed on to other sites and give non-specific staining. Another problem was that the method assumes that, as the enzyme splits the glycerophosphate, precipitation of the phosphate ion will be instantaneous. This is not necessarily true. It was possible that the localization was wrong and that the phosphate ions diffused some distance before being finally precipitated. What was required was confirmation of the result using a totally different technique. This second technique was developed in the form of the azo-coupling technique.

Azo-coupling technique

This uses an artificial substrate, α-naphthol phosphate. When α-naphthol phosphate is hydrolysed by a phosphatase it releases phosphate ions and α-naphthol. The α-naphthol can react with a diazonium salt such as fast red B to form an insoluble azo dye at the site of the enzyme activity:

α-Naphthol phosphate α-Naphthol

α-Naphthol   Diazonium cation
Fast red B

Azo dye

When this technique was used, it was found to give similar results to the metal precipitation method of Gomori. Thus, the α-naphthol phosphate technique confirmed the results from the Gomori technique and the Gomori technique validated the α-naphthol phosphate method. With two techniques giving the same results, it is possible to have confidence in both. In practice, the α-naphthol phosphate method has some advantages over the Gomori technique and is now the more popular technique. It is very simple to perform (see *Box 8.5*) and gives strong reactions, especially using the later modified naphthol derivatives such as the naphthol AS derivatives developed by Burstone.

Box 8.5 Identification of semen

Acid phosphatase is found in prostatic fluid and can be used to localize and identify semen stains in cases of rape. If a semen stain is found in a case of rape, then the sperm can be used for DNA fingerprinting. The difficulty is in locating these stains once they have dried. If a piece of clothing is believed to have been contaminated with semen, it can be very tedious to search it visually to find minute traces of semen. If a damp sheet of paper is pressed against the clothing for a short period, then some of the protein in the semen will diffuse on to the paper, including the acid phosphatase enzyme. The paper can then be sprayed with acid phosphatase reagent. The resulting reaction will show exactly where the semen is, sperm can be located more quickly and the DNA testing can be carried out.

This has also been taken up commercially for a less commendable purpose. A commercial spray was marketed to be used to spray the underclothes of a partner, the logic being that semen stains were an indication of marital infidelity. Unfortunately the logic is faulty. Men suffering from prostate problems will generate a positive reaction even when faithful. The manufacturers earned an 'Ignoble Prize' for their efforts.

General techniques can be adapted for other enzymes

The α-naphthol method is quite adaptable and has been developed for many hydrolase enzymes as well as the phosphatases; for example, naphthol acetate can be used for esterase enzymes and naphthol glucuronate for glucuronidase enzymes. When hydrolysed, these substrates release α-naphthol, which can couple with a diazonium salt as above. In general, provided the natural substrate of an enzyme can be coupled to α-naphthol without stopping the enzyme hydrolysing the compound, then this technique can be adapted for any hydrolase enzyme.

The metal trapping technique of Gomori can also be extended to other hydrolases; for example, lipases split fatty materials and release fatty acids that can form insoluble soaps with calcium ions in the substrate solutions. These insoluble calcium salts can then be visualized using the cobalt/sulphide technique of Gomori. Usually the synthetic detergent Tween is used as the lipid rather than simple soap.

Acetyl cholinesterase can be demonstrated using acetyl thiocholine. The esterase releases the thiocholine, which can be trapped with copper ions, and the copper thiocholine can be blackened with hydrogen sulphide.

Oxidoreductase enzymes

Oxidoreductases are enzymes that affect their substrates by changing the redox potential and often transfer electrons between the reactants. Several types of oxidoreductase enzyme can be demonstrated and they differ in the type of change they produce. Three types will be considered here: dehydrogenases, which transfer hydrogen from a substrate to a carrier molecule; oxidases, in which oxygen acts as the oxidizing agent; and peroxidases, which involve the use of peroxides.

Dehydrogenase enzymes

The action of dehydrogenase enzymes involves the exchange of hydrogen between two substances, the first of which is usually called the substrate and the other the hydrogen acceptor (or sometimes electron carrier). The hydrogen acceptor therefore changes from an oxidized state to a reduced state, whilst the substrate becomes oxidized (dehydrogenated). These changes are described for the forward reaction, but since most of these reactions are easily reversible the metabolism of the cell may well use the opposite direction.

The common hydrogen acceptors in the cell are NAD^+ ($NADH_2$), $NADP^+$ ($NADPH_2$) and FAD^+ ($FADH_2$) with the reduced form of the co-enzyme shown in parentheses.

In the detection of dehydrogenase enzymes, an artificial hydrogen acceptor replaces the natural NAD or FAD. The usual artificial acceptors are tetrazolium compounds, which are converted from a soluble non-coloured form to a coloured insoluble precipitate, called formazan, when they become reduced (see *Colour plate 14*).

There are several forms of tetrazolium, which differ in their redox potential and solubility of the formazan. The different redox potentials of the tetrazolium compounds affect which enzymes each form of tetrazolium will be best suited to demonstrate. The solubility of the formazan is only important in that it determines how the slides should be mounted.

The technique for succinic dehydrogenase works quite well using only the tetrazolium salt (nitro blue tetrazolium) and enzyme substrate (sodium succinate) in a buffer since the enzyme incorporates a molecule of FAD. Many dehydrogenases, including lactic dehydrogenase, do not incorporate a natural hydrogen acceptor and need a soluble natural acceptor to be present in the substrate solution.

The lactic dehydrogenase transfers the hydrogens to NAD, which is its natural co-factor, and the NAD in turn transfers the hydrogens to the tetrazolium. This second transfer is carried out by another enzyme known as either a tetrazolium reductase or a **diaphorase**. These enzymes occur in the mitochondria and this results in lactic dehydrogenase being apparently located in the mitochondria. The reason is that there is a double reaction occurring. The lactic dehydrogenase transfers hydrogen from lactic acid to NAD in the cytosol and the NAD then diffuses into the mitochondria where it is acted on by diaphorases, which reduce the tetrazolium and produce the final colour. Thus, lactic dehydrogenase techniques usually show deposits of blue in the mitochondria, even though the mitochondria do not contain any lactic dehydrogenase. Since diffusion is always going to be a significant factor in dehydrogenases, the location of the enzyme is best considered as accurate enough to identify cells containing the enzyme but not accurate enough to identify the subcellular compartment.

Preventing destruction of reduced coenzymes by the electron transport chain. In cases where soluble cofactors such as NAD (or NADP) are being used, there is usually a need to add extra NAD to the substrate solution. (The reagent dilutes the natural NAD found in the cell and so the concentration is too low to maintain the reaction at a reasonable rate.) On entering the mitochondria, the $NADH_2$ would normally be acted on by the electron transport chain (oxidative phosphorylation). The hydrogens are transferred along the chain and eventually form water by combining with atmospheric oxygen. If this natural reaction is allowed to occur, it would result in very little colour developing as very little of the $NADH_2$ would form the coloured formazan and most would simply produce water. To prevent this loss of $NADH_2$, the cytochromes of the electron transport chain can be poisoned by cyanide; thus, none of the $NADH_2$ is converted to water and it all forms formazan. Azide has a similar function and the same effect can be achieved by removing all of the oxygen and performing the reaction under anaerobic conditions.

Extra electron transport reagents are sometimes added to improve the transfer of electrons to the tetrazolium, e.g. Meldola's blue or phenazine methosulphate. These will speed up the reaction but in some cases of long incubation may give a non-specific deposit of formazan.

Oxidase enzymes

Oxidase enzymes catalyse oxidation reactions that involve oxygen as the hydrogen acceptor. Four atoms of hydrogen are oxidized by one molecule of oxygen. Thus, the reaction is often shown as one molecule of substrate (which loses two hydrogen atoms) and $\frac{1}{2}O_2$:

$$O_2 + 2(\text{Substrate}) \rightarrow 2H_2O + 2(\text{Product})$$

or

$$\frac{1}{2}O_2 + \text{Substrate} \rightarrow H_2O + \text{Product}$$

Although it is possible theoretically to use a tetrazolium salt as a hydrogen acceptor to replace oxygen, in practice the redox potentials for the reactions are not compatible with the redox potentials of the available tetrazolium salts. The methods used to demonstrate the oxidase enzymes therefore tend to be unique to individual reactions, rather than variations on a common theme. Two examples that are important in practice will be considered.

Catechol oxidases. These are a group of copper-containing enzymes that catalyse the conversion of tyrosine to dihydroxyphenylalanine (DOPA) and then the further oxidation of DOPA to DOPA quinone, which then spontaneously undergoes a series of reactions to form melanin. The enzyme may also be called tyrosine oxidase or DOPA oxidase depending on the reaction occurring.

DOPA quinone spontaneously oxidizes and decarboxylates to form indole-5,6-quinone and this polymerizes to melanin. The exact molecular nature of melanin is still uncertain but it is insoluble in all of the usual solvents, and is stable and very densely coloured (it appears black).

In tissues, the enzyme is usually demonstrated by using DOPA, thus demonstrating the second fast reaction rather than the slower first reaction. The sites of activity show up as black as the melanin develops. This histochemical reaction is unusual as it uses a natural substrate (DOPA) and natural product (melanin) rather than an artificial analogue (see *Box 8.6*).

Box 8.6 DOPA in the brain

Melanin normally occurs as a protective pigment in the skin and eyes but it also occurs in the brain in a region called the substantia nigra. The melanin here is related not to protection from UV light but to the inhibitory neurotransmitter dopamine. In Parkinson's disease, there is a loss of these pigmented neurones and loss of dopamine secretion. The chemical L-DOPA is used as a treatment as it can cross the blood–brain barrier, whilst dopamine cannot.

Peroxidases. These enzymes catalyse the conversion of peroxide to water and oxygen. The active oxygen then oxidizes a substrate to a coloured insoluble product. These enzymes are found not only in animal tissue but also in plants such as horseradish (see *Box 8.7*).

$$H_2O_2 + \text{substrate} = \text{oxidized substrate} + 2H_2O$$

Box 8.7 Using horseradish peroxidase as a reagent

Horseradish peroxidase has become a popular enzyme in research. It can be demonstrated using the technique outlined here and gives a brown deposit that can easily be seen in sections. It can be used as a tracer in several different ways.

As it is a protein, it can be used to identify where blood vessel permeability changes in experiments. If the blood vessel is impermeable, then the peroxidase cannot escape, but if the permeability increases, as in an inflammatory condition, then the peroxidase will escape and be trapped in the tissues. By sectioning the tissues and demonstrating the presence of the enzyme by histochemistry, the leaky sites can be seen. It is also used in antibody labelling techniques (see Chapter 10).

Diaminobenzidine $+$ H_2O_2 $\longrightarrow$ Quinone imine derivative $+$ $2H_2O$

The quinone imine then polymerizes to a brown product. The polymerization reaction may also be catalysed by peroxidase as it involves a further oxidation.

Examples of the use of redox and hydrolytic enzymes

An example of the use of redox and hydrolytic enzymes is in the recognition of different muscle types. The nature of a disease affecting muscle can often be recognized in a biopsy by changes in the distribution of the types of muscle cells present. By staining for the enzymes, the muscle types can be recognized (see *Table 8.2*). The myosin ATPase enzymes vary in their activity sensitivity to pre-incubation at different pH levels. The activity of the phosphorylase enzyme is not important in classifying muscle types but is useful in diagnosing McArdle's disease (phosphorylase deficiency).

Quantitation of enzyme activity

The apparent enzyme activity as observed by the colour of the final deposit is not always directly proportional to the actual amount of enzyme. This is

Table 8.2   Enzymes and muscle types

| Muscle type | Succinic dehydrogenase | Myosin ATPase | | | Phosphorylase |
		pH 9.4	pH 4.6	pH 4.3	
Type 1 (red)	+++	+	+++	+++	+
Type 2a	++	+++	0	0	+++
Type 2b	+	+++	+++	0	+++

due to the fact that the usual Beer–Lambert relationship is not necessarily applicable. In the absence of the Beer–Lambert relationship, it is difficult or impossible to relate the density of colour to the activity of the enzyme.

The problems associated with quantifying enzymes in tissue sections include:

1. Loss of enzyme activity during fixation, cutting, etc. All processing of tissues, even just preparing frozen sections, can involve significant loss of enzyme activity. The actual amount of enzyme activity in a section is always less than was present in the original tissue.
2. The rate of an enzyme's activity in a section may be controlled by how rapidly the substrate diffuses into the tissue, rather than the amount of enzyme present. The diffusion of substrate can effectively be one-dimensional, with all of the substrate coming directly down on to the site of the enzyme. Diffusion from the side will always be slower and may be non-existent if there are adjacent enzyme sites, and of course diffusion from below is not possible since sections are normally attached to an impermeable glass slide or coverslip. If the rate of diffusion is slower than the maximal activity of the enzyme, then the amount of colour produced will not follow the usual Beer–Lambert law and enzyme activity will be underestimated.
3. Diffusion rate may be altered by the precipitation of insoluble product. The nature of histochemical demonstration requires the production of an insoluble product at the site of activity. This makes the diffusion process even worse. There may be a maximum colour that is able to develop where diffusion is completely blocked, so again Beer–Lambert relationships are not valid.
4. Section thickness may not be constant. This is a major problem as section thickness determines how much enzyme is present. If the thickness of sections from a microtome fluctuates by as little as 1 μm (1/1000 of a millimetre), it can alter the thickness of the section by as much as 20 or 25% (a nominal 5 μm section could in reality be anywhere between 4 and 6 μm thick). Section thickness is very difficult to measure and fluctuation in section thickness is a common finding. Sections will be alternately thicker and thinner than the set thickness. This may be due to a slightly loose knife or block or due to wear in the microtome producing looseness.

5. Diffusional losses of reaction product. If the final product is even slightly soluble in any of the reagents used in processing the section, then some of the colour will be lost.

SUGGESTED FURTHER READING

Bancroft, J.D. (2002) Proteins and nucleic acids. In *Theory and Practice of Histological Techniques*, 5th edn (eds J.D. Bancroft and M. Gamble). Edinburgh: Churchill Livingstone.

Kiernan, J.A. (2001) *Histological and Histochemical Methods*, 3rd edn. Oxford: Hodder Arnold.

Sheehan, D.C. and Hrapchak, B. (1980) *Theory and Practice of Histotechnology*. St Louis: Mosby.

SELF-ASSESSMENT QUESTIONS

1. How can the basophilic staining of nuclei be controlled to ensure that it is due to DNA and not to other basophilic materials?
2. What is meant by 'intercalation'? Name one dye that stains by intercalation.
3. Outline the principles of the Feulgen technique.
4. Give two different ways that proteins can be stained in tissue sections and indicate how specific they are.
5. Name two ways in which enzyme activity may be lost in tissue sections.
6. What is the reason for adding potassium cyanide to substrate solutions being used to demonstrate dehydrogenase enzymes?
7. How is the naphthol azo-coupling method modified to demonstrate hydrolases other than phosphatases?
8. Why is it better to measure enzyme activity biochemically rather than histochemically?

CHAPTER

9

Histochemistry of pigments, neuroendocrine amines and minerals

Learning objectives

After studying this chapter you should confidently be able to:

■ **Describe the classification of pigments found in sections.**
  Pigments are classified as artefact (caused by tissue processing),
  exogenous (foreign materials from the environment that enter the body
  whilst it is still alive), or endogenous (generated within the body by
  metabolism). Endogenous pigments may be subdivided into
  haematogenous (derived from blood) or autogenous (not directly
  connected to blood).

■ **Describe the formalin-induced fluorescence reaction of
  neuroendocrine amines.**
  Treatment with formaldehyde converts many neurotransmitter amines into
  fluorescent compounds that can be visualized directly with a fluorescent
  microscope. Most amines require freeze-drying and treatment with
  formaldehyde vapour as they are small water-soluble molecules and are
  lost during aqueous formalin fixation.

■ **List the main minerals found in tissue sections and describe how they
  can be identified.**
  Calcium, iron and magnesium are the main minerals in normal tissues.
  Smaller amounts of copper, aluminium and trace elements may be
  present but are normally present in too small a quantity to be
  demonstrated easily. Calcium can be demonstrated by the von Kossa
  technique or by reaction with dyes such as alizarin. Magnesium is usually
  found associated with calcium and is rarely identified separately. Iron in
  the ferric form is usually identified using the Perls technique.

■ **Outline the use of ion-selective dyes.**
  Ion-selective dyes identify soluble metallic salts but are only suitable for
  use in intact cells and not in histological sections. They are used in
  research and are not currently used in routine diagnosis.

9.1 PIGMENTS

Most materials in tissue sections are uncoloured until a stain is applied, but
a few materials are coloured and can be seen in unstained sections. These
self-coloured materials are referred to as pigments. They include a wide
variety of materials from different sources and have differing significance.

Box 9.1 Other pigments

The pigments discussed in the main text are the common ones encountered in tissue sections. Other pigments do occasionally occur but are rarely demonstrated.

   The slight yellow colour of fat is due to fat-soluble plant pigments such as carotenoids. These pigments are of no significance in the usual amounts and I have only heard of one exceptional case of person who was adversely affected by an unusually high amount. He died of a vitamin A overdose. He was taking vitamin A tablets and drinking a lot of carrot juice and turned a bright orange colour. Most people do not suffer from the small amounts present in their bodies.

The presence of some pigments is normal but others can be related to disease, so it is often important to be able to recognize and identify them.

   When identifying pigments, two features need to be borne in mind about the appearance and reactions of the pigments:

1. Pigments generally have a limited range of colour with most being yellow to brown or brown to black. The colour varies depending on how much is present. A brown pigment present as a very heavy deposit may appear almost black, whilst the same pigment present in only small amounts may appear yellowish. Thus, descriptions of the pigment colour are only a guide and not a precise description.

2. The results of a test are affected by the colour of the pigment. Schmorl's test, for example, gives a blue colour as a positive reaction, but if it is applied to a yellow pigment, then a positive result will be greenish (blue + yellow) rather than pure blue. This also means that it may be difficult to see whether a reaction has occurred. How can you tell what has happened if a positive reaction gives a black colour but the pigment is already black?

   Pigments can be conveniently grouped into three major types: **artefact pigments**, **exogenous pigments** and **endogenous pigments** (which can be haematogenous or autogenous). These groups are convenient labels, although some pigments can be put into more than one category.

Artefact pigments

These were not originally part of the tissue but have been added by the processes used to prepare the tissue. The commonest are associated with fixatives.

Formalin (formaldehyde) pigment is most easily seen around old or degenerating blood in tissues fixed in acid solutions of formaldehyde. The formation of this type of pigment can mostly be prevented by using buffered formaldehyde for fixation. The pigment appears as a fine brownish deposit around the old blood and is usually birefringent. Formaldehyde pigment can be identified and removed by treatment with picric acid solutions.

   A similar, sometimes identical, pigment is formed in malaria and is therefore called **malarial pigment**. The mechanism of its production is different and it may be found within red cells infected with the parasite, in the area around infected red cells and even within the cytoplasm of macrophages that have ingested affected red blood cells. The colour is similar to formaldehyde pigment and it will dissolve in picric acid solutions similarly to formaldehyde pigment. The presence of the parasite within the red cells helps to identify the source of the pigment, although large deposits of the pigment may obscure the parasite.

Mercury pigment is a dense black granular (or occasionally globular) pigment, occurring irregularly throughout the tissue. It cannot be prevented if the fixative contains mercuric chloride, but it is easily removed by treating the section with iodine solutions (this also acts as a test to recognize mercury, although all heavy metal-derived pigments will also be dissolved). Mercury pigment is less common in modern histological practice where mercury-containing fixatives are used less frequently, but it is found in tissues stored in archives, as mercuric chloride was once a very common fixative.

Chrome pigment may be found as a brownish pigment in tissues fixed in chrome fixatives and not washed in water before processing. It occurs when the chrome salt reacts with the alcohols used in tissue processing and produces a brown oxide, although the reaction is not easily produced even when it is done deliberately as a demonstration. Chrome pigment is not readily removed once formed, so it is better to avoid it by always washing chromium-fixed tissues in water.

Osmium pigment occurs as a very dense black pigment spread throughout the tissue following fixation in osmium tetroxide (commonly used for electron microscopy specimens). It is not usually a problem since in electron microscopy it acts as a stain and when it is used in light microscopy the blackening is often wanted to identify double bonds. However, it can be removed from sections by oxidation with hydrogen peroxide if required for some stains.

Exogenous pigments

Exogenous pigments were present in the original tissue but are not a normal part of the body and are contaminants that entered the body during life. The pigments were ingested, inhaled or otherwise introduced in life. Their significance varies, with some being pathological and some being indicators of the person's employment (e.g. silica) or lifestyle (e.g. tattoos).

Carbon usually occurs as a dense black pigment. Carbon may be intracellular in macrophages, when it is often seen as a fine powder, or can occur in angular clumps in the extracellular connective tissue. Carbon is very common in the lungs of city dwellers and in particular in the lungs of smokers. It also occurs in regional lymph nodes around the lungs where it has been carried by macrophages (see *Colour plate 15*). It can sometimes be seen in skin from tattoos (see *Box 9.2*) and needle tracks. The carbon itself

---

Box 9.2 Tattoo pigments

A variety of pigments are sometimes used in tattoos. Carbon is one that sometimes occurs, especially in 'amateur tattoos'. In professional tattoos the pigments used can be much more elaborate and of many different colours. The pigments do not usually need to be identified but if you wish to see the colours, then use an incident light microscope rather than the usual transmitted light microscope.

---

is not pathological, although the association with tobacco smoke does have links to smoking-related disease. It may also act as a carrier for more dangerous materials as fine carbon particles adsorb many chemicals on to their surface (this is why 'activated charcoal' is used in many filters). The carbon produced during the burning of tobacco or in badly maintained diesel engines may adsorb carcinogens produced by incomplete combustion and transport them into the lungs.

Carbon is difficult to identify accurately as it is very inert. Usually it can be reliably identified by its location (lungs) and shape. It can be destroyed by micro-incineration but this is not commonly done. It has no pathological significance in itself but it sometimes needs to be distinguished from other black pigments that may be important. This can be done by eliminating the other pigments by testing for each one in turn.

Silica may be brown to black in colour depending on the source of the silica and is found as angular masses in the lungs and lymph nodes of miners, quarry workers, stonemasons and other people exposed to stone dust, especially from power grinding equipment.

Silica is very inert as it is the same material as glass, and it is difficult to identify with specific tests. There are no positive tests and it is unaffected by all histochemical reagents and micro-incineration. Silica may be birefringent (rotates the plane of polarized light) and shows up brightly using a polarizing microscope; this is often a useful indicator.

Silica causes the disease silicosis (see *Box 9.3*), which is a serious and often fatal fibrosis of the lungs. Silicosis is a recognized industrial disease, so that assessment of the amount of damage caused by silica may be important in cases of industrial compensation.

Box 9.3 Silicosis

Silica causes damage to cells by its ability to form hydrogen bonds with membranes. If very fine particles get into the lungs, they will be ingested by macrophages and end up in the lysosomes. Here, the silica particles can hydrogen bond to the lysosomal membrane and cause it to rupture. Lysosomal enzymes are released into the cytoplasm and kill the cell. The enzymes break down both the cell and surrounding tissue. The silica is inert and remains unaffected. The silica will be ingested by another macrophage and the cycle will be repeated. This results in chronic inflammation and scar tissue forms where the tissue is damaged. The cycle will continue to repeat until the silica becomes coated with enough protein or fibrous tissue for it to be ignored by the macrophages. If the silica load in the lungs is large, then large areas of the lungs will be replaced by fibrous scar tissue and this is the cause of silicosis.

Asbestos occurs as a brown pigment found in the lungs but usually appears as fibres rather than the angular masses associated with silica. Inside the body, it becomes coated with an iron-containing protein that forms distinctive beaded asbestos bodies. These asbestos bodies are easily recognized and give a positive Perls reaction for iron (see *Fig. 9.1* and *Colour plate 16*).

Figure 9.1
An asbestos body

The fibres are inert and birefringent (different types of asbestos can be identified by their birefringence). As with silica, asbestos is not destroyed by micro-incineration. Asbestos is often associated with disease and causes asbestosis, which can be very debilitating and is a recognized industrial disease. Asbestos increases the risk of developing lung cancer and is the only known cause of the malignant mesothelioma tumour.

Endogenous pigments

Endogenous pigments are the products of metabolism in the body. They occur naturally within the tissues and so occur in normal tissues. However, they are also associated with disease states when they occur in excessive amounts or in unusual situations. The pigments can come from blood or one of its breakdown products (**haematogenous pigments**) or can be derived from other metabolic processes (**autogenous pigments**).

Haematogenous pigments

These pigments come from the blood or one of its breakdown products.

Haemoglobin is always present in the tissues inside the red blood cells and in this form it is usually ignored as a pigment. It does, however, sometimes occur outside the red blood cells, for example in haemolytic diseases, and then it becomes significant. Haemoglobin has a molecular size that is close to the limit of the glomerular filtration system. Once haemoglobin is released into the plasma, it can pass through the glomerular filter into the renal tubules and this can lead to renal problems (see *Colour plate 17*).

In formalin-fixed sections, haemoglobin is not the bright red colour usually associated with blood but is a brownish colour. Free haemoglobin is an amorphous or globular material that is strongly acidophilic. Haemoglobin can be identified by this strong acidophilia. In a haematoxylin and eosin stain, the eosin gives a more orange/pink colour to haemoglobin than to other materials in the section and this is often sufficiently distinctive to allow haemoglobin to be identified. More specialized techniques have been developed that allow an even better distinction, e.g. the kiton red/almond green stain. Histochemically, haemoglobin can be identified by the peroxidase activity of the haemoglobin molecule (see Chapter 8 for the peroxidase reaction). This peroxidase activity is unusual in that it resists normal processing and often can be demonstrated in paraffin wax sections.

Haemosiderin and ferritin. A whole range of iron-binding proteins occurs in cells and tissues to scavenge and recycle the iron released by the degradation of haemoglobin. Many are present in such small quantities that they cannot be easily visualized by light microscopy. Larger deposits occur as brown granular or powdery deposits, particularly in macrophages of the spleen and liver (where destruction of old red blood cells occurs) and around sites of haemorrhage. These larger accumulations are called haemosiderin by histologists. Haemosiderin is easily identified by the Perls reaction, which detects the iron in the haemosiderin. The iron is detected by potassium ferrocyanide (potassium hexacyanoferrate (III)). This produces a dense blue precipitate, which is the pigment Prussian blue, hence the other names for the test: Prussian blue reaction (PBR) or Perls' Prussian blue reaction (PPBR) (see *Colour plate 18*).

The iron in haemosiderin will not react directly with the ferrocyanide but must be released from the protein by acid hydrolysis. Thus, the Perls reagent is a mixture of 2% potassium ferrocyanide and 2% hydrochloric acid. The iron in haemoglobin is too strongly held within the porphyrin ring to be released in this way and so haemoglobin and red blood cells are negative for the Perls stain.

Other tests are available for haemosiderin (Turnbull's blue and blackening of the free iron with hydrogen sulphide) but are rarely used.

Diseases associated with excess haemosiderin include haemochromatosis and haemosiderosis. It is also an important way of identifying sites of tissue damage (remnants of bleeding), and identification of haemosiderin is useful in identifying some types of cells.

Bile pigments. These are derived from the porphyrin ring of haemoglobin. They vary in colour from red/brown (bilirubin, the commonest form) to green (biliverdin). The range of colours seen in a bruise as it heals is mainly due to the breakdown of these pigments. Bile pigments are slightly soluble in organic solvents, so small amounts are usually lost. Thus, paraffin sections of normal liver cells (the main site of pigment production) are usually free from pigment. Only large deposits can survive processing and appear in wax sections.

Bile pigments are difficult to identify. They can be identified by oxidation, which alters the colour. The Fouchet technique uses ferric chloride as an oxidant in the presence of trichloracetic acid. This gives a bright green colour, which is fairly stable, but not all forms of bile pigment will react.

Gmelin's test uses concentrated nitric acid as the oxidizing agent and reacts with more types of bile pigment but the colour change is fleeting. Sections are examined whilst the test is being applied, but even so the colour changes can easily be missed and the slides cannot be kept or viewed later. A positive result is usually reliable but a negative result with the normal tests should not be considered conclusive. The test involves oxidation of the pigments by irrigation. This means running the reagent under the coverslip whilst viewing the section. The reagents are quite corrosive and the difficulties of looking down the microscope and focusing on the section at the same time as squeezing nitric acid out of a Pasteur pipette mean that it is a cumbersome technique and is best carried out using three arms and two heads. For most people this means getting someone else to help while you do the test.

Excessive amounts of bile pigment are found in some liver diseases or in haemolytic disease. The main confusion likely to occur is between lipofuscin (see Autogenous pigments below) and bilirubin, both of which can occur in the liver. It is often easier to eliminate lipofuscin than to identify bile definitively.

Autogenous pigments

These bile pigments are in many ways quite diverse and are derived from metabolism but not associated directly with blood. Despite their diverse origins, the pigments described here do have one characteristic in common – they are all reducing pigments. This makes them a neat group in practice since a single reducing test allows them to be identified as belonging to this group.

Two reducing tests are in use:

- Masson–Fontana silver reduction (black result);
- Schmorl's ferricyanide reduction (blue result).

The first is more sensitive but is slow (24 h or more) and the black result may be difficult to interpret if the pigment itself is dark brown or black. The Schmorl's test is quicker (5–15 min) but it is often difficult to interpret because the background tissue takes on a greenish tinge.

Melanin. This is a black or brown pigment that is found in the eye (especially the retina), skin (especially negroid skin, tanned skin and around the nipples) and in parts of the brain (substantia nigra) (also see *Box 9.4*). Melanin can be identified by its reducing ability with the Schmorl's test, appearance and the fact that it is bleached by oxidizing agents (hydrogen peroxide, potassium permanganate or potassium chlorate/HCl).

The main pathological significance of melanin is its association with malignant melanoma (see *Colour plate 19*).

Box 9.4 Melanosis coli

In melanosis coli, the gut becomes almost black due to the accumulation of a pigment in the macrophages similar to lipofuscin. This condition is caused by excessive use of purgative laxatives. Despite the name, the pigment is not related to melanin and it is just the sheer amount of pigment that causes the dark colour. The pigment is sometimes called pseudomelanin.

Lipofuscin is a pigment derived from oxidized lipid. It appears as droplets in the lysosomes of cells. It accumulates with age and is sometimes called 'wear and tear' pigment. Levels increase after the use of some poisons (e.g. carbon tetrachloride) and in some chronic diseases. It can be found in any tissue but is often prominent in heart muscle (see *Colour plate 20*), liver and brain.

Lipofuscin is the most easily identified of the autogenous pigments as there are several good tests, which, whilst individually not conclusive, become highly selective when two or three are used in combination:

1. It is basophilic: methylene blue and aldehyde fuchsin both give good strong staining (see *Colour plate 20*).
2. It is periodic acid–Schiff (PAS)-positive, but this is less useful as there are many other substances in the tissues that are also PAS-positive. It is useful to remember that this may be the cause of an unidentified PAS-positive reaction.
3. It stains as a lipid with some fat-soluble dyes, especially Sudan black.
4. It is peracetic acid–Schiff-positive and performic acid–Schiff-positive (typical of unsaturated lipids). However, as these are dangerous methods, it is always better to use a simpler and safer technique.
5. It stains positive by the Ziehl–Neelsen technique. This is usually used for the acid-fast mycobacteria associated with tuberculosis and leprosy but is a useful method for lipofuscin.

Chromaffin pigment is a brownish intracellular pigment that is found in adrenaline-producing cells (adrenal medulla and sympathetic ganglia). The pigment is not entirely natural as it only occurs after an oxidizing fixative such as chrome fixatives (hence the name, from 'chrome affinity') and is not seen in formaldehyde-fixed tissues. Chromaffin pigment represents the oxidized precursor of adrenaline.

It is often considered not to be a pigment as it is a part of normal metabolism. It can be considered along with the other neurotransmitter amines and demonstrated by the formalin-induced fluorescent technique on freeze-dried tissue (see below). It can also be considered as an artefact pigment since it only occurs after fixation in chrome fixatives and is not a natural pigment. However, it has traditionally been included as a pigment and has been retained in this section as it is often easier to demonstrate it by fixing a piece of tissue in a chrome fixative than to carry out the full formalin-induced fluorescent technique on freeze-dried tissue. It is a basophilic pigment and produces green colour when stained with Giemsa.

Excessive chromaffin is found in phaeochromocytomas, which are tumours of the chromaffin or adrenaline-secreting tissues.

Argentaffin. This pigment is the strongest reducing pigment and will react strongly with silver reagents (hence its name). It is found in the endocrine-secreting cells of the gut (argentaffin cells) (see *Colour plate 21*). Again, this pigment only occurs after the use of certain fixatives, particularly formaldehyde, and is strongly fluorescent (formalin-induced fluorescence; see below). It also reacts with diazo salts such as fast red B giving a red deposit.

Argentaffin pigment also gives a chromaffin reaction if fixed in chrome fixatives and can be called enterochromaffin pigment (hence, the alternative name for argentaffin cells is enterochromaffin or EC cells).

Other pigments also occur but are less commonly encountered (e.g. ochronosis pigment) and will not be considered here.

9.2 NEUROENDOCRINE GRANULES

The neuroendocrine cells are a scattered group of cells that secrete biologically active amines as hormones. These amines are more commonly thought of as neurotransmitters, but in these cells they are secreted into the bloodstream rather than into the synapses between nerve cells. They also secrete characteristic neuropeptides that act as hormones. This set of cells is also known as the 'diffuse endocrine system' and the amine precursor uptake and decarboxylation (APUD) system from their metabolic activity (see *Box 9.5*). Amines are formed by the decarboxylation of precursor materials such as tryptophan to form serotonin (5-hydroxytryptamine).

Box 9.5 APUD cells

The neuroendocrine cells form a useful system but their embryonic origin is disputed. They may not even all come from the same original embryonic layer, but the difficulty of tracing cells as they migrate in embryonic development means that no one is certain of their origin. They form a coherent set of cells in functional terms and also have a characteristic set of tumours, apudomas, which continue to secrete their peptides and can result in clinical syndromes from this secretion.

Carcinoid tumours are tumours arising from the gut or respiratory tract APUD cells but do not secrete any identifiable peptide hormone.

Staining techniques for neuropeptides

Neuropeptide secretions are reasonably well preserved in fixed sections and can usually be stained using dyeing techniques. There are many reasonably selective methods that will stain different cells within the same neuroendocrine organ in different colours. Methods for the pituitary and pancreas are available to distinguish the main cell types on the basis of their acidophilic and basophilic characteristics. These stains are usually quite attractive with clear bright colours but require a fair degree of skill to get good results. These methods are largely empirical and so do not have any particular theoretical interest. The peptides can also be specifically demonstrated by using immunotechniques. The main interest in neuropeptide identification is in their role in the diagnosis of tumours of the diffuse endocrine system.

Demonstrating neuroendocrine amines

The other secretory components of the neuroendocrine cells are much more difficult to demonstrate because of their low molecular weight and solubility. Substances such as adrenaline and histamine are usually lost during processing as they readily diffuse and are quickly destroyed by enzymes. The only efficient way to preserve amines is to freeze-dry the tissues. The snap freezing prevents diffusion and sublimation of the water prevents their loss. Some amines can be detected in routine paraffin sections if they are bound to a larger tissue component. This seems to occur with serotonin (5-hydroxytryptamine) in argentaffin cells (and rat mast cells) and histamine in mast cells granules (see *Box 9.6*).

Box 9.6 Mast cells and amines

Although amines are difficult to demonstrate in tissues, they are very important in disease. They play a crucial role in the inflammatory response. Mast cells are the main cells that produce these amines, but the amines that are present vary with species. Human mast cells, like all mammalian mast cells, contain histamine, but rat mast cells also contain serotonin and ruminant mast cells contain dopamine.

Individual methods for some amines

A number of demonstration methods have been developed to detect individual amines. The specificity of some of these methods is not very high but they can be useful for tumours to demonstrate that a substance is present. An example of this is silver reduction by argentaffin cells. The method is not specific for serotonin in these cells but is a useful histological method and can be helpful in the recognition of carcinoid tumours. Similarly, the chromaffin method can be used for catecholamines in the adrenal medulla using an oxidizing fixative to preserve the adrenaline and noradrenaline. Serotonin can also be demonstrated using the azo-coupling method, which reacts with the phenolic group of serotonin.

Formaldehyde-induced fluorescence

Amines will react with formaldehyde to give a fluorescent product. This is known as the formalin-induced fluorescence (FIF) technique. The reaction does not occur readily in solution (the amines will rapidly diffuse away) and instead it must be done on freeze-dried sections using formaldehyde vapour. The tissues are freeze-dried and then transferred to a closed container along with some paraformaldehyde and heated to generate formaldehyde vapour. The temperature and humidity are critical factors for maximum fluorescence. The temperature and humidity may need to be altered slightly to adjust for differences in tissues and preparation. Generally a temperature of between 60 and 80°C for 1 h is used at a relative humidity of 50–75%.

The tissue can then be embedded in paraffin wax. This does not need any processing since the tissue is freeze-dried; simply put the tissue into molten wax and gently reduce the pressure to remove air bubbles. The tissue can be blocked out and sectioned, but water must be avoided so they are not floated on a waterbath to flatten them. The tissue is dewaxed, but not rehydrated, and mounted. Fluorescence can be seen if the specimens are irradiated with blue-violet light of 410 nm wavelength. Dopamine and noradrenaline fluoresce green, whilst serotonin gives a yellower colour.

Glyoxylic acid can replace formaldehyde

Instead of using formaldehyde, a similar reaction can be produced using glyoxylic acid. Glyoxylic acid can be used to perfuse the animal, thus generating a weakly fluorescent compound before removing the tissue from the animal. Glyoxylic acid will react with cryostat sections and this is more convenient than the block method used for FIF and can give a brighter result. The fluorescence is intensified by heating or treating with formaldehyde vapour. The sensitivity of this method is very high and it has been estimated that 10^{-7} picomoles of adrenaline can be detected in cells.

Other fluorescent methods

Although formaldehyde and glyoxylic acid are the most commonly used forms of induced fluorescence, it is possible to get condensation reactions with other substances such as *o*-phthalaldehyde (histamine), hydrochloric acid (dopamine), acetaldehyde, glutaraldehyde and acetic acid (similar to FIF).

FIF and related methods have been used in research mainly to identify and locate nerves using the amine neurotransmitters. FIF has been replaced to some extent by antibody techniques using antibodies against the enzymes producing the amines. Immunocytochemistry is more convenient as routine paraffin sections can be used, but these methods only show which cells are producing amines and not how much is present. In some cases, it is useful to detect which nerves are depleted of their transmitters, as well as which ones are capable of producing the transmitters. The depletion can only be seen using FIF or a related method.

9.3 METALS AND THEIR COMPOUNDS

The histochemistry of metals and their salts is partly dependent on their solubility. In most cases of sectioned material, the only metallic substances that are likely to be present are those that are insoluble. Metal-containing compounds can be divided roughly into four different types:

- elemental metals;
- soluble metal salts;
- insoluble metal salts;
- organically bound metals.

> **Box 9.7 Many trace elements and poisons are difficult to demonstrate histochemically**
>
> Metals are extremely important in metabolism and there are a huge number of 'trace elements' that are needed by the body. However, these are often present in such minute quantities that there is no method sensitive enough to detect them in single sections. These include elements such as cobalt (found in vitamin B12) and zinc (found in the zinc-finger structures of proteins).
>
> Many metals are also poisonous but even in toxic amounts they may still be difficult to demonstrate histochemically. Some metals are always toxic, e.g. cadmium, mercury and lead. The role of other materials is less certain, for example arsenic, which is certainly highly toxic, yet some evidence exists that it may be used by the metabolism, although only in minute amounts.

Elemental metals

Elemental metals are found as the solid element and not combined with any other subtsance. Such metals are uncommon in sections except as contaminants or exogenous implants. Metals are used in medicine in the form of dental fillings, radiotherapy implants and metal prostheses such as replacement joints, pins and plates in bones, and metal implants in arteries used to open out the narrowing lumens ('stents'). The identification of the metal is rarely a problem in these cases. Preparing sections of these substances, however, can be extremely difficult. Radiotherapy implants may be left in place permanently and the tissues may not be removed until much later. They can ruin a knife-edge if they are unwittingly left in the paraffin wax block and may rip through the tissues at the same time, damaging the tissue itself. Occasionally sections are required, usually for research, with the implant in place and the tissue still adhering to it. Depending on the metal used, sectioning can be near to impossible but histochemical identification is not a problem.

Soluble metal salts

The soluble metal salts are ionic and are not able to be demonstrated or localized in sections produced by any method since they will rapidly either be lost or relocated by any technique. Metal salts are ionic and very mobile. Simply cutting the tissue will allow them to diffuse. Frozen sections are not necessarily any better as the section often thaws briefly during cutting and then refreezes and relocation can occur in that brief instant. Even freeze-drying may not prevent movement since the salts may be soluble in wax or plastic monomers. It is sometimes possible to precipitate the metal by some means, but even then relocation is more likely than accurate localization. The only method of localizing these materials is to examine intact living cells without sectioning using ion-sensitive dyes (see below); however, this is not always a reasonable method to apply.

Insoluble metal salts

Insoluble metal salts are found mainly in the minerals of bone, but other insoluble calcium salts such as calcium oxalate do occur. As with the first group, it is also possible to have contamination with metal salts. The metals may even be introduced by the processing. Rust in tap water is not unknown and may contaminate tissues during a washing step in the preparation.

Organically bound metals and their unmasking

The final group, where the minerals are bound into organic form, is the most important group and includes the iron in haemoglobin and the cytochromes.

There are several methods available for releasing such organically bound metals. Minerals need to be soluble and ionic before they can be demonstrated since it is only the ions that react. Many of the difficulties with the techniques are related to releasing or unmasking the minerals without losing or relocating them. Releasing the minerals can sometimes be done by chemical treatments such as acid hydrolysis with hydrochloric acid or oxidation by hydrogen peroxide. If these can be shown to release all of the metal, then they are certainly the simplest solution.

Micro-incineration can unmask many metals

As an alternative to chemical unmasking, the release of metals can be achieved by burning off all of the organic matter using **micro-incineration**. This changes all of the organic minerals into salts and so the total content of metal can be seen. Incineration is done in a laboratory furnace at 500–600°C. Glass slides cannot withstand this high temperature, so sections need to be mounted on quartz slides. For the best results, oxygen needs to be excluded whilst the temperature is low (<500°C) and only then is air admitted. Oxidation then occurs rapidly and completely. The exclusion of air helps to remove the organic matter by preventing incomplete combustion products forming that then resist further oxidation. The slide is then carefully removed and cooled. The pattern of ash is quite extensive and usually the main tissue structures can be seen in outline. The pattern of ash is sometimes known by the somewhat grand name of a **spodogram**. It is very fragile and must be protected with a coverslip and then ringed. An alternative is to coat it gently by gently dipping into a solution of celloidin. The celloidin then hardens and protects it, whilst still allowing reagents to penetrate and react with the released salts.

Micro-incineration can also be done more crudely with a standard Bunsen burner. The tissue section on an ordinary slide is placed on an asbestos mat. A Bunsen burner is then picked up and the hot blue spot of the flame is played over the section so that the section passes through the bright blue edge of the flame where it is hottest. The section will turn brown initially and then turn from brown to white as the organic material burns off. There is no need to dewax paraffin sections as the wax will also burn off. Once the section has turned white, it consists of only the mineral salts.

The slide should then be covered to slow down cooling as the slide is likely to shatter if cooling is rapid. The final ash can then be protected as before.

Micro-incineration is very rarely done. It is not suitable for all minerals; for example, mercury will evaporate. It is a simple way of distinguishing pure carbon deposits from silica as carbon will be burnt off in the process but silica will remain. It is also very difficult to locate minerals precisely within the tissue as by the time you have incinerated the section there is no tissue left and accurate location is not possible.

Spot test sensitivity and contamination

One further problem with mineral identification is contamination during preparation of the sections. Many of the histochemical spot tests are so sensitive that they will pick up contamination at very low concentrations. For the best and most reliable results, ALL reagents should be completely free of the ions that are going to be demonstrated. This can be surprisingly difficult since some reagents will pick up ions very easily. Copper contamination from wax baths is not unknown and sections can be contaminated from metal forceps, scalpels and even microtome knives. Contamination should always be considered if results seem at all unexpected. If the wax block is prepared before you know that a histochemical test for minerals is needed, it may be too late and contamination may already have occurred. The opposite problem is the loss of minute deposits during processing, especially in acidic reagents. More materials are soluble at acid pH than in alkaline solutions but ideally neutral pH should be used.

Calcium

Calcium deposits in the body come in a few main forms. Hydroxyapatite is the main mineral in teeth and bone. Mineralization in bone is critical for health, whilst for some diseases the measurement of calcification is an important diagnostic aid (see *Box 9.8*). Strictly, calcification should be called mineralization as it includes metals other than calcium.

The von Kossa technique is useful for calcification but is not specific for calcium

The von Kossa technique using silver to demonstrate mineralization has been explained in Chapter 6 and, although important, this technique is not specific for calcium itself (see *Colour plate 22*). Other forms of calcium often do not react using the von Kossa technique, for example crystalline calcium carbonate and the calcified materials in invertebrates, so it is best regarded as a measure of bone mineral and not as a method for calcium detection.

Some dyes will complex with calcium

Some dyes can bind selectively to calcium and are more specific methods for calcium than the von Kossa method. They are also equally good at

---

Box 9.8 Calcium deficiency in bone

Diseases in which calcium is deficient include rickets and osteomalacia, which are caused by lack of vitamin D. Although dietary deficiency is now quite rare in developed countries as vitamin D is added to many foodstuffs, these diseases can still occur due to malabsorption in Crohn's disease.

Vitamin D can be synthesized in the skin by the action of UV light but the darker skins of some races prevent this formation of vitamin D in the skin. There is an occasional case of vitamin D deficiency in some Asian communities in Britain. Some chapatti flours also seem to inhibit the absorption of calcium and this exaggerates the disease. Bone biopsies may be used to confirm the diagnosis.

Osteoporosis is a very important disease in post-menopausal women and causes skeletal deformities, bone pain and fractures. In the years immediately following the menopause, bone mass may reduce by as much as 3% per year. Osteoporosis is usually diagnosed from the radiographic appearance rather than by bone biopsy.

---

determining mineralization. Simple haematoxylin staining as with haematoxylin and eosin gives a distinctive blue colour with mineralized bone compared with the pink colour of osteoid. This is seen even more clearly with an unmordanted haematoxylin when only the calcified material will stain. Alizarin red sulphonate (alizarin red S) is probably the most used of the simple dyes. Alizarin is not absolutely specific for calcium and also reacts with aluminium, barium and strontium. Aluminium and barium, however, give a slightly different colour but strontium is usually mixed with the calcium and is indistinguishable from it.

Alizarin can be used to show bone development in embryos

One use for alizarin is in the Dawson technique for examining bones in embryos. This is a method of treating whole embryos so that the bony structures can be seen through the body tissues. The soft tissues of the embryo are macerated by treatment with strong hydroxide. This renders them softer and less likely to take up the stain. The bones are stained with alizarin and the soft tissues are then made transparent by soaking in glycerol, which has a high refractive index and, like the organic clearing agents, makes soft tissues almost transparent. The stained bones can then be seen clearly through the translucent soft tissues (see *Colour plate 23*).

Drug and dye incorporation into bone during normal bone growth

Xylenol orange is another dye that can be incorporated into bone but is usually used as a vital stain when it is incorporated into new bone as it mineralizes. This is a useful way of locating where new bone is being formed but is of course limited to animal studies. An alternative to the xylenol orange dye is the use of tetracycline antibiotics. These work in the same way and fluoresce quite strongly when bound to calcium in bone. Different tetracyclines fluoresce in different colours, so, depending on the tetracyclines that have been used, it is possible to identify when particular parts of calcified structures have formed. This can be useful even in humans – tetracyclines are used as antibiotics for the treatment of infections, so some samples may include tetracyclines from their clinical use. This technique can be used in a pulsed delivery with a short dose given to label newly formed bone and then a gap before a second dose. The doses rapidly localize in the newly forming bone as discrete lines and the distance between them represents the rate of bone growth in the period between the two pulses. I have even seen the same effect in the tooth of a child who had had three courses of tetracycline – the tooth showed distinct lines corresponding to the growth between the tetracycline treatments.

Magnesium

Magnesium is often found along with calcium in mineralized tissues but it can be identified as an independent ion by chelation with dyes. The dyes are thiazol yellow G and 4-(*p*-nitrophenylazo)-resorcinol (Magneson). Thiazol yellow gives a red colour to magnesium deposits, whilst Magneson gives a blue colour.

Iron

Iron occurs in haemoglobin, myoglobin, cytochromes, ferritin and haemosiderin, in all of which it is organically bound. Iron is constantly recycled by the body, with only small amounts being lost or gained under normal circumstances. Iron is poorly absorbed from the diet, particularly from vegetable sources, and women can become iron deficient due to the monthly losses of iron in the menstrual blood flow. Many women are prescribed iron tablets to supplement their dietary sources. If large amounts are absorbed, it can prove toxic and iron poisoning has been a problem with children taking their parents' iron pills (see *Box 9.9*). This toxicity may be due to the iron generating free radicals, which then damage the tissue.

Haemochromatosis is caused by excessive iron uptake

In the disease primary haemochromatosis, there is an excessive absorption of iron and the iron deposits as haemosiderin in many organs. In the liver, the deposits may lead to cirrhosis following hepatocyte death. In the heart, it may cause cardiac myopathy leading to heart failure, and in the pancreas, it can cause diabetes mellitus. The disease is inherited as an autosomal recessive disorder, so it will appear suddenly in families rather than showing a strong familial inheritance.

Box 9.9 Iron and toxicity in children

Iron poisoning is one of the commonest causes of poisoning in children. In the USA, there were 110,000 cases between 1986 and 1992 of whom 33 died. The immediate effects of iron overdose are vomiting, diarrhoea and gastrointestinal bleeding. If the child recovers from these problems, there may be liver damage, heart failure and coma within 1–2 days. If the child survives and recovers from the initial toxicity, there may still be problems including liver damage up to 6 weeks later.

Haemosiderosis occurs following repeated blood transfusions in thalassaemia

In secondary haemochromatosis or haemosiderosis, there is a similar accumulation of iron but this is not due to a genetic defect and instead is the result of other problems such as alcoholism or thalassaemia. Thalassaemia patients need regular blood transfusions as their own red cells are destroyed rapidly. The constant influx of blood overloads their iron excretion system, so iron will build up unless it is removed constantly using drugs.

Iron is difficult to unmask when bound in a porphyrin ring

Iron is usually only detected as the protein-bound forms of haemosiderin and ferritin, both of which give positive Perls reactions. The use of the Perls reagent for detecting haemosiderin has been covered in the section on pigments earlier in this chapter. In haemoglobin, myoglobin and the cytochromes, iron is not simply attached to protein but also complexed into a porphyrin ring to form the haem group. This stronger link makes it resistant to removal and the simple use of low pH in the Perls reaction will not allow it to be released; thus, any compound with the iron bound in this way will usually be Perls-negative. The iron can be detached from the haem using an alkaline solution of peroxide, but this is less reliable as a method than the usual Perls reaction and is not often used.

Ferrous iron can be detected with Turnbull's blue reaction

The Perls method only detects ferric iron, but since this is the main form in the body this is not a major limitation. If ferrous iron needs to be detected specifically, then a modified Perls reaction should be used. This uses potassium ferricyanide instead of the potassium ferrocyanide used in the standard Perls reaction. The final pigment produced by the reaction is the same deep blue colour and is usually called Turnbull's blue, although it is probably exactly the same material as the pigment in the Perls reaction. Usually Turnbull's blue reaction does not detect much ferrous iron in tissues unless there is a deposit of exogenous ferrous material.

If all of the iron present in a piece of tissue is required, regardless of the ionic form, then the section can be treated with hydrogen sulphide or ammonium sulphide. All of the iron will be converted to ferrous sulphide, which is black, and this can then be stained using Turnbull's blue reaction. The result is usually little different to a simple Perls reaction. Iron, which is resistant to most methods of unmasking, can usually be detected by micro-incineration, followed by a sulphide/Turnbull's blue reaction.

Other (rarely used) methods for detecting iron

There are also various methods of detecting iron using chelating agents. Unoxidized haematoxylin will give a blue/black colour but is not very specific. A more specific chelating agent is 4,7-diphenyl-1,10-phenanthroline, which gives a red colour with iron and a yellow colour with cobalt. The copper chelate is uncoloured. Ferric iron chelates only slowly, so if the reaction is being used specifically for ferrous iron the treatment should be kept short. If both ferrous and ferric iron are required to be demonstrated, then adding some thioglycolic acid will reduce the ferric ions in haemosiderin and unmask it from the protein without the need to add hydrochloric acid as in the Perls reaction.

The detection of non-haem iron is very important and frequently done, but despite the variety of methods available, it is the oldest method, Perls, that has proved to be the simplest, most reliable and most sensitive.

Copper

Copper is an important ion in metabolism but is present in only in small amounts in a normal person and these amounts are below the detection limit of histochemical tests. Copper is normally handled efficiently by the liver, with copper from the diet being linked to caeruloplasmin for transport. Copper caeruloplasmin is recycled by the liver and free copper can be excreted into the bile. Copper accumulates in the liver in Wilson's disease, which is a rare autosomal recessive genetic disorder. In Wilson's disease, the copper and caeruloplasmin are not secreted into the plasma and there is an accumulation in the liver cells. Free copper may then appear in the blood and can deposit in the brain and cornea. The excessive levels of copper in Wilson's disease can be detected histochemically, although it may need unmasking if it is associated with protein. It can be unmasked by treating the section with hydrogen peroxide or hydrochloric acid.

Copper can be detected with rubeanic acid

The best detecting agents for copper are rubeanic acid (dithio-oxamide) and *p*-dimethylaminobenzylidine rhodanine (DMABR). Copper can be detected using an unmordanted haematoxylin solution but this is less sensitive and is non-specific.

Lead

Lead was at one time a widespread material used in plumbing (hence the name, *plumbum*, which is Latin for lead), paints and as a petrol additive. The average total body load is estimated at around 120 mg. Environmental exposure to lead compounds can result in significant problems with anaemia, motor neuropathy and deposition of lead in bone but it is rarely diagnosed on tissues (see *Box 9.10*). Lead poisoning can be recognized in blood samples by the stippling of red cells or can be measured chemically in serum samples. It is rare that there is sufficient lead in a normal person to be detectable by histochemical methods. The most sensitive method of detection is the sodium rhodizonate method, which produces a red chelate with lead ions.

Box 9.10 Toxic metals in diet

Both copper and lead have been used in water pipes but only lead seems to dissolve significantly in the water and cause poisoning. Lead will only dissolve significantly in soft water areas. In hard water areas, the pipes rapidly become lined with a deposit of calcium salts. This furring causes problems of blockages and narrowing of the pipes but protects humans. Lead pipes are being gradually replaced but the vast numbers of these pipes in older houses means that it will be many years before they are all completely replaced.

Soft water is generally slightly acid due to dissolved carbon dioxide and it is this acidity that allows metals to dissolve more rapidly. Acid solutions will generally dissolve more metals than neutral or alkaline solutions. In cooking it is not wise to allow any acidic material (such as fruits and fruit juices) to stay in contact with anything containing potentially dangerous metals. This includes pans (copper, iron and aluminium are all toxic), glazed pots (many coloured glazes contain dangerous metals including uranium) and enamel containers (again it is the coloured pigments that are the problem).

Aluminium

Aluminium accumulates in the bodies of patients on haemodialysis and can cause an osteomalacia-like condition that resists normal treatment. In the brain, aluminium causes encephalopathy, which again is found in some long-term dialysis patients. Aluminium is commonly used in normal life (see *Box 9.11*) in the form of cooking utensils and aluminium foil. Aluminium hydroxide is also used in some antacid remedies. Aluminium has also been reported in the neural plaques found in the brains of patients with Alzheimer's disease but it is not thought to be the cause of Alzheimer's.

Aluminium can be detected in sections using solochrome azurine, which forms a chelate complex with a deep blue colour. This reaction is also given by **beryllium**. Beryllium is used in fluorescent lights and may get into the body by inhalation or through cuts. Even quite small amounts produce accumulations of macrophages forming a **granuloma**.

Other heavy metals

Other heavy metals will also sometimes be seen but are not common. Silver and mercury are seen in the form of dental amalgam, which can become

---

Box 9.11 Aluminium and tap water

Aluminium can occur in tap water naturally and the World Health Organization recommends that aluminium concentrations should not exceed 0.1 parts per million. Some parts of the world have much higher levels; for example, a survey in Malawi found levels up to 100 times higher.

Aluminium is also used as a flocculating agent to clarify drinking water. Normally the levels of aluminium are very low but in the town of Camelford there was an accident in which a delivery of aluminium salts was put into the wrong manhole and ended up being pumped directly into drinking water. The local inhabitants were severely affected by this release. The long-term effects of this release are not known and the affected people will no doubt provide more information about the effects of aluminium on humans.

impacted into soft tissues during dental treatment. Silver is associated with silver earrings in badly pierced ears (or other pierced organs). Both metals are removed by iodine and hypo treatments as for the mercury artefact pigment

Another method of identifying minerals is the use of X-ray analysis. This topic will be dealt with in Chapter 16.

9.4   ION-SELECTIVE DYES

These are a group of specially designed reagents that alter their fluorescent characteristics depending on their immediate local environment (see *Box 9.12*). The fluorescence change is related quantitatively to the concentration of particular ions in the fluid surrounding them. The change in concentrations of the ion can be followed dynamically in living cells. These dyes are quite different to most of the histochemical methods in the rest of this chapter in that they do not produce a coloured precipitate in slices of dead tissue but instead measure minute changes in the cytoplasmic concentration of selected ions. The dyes are only suitable for use inside living cells; they are not conventional stains and cannot be used on fixed sections. They are a research tool for examining metabolism, particularly in cultured cells.

Ion-selective dyes can be used to monitor metabolism in living cells

By introducing these dyes into cells, it is possible to see and measure directly how particular ions alter with time or to following specific events. The cytoplasmic changes in calcium concentration are critical in the control of many activities. It is the release of calcium ions into the cytoplasm that triggers muscle contractions, changes in the ovum following fertilization and the response of cells to many other stimuli. The calcium-selective dyes fura and quin-2 allow direct observation and measurement of these calcium

---

Box 9.12 Aequorin

The ion-selective dyes are a masterpiece of synthetic chemistry since many of these compounds have been designed specifically to identify one particular ion. The chemists start with a relatively crude ion-sensitive dye and alter it to make it more selective and more sensitive. This designer approach requires great knowledge of the interaction of molecules and ions and relies on the use of computer modelling to determine the best configuration. The improvements are still continuing.

There is also a range of ion-selective compounds that have been produced by nature that are also useful probes. Aequorin (a bioluminescent tracer from a jellyfish) and luciferase (an enzyme used to detect ATP) can both be used as tracers but such biological molecules are difficult to load into cells and are often more useful in cell-free extracts.

One advantage of biological molecules is that the genes for these molecules can be incorporated into cells and animals, so that all of the cells will exhibit fluorescence without the need to introduce the probe molecules. This has already been done with mice that glow green in the right light.

Table 9.1 Examples of ion-selective dyes

Ion or process measured	Example of a selective probe	Concentration range
Calcium	Fura	14–1450 nM
Magnesium	Mag-fura	2–200 nM
pH	SNAFL (seminaphthofluorescein)	pH 7.2–8.2
pH	BCECF (bis-carboxyethylcarboxyfluorescein)	pH 6.6–7.5
Sodium	Sodium green	0.6–600 mM
Chloride	MQAE (*N*-(ethoxycarbonylmethyl)-6-methoxyquinolinium bromide)	1–100 mM

fluxes. Other dyes of the same type can be used to measure a variety of changes, but each is more or less selective for a particular type of ionic change. These ion-selective dyes have enabled visualization of many internal processes within the cell.

A list of some of the changes that can be measured and examples of the probes used are given in the *Table 9.1*.

Introducing ion-selective dyes into cells

Ion-selective dyes need to penetrate the living cells before they can be used to measure the internal concentrations of the ions. This is termed 'cell loading' and can be done in two ways:

■ **Bulk loading**, where a suspension of living cells is treated so that many cells are labelled at once. One of the more popular ways of achieving this is to use the acetomethoxy ester (AM derivative) of the dye, which is able to penetrate through the cell membrane. Once inside the cell, these esters are hydrolysed by the cell's esterase enzymes releasing the active dye. The active dye is polar and cannot move out of the cell, so it is trapped in the cytoplasm. Other bulk loading methods include the use of osmotic shock or liposome delivery. Liposomes are membrane vesicles containing solutions of materials. They can be made in the laboratory and fused with cell membranes to deliver their contents into the cytoplasm.

■ **Single-cell loading** involves directly injecting the dye through the cell membrane using a micro-pipette or micro-electrode.

Measuring the change in fluorescence

The change in fluorescence needs to be measured and calibrated. The method varies with the dye being used but two methods are commonly used:

■ **The ratiometric method.** The dye has two emission peaks and the ratio between the heights of the two peaks measures the concentration of the selected ion. This method is used to measure calcium concentrations using fura-2. The advantage of this technique is that it is self-calibrating for the amount of dye since both peaks are measured and if the dye concentration changes, then both peaks change in parallel.

■ **Single-wavelength change.** Here only a single wavelength is measured and the system needs to be calibrated using a buffer and an ionophore. At the end of the experiment, the cell is immersed in a calcium buffer with a constant and known concentration of calcium ions. The cell membrane is made fully permeable to calcium using an ionophore. The calcium concentration inside the cell will be in equilibrium with the buffer, so the system can be calibrated from the readings of the equilibrated cell.

The measurements are often made using a confocal microscope, which allows accurate measurements not only within a single cell but also within compartments of the cell. This system of measuring inside living cells in a dynamic manner is extremely useful in research but as yet has no real use in diagnosis. The only drawback to the technique is the capital cost of the equipment needed to carry out these techniques and the cost of the ion-selective dyes.

SUGGESTED FURTHER READING

Churukian, C.J. (2002) Pigments and minerals. In *Theory and Practice of Histological Techniques*, 5th edn (eds J.D. Bancroft and M. Gamble). Edinburgh: Churchill Livingstone.

Kiernan, J.A. (2001) *Histological and Histochemical Methods*, 3rd edn. Oxford: Hodder Arnold.

Lyon, H. (1991) *Theory and Strategy in Histochemistry*. Berlin: Springer.

Sheehan, D.C. and Hrapchak, B. (1980) *Theory and Practice of Histotechnology*. St Louis: Mosby.

SELF-ASSESSMENT QUESTIONS

1. What are the three most common exogenous pigments in sections?
2. How does the occurrence of lipofuscin vary with age?
3. Which pigment(s) are positive with the Perls test?
4. Which pigments act as reducing agents and will give a positive Schmorl's test?
5. What are the two main types of secretion from APUD cells?
6. An excess of iron in the tissues causes which disease(s)?
7. How can calcium salts be demonstrated in sections?
8. Which metal accumulates in Wilson's disease and how can the metal be demonstrated?
9. What is the difference between ratiometric and single-wavelength ion-selective dyes?

Immunological techniques

Learning objectives

After studying this chapter you should confidently be able to:

■ **Describe how antibodies can be used as histological reagents.**
Antibodies are specific and can be used to identify individual proteins in tissues. The antibodies can be labelled in a variety of ways including the use of fluorescent dyes and biotin or can be used in bridging techniques, which do not need the antibodies to be modified.

■ **Outline the principles of the direct and indirect immunofluorescent techniques.**
In the direct technique, only one antibody is needed and this antibody is labelled with fluorescent dye. The antibody can be applied directly to the section and will bind to its specific antigen, which can then be localized by the fluorescence. In the indirect technique, the primary antibody is not labelled fluorescently. A second antibody capable of binding to the primary antibody is needed and this needs to be labelled with fluorescent dye.

■ **Outline the use of enzymes as labels and the advantages of immunohistochemistry.**
Enzymes can be used instead of fluorescent dyes as labels. They can be detected using enzyme histochemical techniques. They can give greater amplification of the signal than simple fluorescence, they can be viewed without the need for a fluorescent microscope and it is possible to use unlabelled bridging techniques. All of these make immunohistochemistry more popular than immunofluorescence for histological sections.

■ **Describe the reasons for antigen retrieval techniques and name the common methods of antigen retrieval.**
Antigen retrieval is needed to allow antibodies to bind to antigens in fixed tissues as the fixation effectively masks the antigen. Antigen retrieval can use enzymes, microwave heating or pressurized heating in an autoclave or pressure cooker.

■ **Outline the use of lectins in histochemistry.**
Lectins can be used in a similar way to antibodies but bind to specific sugars rather than antigens. Lectins are non-immune proteins and do not need to be elicited by immunization.

10.1   USE OF ANTIBODIES AS HISTOLOGICAL REAGENTS

Animals are constantly threatened by pathological bacteria, fungi and viruses that cause infective diseases. As a defence against these organisms, evolution has produced the vertebrate immune system. The immune system of animals has two major parts, one of which is the cellular immune system and is concerned with the killing of invading cells by direct cellular action. The cell types involved are the T lymphocytes and macrophages. The second type of immunity is humoral immunity, which depends on antibodies produced by B lymphocytes and plasma cells. Antibodies are glycoproteins that react with the invading organisms and bind strongly to them. Antibodies are also known as immunoglobulins and can be extracted from the blood of an immune animal or human being. The binding of the antibody to the foreign cells either inactivates the invading cells or coats the cells and makes them more likely to be attacked by the cellular immune system.

As antibodies are soluble proteins, they can be used as biochemical and histochemical reagents. Immunological methods have become very important in histology because of their specificity, sensitivity and reliability.

Antibody production

Antibodies are specific proteins produced in response to antigens. The trigger for the immune system to produce antibodies is the presence of a foreign material called an **antigen.** Antibodies are produced by B lymphocytes and each B lymphocytes is specific for one antigen and has on its surface a receptor that is specific for the antibody it produces. When this receptor is simulated by the specific antigen, it causes the cell to divide rapidly and produce a clone of identical cells, all producing exactly the same antibody. This proliferation produces a large number of cells and hence increases the production of antibody.

An antigen is any material that can be recognized by the receptors on the immune cells. Antigens can be solid particles such as cells or bacteria, but they can also be soluble materials such as foreign proteins or certain other complex molecules. It requires a fairly large molecule to trigger the response and small molecules are not usually antigenic. An antibody that has been triggered in this way is very selective and will react only with the antigen that stimulated its production. Other antigens will not be bound by the antibody, i.e. it is highly **specific**. Antibodies are also extremely active in binding to their antigen and are not easily dislodged by washing or by minor changes in the fluid environment i.e. they have high **avidity**. It is this specificity and the high binding strength that make antibodies so popular as reagents.

Antibodies used in histology

There are a number of different types of antibodies (see *Box 10.1*) but the main ones used in immunotechniques in histology are immunoglobulin G (IgG) and immunoglobulin M (IgM). They differ in the number of binding sites they have for antigens. IgG has two identical binding sites and consists

---

Box 10.1 Immunoglobulins

Antibodies are found in the blood and form part of the **globulin** fraction: they form the γ-globulins, which can be identified by electrophoresis. Since they are a part of the immune system, they are also termed **immunoglobulins**, which is abbreviated to Ig. There are several subtypes of immunoglobulins. IgG and IgM are important in the normal immune reaction in blood. IgA is found in secretions such as milk and saliva and IgD is found as membrane receptors on B lymphocytes. IgE is important as it is the cause of allergies but its normal function is not understood. For histochemistry, only IgG and IgM are used as reagents but detection of other immunoglobulins is sometimes needed.

The antibodies form the **humoral** response of inflammation. The term humour, in this context, comes from the ancient theory of health in which there were four body fluids or **humours** (blood, phlegm, green bile and black bile) that needed to be kept in balance for health. Any material found in body fluids was described as humoral. The second form of immune response is the **cellular immune system**; this is less important in histochemistry although vital for health.

---

of a Y-shaped molecule with a binding site at the end of each arm of the Y. IgM is a larger molecule and resembles five IgG-like molecules bound together to form a pentamer. IgM is usually produced early in the immune reaction, with IgG being produced later. There are some differences in these two proteins and this can sometimes be relevant, but for most purposes in histology the differences between the major types are minor and either type will work as a reagent.

Animals do not usually produce antibodies against their own proteins

Antibodies are not usually produced against the body's own proteins as this would cause the body to attack itself. If the method of controlling the production of antibodies fails to prevent this happening, then this results in autoimmune disease. The diagnosis of autoimmune disease is one of the areas in which immunotechniques is important. The fact that an animal does not react to its own proteins does not mean they are not antigenic. If the protein is injected into a different species of animal, then it will act as an antigen. Some proteins are very similar in all species of animal and will not be recognized as being different and will not produce an immune response and antibodies will not build up in the blood. It is for this reason that insulin from other species such as pigs or cattle can be used to treat human diabetes. Insulin is a small protein and is not sufficiently different in the different species to trigger antibody production (at least in most people), even with many years of use. This low antigenicity of some proteins sometimes causes problems when scientists try to produce antibodies for use in immunotechniques.

Raising antibodies in animals can be difficult

Often it requires ingenuity and persistence to produce some of the antibodies that are commercially available. Once an animal is immunized

---

Box 10.2 Problems of immunization

Raising antibodies often requires adding **adjuvants** to improve the reaction. Adjuvants include a variety of nasty materials such as killed bacteria, oil droplets or irritant chemicals. The method of preparing these adjuvant cocktails is often little more than guesswork or trial and error.

The raising of antibodies is also an 'experiment' using a live animal and in the UK this requires a special licence from the Home Office. The actual interference with the animal is usually comparatively minor (one or two simple injections and taking samples of blood) but it is still strictly controlled. These two difficulties are the reason why most people prefer to buy antibodies and so save themselves considerable trouble.

---

against an antigen, it is then kept immune or hyperimmune by regularly challenging the animal with fresh antigen injections. This keeps the concentration of antibody high in the blood and helps to make an efficient reagent. The complexities of immunizing the animal (see *Box 10.2*) and keeping it immune mean that it is unusual for most scientists to produce their own antibodies and instead they rely on commercial firms to produce and test them.

The immune system often produces many antibodies against the same protein

The actual binding site between an antibody and an antigen is quite small compared with the size of the actual protein. If a large antigen is injected into an animal, then it is common for more than one antibody to be produced. Each antibody will be specific for its own binding site but a range of antibodies will be produced that react with different parts of the antigen molecule. Some of the antibodies will react only with the ends of the antigen molecule, whilst others will only react with the centre. Each antibody will come from a different clone of lymphocytes so the antibody is referred to as a **polyclonal antibody**.

Polyclonal antibodies are not specific

Antibodies may react with proteins other than the specific antigen used to trigger their production. Usually these will be closely related proteins that share a sequence of amino acids but this cross-reactivity with other proteins can be a problem. The antibodies prepared in an animal may also contain small amounts of natural antibodies other than the specific hyperimmune antibody. This impurity is usually only a theoretical problem as the antibody solutions are used at high dilutions. The hyperimmune antibody will still be active because of its high concentration, but most other antibodies will be too weakly represented to cause difficulties. There is, however, always the possibility of a contaminant antibody giving a false reaction.

Monoclonal antibodies are more specific

A second type of antibody is now available and these are produced by growing cells in tissue culture. Lymphocytes generally do not grow well or for long periods in culture, so the antibody-forming cells are fused with a lymphocytic tumour cell. The hybrid cell can grow well and still produces antibody. Since the cells are all produced from a single original cell they are called **monoclonal antibodies**. Monoclonal antibodies have several advantages:

- They are much more specific and react with only one small part of an antigen.
- They have less likelihood of cross-reacting with other proteins.
- They are not contaminated with any other antibodies and can be purified more easily.
- They will always be identical, whereas polyclonal antibodies will vary depending on the animal.

Monoclonal antibodies are so precise that they are usually able to react with just one part of the antigen and will be designated as reacting with a particular part of the molecule (e.g. the Fc portion of the immunoglobulin heavy chain). Many monoclonal antibodies are designated by simple codes that make them almost unintelligible unless you are familiar with them.

Monoclonal antibodies can sometimes be too precise

Although monoclonal antibodies are more precise and consistent since they can be cultured under highly controlled conditions, they do suffer from the problem that they are absolutely monospecific and only react with a single binding site. A polyclonal antibody, on the other hand, is composed of different antibodies each of which reacts with a different binding site on the target molecule. Although polyclonal antibodies are less specific, they are sometimes more effective for detecting particular proteins since their specific sites of binding differ. For example, in an autoimmune reaction, it may not be known which type of immunoglobulin is acting. It might be IgG, IgM, or even one of the less common antibody types. With monoclonal antibodies, it might be necessary to use several monoclonal antibodies to detect whether there was any antibody. A negative reaction with any single reagent would simply indicate that the specific immunoglobulin was not present but not that there were no immunoglobulins. A less-specific polyclonal antiserum prepared against immunoglobulins in general rather than a specific type could detect the binding with a single reagent. For this and other similar reasons, polyclonal antibodies are still used for some tests. When more detailed information is needed, however, it is usually better to use monoclonal antibodies to provide precise information about the target being stained.

Fluorescent antibody techniques

Although antibodies are very precise reagents, they are not visible even with high-power microscopes and need to be labelled in some way to allow their binding to be localized. Historically, the most widely used method of labelling has been with fluorescein, a fluorescent dye, and the technique is

---

Box 10.3 Antibody inactivation

Chemical labelling could potentially affect the ability of the antibody to bind to its antigen. In practice, this is not a major problem. The term **epitope** or **antigenic determinant** is used to describe the part of an antigen that is directly bound by the antibody. The binding site is quite small and the binding region of the antibody is believed to be only 20–30 amino acids in size. Provided that these critical amino acids are not altered by the labelling process, then the binding ability of the antibody will remain unchanged. In normal labelling conditions, only a few labelling molecules, perhaps four to six, are added to the antibody. The binding sites are only a very small part of the antibody (perhaps 5%), so the chances of the label attaching to the binding sites are small and the majority of the binding sites are unaffected.

---

therefore called **immunofluorescence**. Other labelling techniques have become popular since their introduction in the 1960s and are now probably more common in histology. These methods usually involve the use of enzymes and are collectively called **immunohistochemistry** or **immunocytochemistry** (discussed later in the chapter) as a histochemical or cytochemical test is used to visualize the enzyme.

Labelling with fluorescein

Fluorescein is a highly fluorescent dye related to eosin and is used as a fluorescent label. It can be detected even in minute amounts using fluorescent techniques. The dye must be attached firmly to the antibody. Simple ionic staining (see Chapter 6) of the protein is not satisfactory since the fluorescein could dislodge readily during simple washing and mounting. By using the isothiocyanate derivative of fluorescein (FITC), it is possible to attach the dye permanently. FITC forms covalent links with amino groups in the antibody protein forming a strong bond that does not break easily and resists removal during staining and processing (see *Box 10.3*). Attachment of the dye by this method is termed conjugation to distinguish it from simple staining.

The steps involved in producing a fluorescently labelled antibody are:

1. Prepare a pure antibody solution against a known antigen (e.g. antibody against actin is prepared by injecting purified actin into an animal).
2. Treat the purified antibody with FITC to conjugate the dye and label the antibody.
3. Wash the labelled antibody solution to remove unbound FITC. This can be done by dialysis or gel filtration.

Labelled antibody will react with its specific antigen in the tissues

Labelled antibody can then be used at a suitable dilution to stain sections. Careful washing is needed but the technique is quite simple. The section can then be viewed with a fluorescent microscope, when any bound antibody will fluoresce showing the sites of antibody binding and this in turn identifies the sites of the antigen. Using the example of actin, the binding sites for

> **Box 10.4 Autoimmunity**
>
> Anti-nuclear antibodies are found in a variety of disorders including rheumatoid disease, lupus erythematosis, mixed connective tissue disease and some liver disease. The antibodies are classed as autoimmune antibodies since they will react with antigens present in the patient. Autoimmune diseases can be diagnosed by detecting the free antibody in the patient's blood or by detecting bound antibody on the patient's cells.
>
> Other autoimmune antibodies are also found and many seem to react with endocrine tissues, although the significance of this is not known.
>
> In some cases, autoimmune antibodies are directed against a single organ (e.g. Hashimoto's thyroiditis) or against a whole number of different organs (e.g. systemic lupus erythematosis). The damage to the tissues may be caused directly by antibody or indirectly by cellular immunity but can also occur by the production of immune complexes in the tissues. An immune complex is a combination of antibody and antigen, which can become deposited in delicate tissues such as the kidney. The precipitated complex then causes the damage.

anti-actin antibody would indicate the location of actin. This simple technique involving just one antibody conjugated to FITC is called the **direct immunofluorescent technique**.

Detection of anti-nuclear antibodies in rheumatoid arthritis

In some diseases (e.g. rheumatoid disease), the patients produce an abnormal antibody that reacts with nuclear material (see *Box 10.4*). This anti-nuclear antibody is important for the diagnosis and prognosis of the disease. The antibody is present in the patient's serum and can be identified using tissue sections or cell smears and staining by immunofluorescent methods. The antibody will react with the nuclear proteins of several species and is not limited to human nuclei. Frozen sections of rat tissue or cells cultured *in vitro* can be used as test slides to detect whether there is any antibody present in the patient's serum.

Human antibodies are antigenic in other animals

Detection of immunoglobulins requires an antibody directed against immunoglobulin. This is an antibody against an antibody. This production of antibodies against antibodies is a little difficult to understand and follow the first time you come across it but it is a very useful technique. Human antibodies are proteins and can therefore act as antigens in a species other than humans. The animal produces, as usual, an antibody that will bind with its specific antigen, which in this case is human antibody. Antibodies are immunoglobulins, so the reagent is called anti-human immunoglobulin; if the animal it was prepared in was a rabbit, it would be called rabbit anti-human immunoglobulin.

Human antibodies can be detected using anti-immunoglobulins

To detect whether there are any anti-nuclear antibodies in a patient's serum, the following steps are needed:

1. The first step is to apply the patient's serum to frozen sections. If there is any anti-nuclear antibody present, it will bind to the nuclei.
2. The patient's serum is then washed away.
3. The section is treated with FITC-conjugated anti-human immunoglobulin. The anti-human antibody will only bind to human antibody. In a rat section, the only way that human antibody could be present would be if there were anti-nuclear antibodies in the test serum that had bound to the rat nuclei.
4. Finally, it is necessary to wash away any unbound FITC-labelled antibody and examine the section for fluorescence. If the nuclei fluoresce, then the patient's serum contained anti-nuclear antibodies (see *Colour plate 24*).

Measurement of antibody concentration

The immunofluorescent technique can be used to estimate the concentration of antibody by preparing a series of dilutions of the patient's serum and testing each one for binding. The dilution that just gives a detectable positive reaction is called the **titre** of the serum. A serum that has a titre of 1/512 means that if the serum is diluted to 1 part of serum in 511 parts of buffer it will still give a detectable reaction, but if diluted to 1/1024 (twice as dilute) then no reaction can be detected.

Direct and indirect immunotechniques

The anti-nuclear antibody technique uses two antibodies, the first or primary antibody is in the patient's serum and the second is prepared as an anti-antibody. Only the second antibody is conjugated. This is an example of an **indirect technique** (see *Fig. 10.1*) and can be used to detect any antibody, not just anti-nuclear antibodies in disease states. When a primary antibody is prepared by immunizing an animal, as for direct immunofluorescence, there is no need to conjugate this primary antibody. Instead a second antibody is prepared in a different species against the immunoglobulins of the first species and this secondary antibody is conjugated with FITC or another label (see *Box 10.5*).

Box 10.5 Other fluorescent labels

Fluorescein labelling is the most common method of fluorescently labelling antibodies but other fluorescent dyes are also used. Rhodamine and Texas red both have a red fluorescence and can be used as a second label when two different antigens are to be demonstrated in the same preparation. This double staining is useful for seeing how two materials are distributed and the relationship between them. The plant pigment phycoerythrin has also been used as it has a high fluorescent capability.

As well as labelling using the isothiocyanate derivatives, it is also possible to use succinimidyl esters and sulphonyl halides as reactive forms of the dyes and these will also react with amine groups. These are more stable but are more difficult to produce and are used less often.

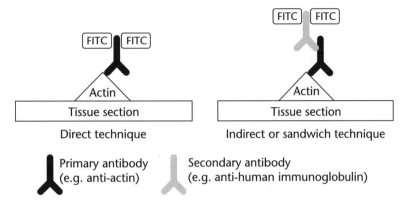

Figure 10.1
Diagram illustrating direct and indirect antibody techniques

Indirect techniques can be used for any antigen

The idea of an indirect technique is perhaps easier to understand if the individual species are named. Anti-actin antibody can be prepared from a rabbit by immunizing it with pure actin. This antibody is not conjugated with fluorescein. Anti-rabbit antibody can be prepared by immunizing a goat with purified rabbit antibody. This is called **goat anti-rabbit immunoglobulin**. The antibody used to immunize the goat does not need to be the specific anti-actin antibody – any rabbit antibody will produce the same effect. The goat anti-rabbit antibody will react with any antibody from any rabbit. This antibody is conjugated and will be a general reagent for any rabbit antibody. Thus, if we need to identify keratin, all that is needed is to prepare a new first antibody. This would mean raising anti-keratin antibody in a rabbit and this could then be detected using the same goat anti-rabbit immunoglobulin that was used with the anti-actin antibody.

The indirect technique has many advantages

The indirect technique is a better method than the direct technique for the following reasons:

■ As just explained, it is not necessary to conjugate every antibody. This makes it cheaper since conjugation adds to the cost of an antibody.
■ It is more sensitive since there can be more than one conjugated antibody bound to a single antigen site. In the direct technique, only one conjugated antibody can be bound to an antigen site. In the indirect technique, although there can still only be one primary antibody bound to the antigen site, there can be several secondary antibodies bound to the primary antibody. Each of the secondary antibodies will have fluorescein attached to it. This increases the intensity of the fluorescence, so smaller amounts of antigen can be detected. This increase in intensity is termed **amplification**.

■ The increased sensitivity means that the antibodies can be used in a more dilute solution, which means that the same amount of serum will be able to treat more sections. This reduces the cost of preparing a large number of slides.

Disadvantages of fluorescent labelling

Fluorescent labelling is widely used, not only in histology but also in microbiology and haematology. However, it is less suited to staining sections than other types of specimen. The main disadvantages are:

1. Observing fluorescence requires a special fluorescence microscope with a high-power lamp and this is usually significantly more expensive than a simple microscope using visible light. This cost is both in the initial cost and in the cost of replacement lamps.
2. Fluorescence is always quite dim and in order to observe the faint glow a darkened room is required and the observer needs to allow their eyes to become adjusted to the dark before looking at the slides.
3. It is difficult to counterstain the section with a dye since any fluorescence of the background might mask a dim positive reaction. In the absence of a counterstain, it is therefore more difficult to locate the position of the fluorescent material accurately in relation to other structures.
4. The fluorescence is not permanent. The dye will start to fade or bleach in a few days and will fade more quickly if it is examined under the microscope. Fading under the microscope illumination can be sufficiently fast that it will become lost in minutes.
5. It is difficult to photograph fluorescence. The image is dim, so a long exposure is needed but the dye fades with long exposures making photography difficult.

Immunohistochemistry

The problems with fluorescein labels led to a search for other antibody labels including the use of enzymes and the use of these histochemical labels is termed **immunohistochemistry**. Immunohistochemistry uses enzymes to label the antibodies and histochemical tests to identify the sites of binding.

As explained in Chapter 8, enzymes can be demonstrated in tissues and can produce highly coloured insoluble reaction products. An enzyme can also produce large amounts of coloured product if the incubation time with the substrate is long enough. This allows visualization of very small amounts of enzyme. This makes enzymes an excellent labelling material provided some way can be found to link the enzyme and the antibody together. Although there are many enzymes that could be used, the ones that have proved most popular are horseradish peroxidase (HRP) and alkaline phosphatase (AP).

Initially chemicals were used to link the enzyme to the antibody

Having chosen an enzyme, the next step is to link the enzyme and the antibody together. One of the first techniques used glutaraldehyde, which is a bifunctional aldehyde. One aldehyde group can react with the protein of the antibody, whilst the other reacts with the protein of the enzyme:

Thus, glutaraldehyde cross-links the antibody and enzyme in the same way that it cross-links tissue proteins when it is used as a fixative. This technique worked quite well but there was a lot of waste of antibody since simply mixing the glutaraldehyde with a mixture of antibody and enzyme resulted in a variety of combinations (see *Fig 10.2*).

■ The antibody can be cross-linked to another antibody. This combination could bind to the antigen but would not be able to be visualized since there is no enzyme present.
■ The enzyme could be cross-linked to another enzyme. This combination could not bind to the antigen.
■ Larger aggregations of several cross-linked proteins could form. These would either precipitate out of solution or would simply be too large to approach the antigenic site and would not bind because of steric hindrance.
■ Finally, there would be a mixture of an antibody linked to an enzyme in small enough aggregations to be useful. This group is the only type of reactant that could be used. The previous three types of combined proteins were not wanted and had to be removed from the solution.

The various forms could be separated effectively using gel filtration techniques so that the antibody could be prepared in a pure form. This was

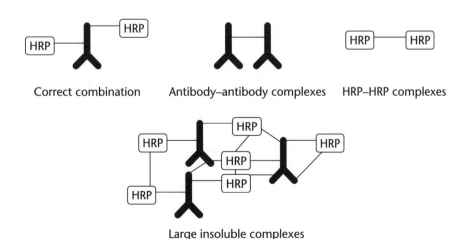

Correct combination   Antibody–antibody complexes   HRP–HRP complexes

Large insoluble complexes

Figure 10.2
Unwanted reactions between enzymes, glutaraldehyde and HRP

Box 10.6 Terminology of antibodies

The terminology of antibodies often hinders understanding. The terms antibody and antigen are fairly well defined. An antigen is a foreign material that, when introduced into the body, stimulates the production of an antibody. The terminology for naming antibodies is to prefix their antigen with 'anti-'. Thus, anti-actin is an antibody against actin. In some cases (as in the accompanying text), it is important to know the animal in which the antibody was prepared. Thus, if an anti-actin antibody was prepared in a rabbit it is termed rabbit anti-actin. If the antibody is prepared against an immunoglobulin (i.e. anti-antibody), then two species are needed. The one in which the antibody was made and the species from which the antigen (an immunoglobulin) came. Injecting rabbit immunoglobulin into a goat will produce goat anti-rabbit immunoglobulin. The first species is the species used to make the reagent, the second is the name of the antigen (in this case rabbit immunoglobulin).

The term serum is also in common use and can cause confusion. Serum is the protein-rich fluid left after plasma has been allowed to clot and the clot has been removed. Serum contains all the antibodies but has lost the ability to clot. Serum has been the traditional material for immunology and the subject is often referred to as **serology** from the widespread use of serum. Unfortunately a serum containing antibodies is referred to as an **antiserum**. This does not mean that it necessarily has antibodies against serum, just that it contains antibodies. The term antiserum is also loosely applied to monoclonal antibodies, which are not serum at all but antibody solutions from cell culture media.

---

very wasteful of reagent since significant amounts of the antibody were being discarded and lost.

The purified antibody–enzyme combination could be used by either the direct or the indirect method, as for fluorescein labelling. In this case, indirect techniques are even more favoured since the labelling technique is so wasteful.

The major steps in the indirect enzyme-labelled antibody method using HRP are:

1. Apply the primary antiserum (see *Box 10.6*) to the sections. If there is any antigen present, then the antibody will bind to it.
2. The primary antiserum is then washed away.
3. The section is then treated with enzyme-linked anti-immunoglobulin. This will bind to any primary antibody held in the section.
4. Wash away the excess labelled antibody.
5. Treat the section with the appropriate enzyme demonstration technique to develop the final colour. For HRP, this could be a mixture of hydrogen peroxide and diaminobenzidene in buffer.
6. Counterstain the tissue to show the general structure.

The sites of the enzyme will show as deposits of brown chromogen and these sites will be the position of the antigen.

Unlabelled antibody techniques

Since both the enzyme (e.g. HRP) and the antibody are proteins, they can both act as antigens. It was realized that it was possible to link these compo-

Figure 10.3
Diagram of the unlabelled antibody method

nents together by using a third antibody. This requires two different species of animal and three antibodies.

The three antibodies needed are:

1. The primary antibody against the antigen prepared in a stated species (e.g. rabbit anti-actin).
2. An anti-HRP antibody prepared in the same species (e.g. rabbit anti-HRP).
3. A bridging antibody against the immunoglobulin of the species used to prepare steps 1 and 2 (e.g. goat anti-rabbit immunoglobulin).

These are applied in sequence to the section (see *Fig 10.3*).

The primary antibody (rabbit anti-actin) is applied first and binds to the antigen. After washing away the excess antibody, the goat anti-rabbit immunoglobulin is applied and will bind to the rabbit anti-actin antibody. As there is a large amount of the goat anti-rabbit immunoglobulin, the binding will only use one of the binding sites available on the secondary antibody. When the final rabbit anti-HRP antibody is applied, it will be trapped by the unused binding sites of the secondary antibody. The secondary antibody thus binds the primary antibody and the tertiary antibody by acting as a bridge between them.

The next step would be to add HRP, which would be trapped by the anti-HRP antibody. The enzyme can then be demonstrated as before and a brown chromogen deposit will indicate the sites of actin within the tissue. The process can be repeated to increase the amount of enzyme (see *Box 10.7*).

The peroxidase–anti-peroxidase technique

Variations on this technique became some of the most popular techniques in immunohistochemistry. The HRP enzyme and the anti-HRP antibody can be prepared as a single ready-prepared complex (peroxidase–anti-

---

Box 10.7 Increasing the amount of bound enzyme

With the unlabelled antibody technique, it is also possible to repeat the processes involving the anti-HRP and HRP. By adding extra anti-HRP after the HRP has been added, the anti-HRP will bind to the HRP. By using a lot of anti-HRP, it is possible to ensure that only one of the two binding sites is used. The other binding site can now bind more HRP. Thus, by alternating anti-HRP and HRP solutions, the amount of HRP can be greatly increased. In practice, the process is limited since there is also an increase in the background staining.

---

peroxidase, or PAP) rather than having to add the final antibody and the enzyme as separate steps. The PAP complex consists of two antibodies and three peroxidase molecules in an almost cyclical structure. The complex is soluble and, even though the enzyme is bound by the antibody, its activity is not inhibited.

The PAP reagent can easily be purified

The PAP complex has another advantage. Since the PAP complex is prepared separately, it can be purified more easily and this gives greater sensitivity and less background staining. The anti-peroxidase antibody needs to be very pure. If it is prepared in an animal, it is likely to be contaminated with non-specific antibodies. These antibodies will compete with the anti-peroxidase antibody for binding on to the bridging antibody and this will reduce the final colour. It is almost impossible to separate the specific and non-specific antibodies whilst they exist as individual molecules but the PAP complex is easier to purify.

If an impure serum from a rabbit immunized with peroxidase is mixed with peroxidase it will form the complex. The complex is now much larger than the other antibodies and can be separated by gel filtration to give a much purer preparation. The same technique can be used with alkaline phosphatase and is referred to as the APAAP (alkaline phosphatase–anti-alkaline phosphatase) method. The PAP and APAAP techniques have almost completely replaced the simple unlabelled bridge technique from which they were originally developed.

The PAP technique is very sensitive but is longer and more complex to perform than the simple direct immunofluorescence technique (see *Colour plate 25*).

Endogenous enzymes may cause background reactions

One possible disadvantage of using enzymes as labelling reagents is that the tissue may contain similar enzymes. Alkaline phosphatases and peroxidases are common in tissues. The enzymes within the tissue are **endogenous** and if they are allowed to react with the substrate they will produce the same chromogen as the exogenous enzyme used to label the antibody.

The presence of endogenous enzyme can be seen if a section is treated with the same technique as the test section but omitting the enzyme-labelled antibody step. Any colour produced can only be due to the tissue enzymes.

This background is a nuisance and needs to be suppressed. One method is to inactivate the endogenous enzyme before performing the immunocyto-chemistry reaction and this is probably the best way if it can be done conveniently.

Blocking may be specific for the enzyme, e.g. using methanol containing 0.3% hydrogen peroxide will inhibit peroxidase enzymes. Alternatively, the enzyme may be blocked non-specifically, e.g. using formaldehyde or other fixatives. This works quite well for the APAAP method and since the technique is often carried out on paraffin wax-processed tissue there is no need to deliberately inactivate the enzyme. The peroxidases in tissues are less easily inactivated in this way and even paraffin wax-processed tissue may still retain significant peroxidase activity and may need to be inactivated specifically using methanol/hydrogen peroxide.

Antibodies may be adsorbed non-specifically on to the tissues

The high sensitivity of the PAP method may itself cause difficulties if the bridging antibody is absorbed or adsorbed on to the tissue at sites where there is no antigen. The bridging antibody will then bind the PAP complex and give a non-specific background colour. This non-specific background can be eliminated by treating the section with a normal serum from the same species as the bridging antibody. Thus, if the bridging antibody was goat anti-rabbit immunoglobulin, then the section would first be treated with diluted normal goat serum. Any binding sites capable of non-specific reaction with goat serum will bind the non-immune serum and be blocked. The immune serum will not be bound and as a result the background will be cleaner.

Box 10.8 The PAP method has some limitations

The PAP and APAAP methods are better for most purposes in histology but fluorescent methods still have their advantages. Firstly, the fluorescence can be easier to locate if there is not a great deal of antigen present, for example trying to locate a few bacteria in a large section. Secondly, the method can be quantitative by measuring the fluorescence. Finally, the fluorescence shows where the antibody is located and can move with the antibody. Enzyme labelling only shows where the antibody occurs if the antibody does not move. If the antibody can move, then it will show where the antibody was at the time the chromogen was being produced. This can be important in some applications. For example, the membrane of a cell is constantly being recycled and the recycling can be demonstrated by 'capping'. An antibody against a cell membrane protein is applied to living cells. The membrane will be evenly labelled all around the membrane. As the membrane is recycled by being drawn into the cell, the membrane proteins form a cap just above where the membrane is being drawn back into the cytoplasm.

Initially even labelling   'Capping' of the label

The PAP technique is not reliably quantitative

Enzyme labelling techniques, and particularly the bridging techniques, are not quantitative (see *Box 10.8*). The method produces such high amplification that even small amounts of antigen can give strong results for very little antigen. If the antigen is highly concentrated in the tissues, then it may even give a weaker response.

High concentrations of antigen can block the adsorption of the PAP

This incongruous result is due to the bridging antibody effectively being blocked by the high concentration of primary antibody that is bound when there is a lot of antigen in the tissue.

   Following the previous example, the goat anti-rabbit IgG antibody is divalent and can bind two rabbit antibodies. Provided the rabbit antibodies are well separated within the tissues and there is a large excess of goat antibodies, then each goat anti-rabbit IgG molecule will only have one of its binding sites attached to the primary rabbit antiserum. The second binding site will then attach to the PAP complex. However, if there is a lot of antigen, then the antibodies will be closer together and the concentration may be higher locally than the concentration of the goat anti-rabbit immunoglobulin. This results in many, or indeed most, of the bridging antibodies binding with *both* of its binding sites to the primary antiserum (see *Fig. 10.4*). There will be few or no free binding sites to bind the PAP, so the final colour will be less. This mechanism also explains why using a more dilute reagent will give a stronger result when there is a lot of antigen in the specimen. The PAP technique should therefore be used to detect the presence of antigen but not used to attempt to quantify the amount, even approximately.

□ Primary antibody   ▶━ Bridging antibody   PAP PAP complex

Figure 10.4
Effect of high antigen density on staining. On the left, the primary antibodies are widely spaced, so the bridging antibody is not saturated and has free binding sites to bind the PAP complex. On the right, the primary antibodies are close enough to allow the antibody to bind to the antigen using both binding sites, resulting in no free binding sites for the PAP complex

Controls are needed to ensure specificity and correct technique

To ensure the technique is working correctly, a minimum of three controls is needed. These must be done at the same time and in the same way as the test section:

1. A known positive control (weakly reacting is best). This control must show a positive reaction. A negative shows a failure to react, indicating that a negative result in the test section is unreliable.
2. A known negative control. This should be negative. Any positive result shows whether there is a non-specific result. Any positive reactions in the test section would be unreliable.
3. A control using the test section but omitting the first (primary) antibody. This control should be negative. If this is positive, it may indicate an endogenous enzyme in the test section, or non-specific adsorption of one of the other reagents.

The above three controls should detect any discrepancies. If any unexpected results are seen, they must be investigated further by using extra control steps to determine the nature of the discrepancy (e.g. blocking controls, no application of any antibody, pre-treatment with HRP).

Avidin–biotin methods

Avidin is a glycoprotein found in egg white (see *Box 10.9*) that binds strongly to the vitamin biotin. This binding is much stronger than the usual antibody binding and is very difficult to disrupt. By linking biotin to the antibody, a complex can be formed that is very stable.

Box 10.9 Avidin

Avidin was originally discovered when rats that were fed a diet rich in raw egg whites began to suffer from biotin deficiency. The avidin was holding the biotin so effectively in the rat gut that the animals became deficient. The investigation of this 'toxicity' of egg protein led to the discovery of avidin. It is unlikely that eggs will have the same effect in humans as the eggs are usually cooked and the number of eggs eaten is usually quite small. Biotin is produced in quite large quantities by the normal gut bacteria and deficiency in humans is extremely rare.

Proteins can be labelled with biotin

Biotin can be conjugated to most proteins, carbohydrates and nucleic acids by using an active derivative. For proteins, this is usually sulpho-*N*-succin-imidobiotin, which can add the biotin on to free amino groups. Biotin is a small molecule and does not usually interfere with the activity of the protein. Biotinylation of antibodies is therefore an alternative method of labelling.

Avidin is used to bind on to the biotinylated protein

The biotin is then detected by using avidin, which binds to the biotin. The avidin itself has a label attached, which can be fluorescent or an enzyme. The most popular of these techniques uses an avidin–biotin complex

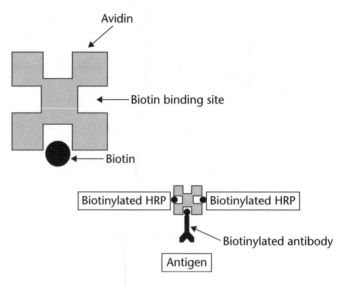

Figure 10.5
Avidin–biotin method. The avidin acts as a bridge between the biotinylated antibody and the biotinylated HRP. The avidin in the lower diagram shows a free biotin binding site, which can be used to bind the 'ABC' reagent

('ABC'), which combines several avidin molecules and several peroxidase molecules. The enzymes are biotinylated so that they will bind to the avidin molecule (see *Fig. 10.5*). This complex is much larger than the PAP complex and contains more peroxidase, but despite this the ABC method is about comparable in sensitivity to the PAP method.

The ratio of biotin and avidin can be varied

A biotin-rich complex, known colloquially as 'CBA', can be used to boost the activity. The CBA is used after the ABC reagent and is bound to the ABC complex by its extra biotin, thus adding an extra layer. The CBA can then be followed by an extra treatment with the ABC reagent, which can bind to the excess biotin in the CBA. This in turn can be followed by ABC and so on. This alternation of biotin-rich and avidin-rich layers could be compounded to give a number of repeats but this is pointless as beyond two or three extra steps the added sensitivity will be counterbalanced by a loss of specificity.

The avidin in all of the above techniques can be replaced by the protein **streptavidin,** which is extracted from the bacterium *Streptomyces* and has similar binding properties. It is preferred by many workers because it gives less background staining.

The use of biotin as a label also has its own problems as many tissues, including liver and kidney, have significant amounts of endogenous biotin and can give false-positive results.

Immunogold labelling

Immunogold labelling uses particles of colloidal gold to label the antibody. The colloidal gold is adsorbed on to the protein and acts as a visible label. This is very popular with electron microscopists as the spherical gold particles are easily seen in the electron microscope. The colloidal gold can be made in differing particle sizes so that it is possible to use two different-sized labels to identify two antigens in the same preparation. Although mainly used for electron microscopy, colloidal gold can be made visible for light microscopy using silver solutions. The silver reagents react with the gold and produce an enhanced blackening easily seen by light microscopy.

Polymer-conjugated systems (EPOS and EnVision patented systems)

This system uses a polymer spine (dextran) with multiple (e.g. ten) antibodies and multiple enzymes (up to 70) attached. This acts in a similar way to PAP but with much higher levels of enzyme giving a strong response. To what extent the spine interferes with penetration is still uncertain.

Polymer-conjugated systems have several advantages. The inert dextran backbone has no great affinity for tissue protein or other components, so there is little endogenous binding (unlike the avidin technique, which binds to biotin in the tissues). There is possibly some increased sensitivity compared with basic streptavidin methods. It is much quicker as there are fewer steps than alternative techniques. There are some disadvantages including the possibility that the size of the polymer may impede penetration into the tissues and thus reduce binding. The reagents are also more expensive than the reagents used in simpler techniques.

Antigen retrieval methods

The fluorescent antibody technique usually only works well on fresh frozen tissue but the high sensitivity of the PAP and ABC methods allows them to be used on paraffin-embedded sections. This has probably been one of their major advantages as the method can be applied to routine blocks with no need to plan in advance for the use of immunostaining and old blocks from the archives can be used quite effectively. Indeed, it is even possible to perform the techniques on stained sections from which the coverslips have been removed. The results from paraffin sections can, however, sometimes be disappointing as the fixation and processing can alter the antigens. To restore the full immunoreactivity of the sections, various techniques have been tried. These techniques are referred to as unmasking of the antigen or **antigen retrieval methods**.

Enzyme retrieval

The first method involved the use of enzymes to digest away some of the protein to expose the masked antigenic sites. Usually it is a proteolytic enzyme, such as trypsin or pepsin, that is used to remove protein. The enzymes need to be prepared freshly as they lose activity once in solution. This works well in most instances, but can be very sensitive to the conditions of incubation. Too long an incubation may remove excess protein and associated antigen, whilst too short an incubation may not unmask the antigen fully. The timing is also very dependent on fixation. This dependency is on both the type of fixative used, with formaldehyde generally being preferred, and also on the length of fixation, with long fixation times needing longer subsequent digestion. Because of these variables, it is usually necessary to test the timing and the technique for each batch of enzyme and sometimes for each individual specimen to get optimal staining.

This variability has led to some workers questioning the validity of the technique and arguing that some of the results may represent an artefact of the digestion process rather than the site of preformed antigen. However, the technique does seem to give reliable and useful results if well controlled and has been widely adopted for paraffin sections; it is less useful for fresh tissue.

Heat retrieval

An alternative to using enzymes is to heat the section. Simple heating is insufficient (see *Box 10.10*) and it requires prolonged exposure to boiling or superheated fluid to achieve the retrieval. Usually a sodium citrate solution buffered to a slightly acid pH is used and the heating can be achieved using a microwave oven or a pressure cooker. The sections do have a much greater tendency to detach from the slide, so the use of adhesives such as silane for coating the slides is needed (see Chapter 3).

Box 10.10 Antigen retrieval needs superheated water

Dry heating of sections does not seem to unmask antigens in the same way as wet heat. It seems likely that there is a hydrolysis effect and the energy needed to activate this is quite high. Simple boiling of the section is less efficient. Microwaves probably produce temperatures above the normal boiling point within the solution and pressure cookers also have a higher temperature than the standard boiling point of water.

Microwave retrieval. In the microwave method the dewaxed sections are placed in buffer in a microwave oven and heated at full power for 10–30 min depending on the antigen to be unmasked, the power of the microwave and the fixation of the tissue. The fluid rapidly boils and if this is being done in a Coplin jar, which hold about 50 ml of fluid, it results in boiling of the fluid and often the buffer spills out, so the fluid needs to be constantly replenished. By using larger containers with an excess of buffer, it may be possible to have sufficient fluid to avoid the need to replenish. The sections are allowed to cool in the buffer and then transferred to distilled water. If the sections are removed whilst still hot, this may result in loss of reactivity to the antibodies This method is rapidly gaining popularity as it does not need to be optimized for different batches of enzyme.

Pressure cooker retrieval. Pressure cookers are an alternative way of heating the sections and use higher temperatures since water boils at a higher temperature at higher pressures. An ordinary stainless steel domestic pressure cooker is used. It is partially filled with citrate buffer and brought to the boil at normal pressure (the cooker is not sealed) before putting in the slides. The pressure cooker is then sealed and brought back to the boil at raised pressure. Most pressure cookers work at 1 atmosphere above normal pressure and this raises the boiling point of water to about 120°C. The increased temperatures reached mean that antigen retrieval times are much shorter, typically 2–4 min once the full pressure is reached. Pressure cookers can also treat many more slides at once than a microwave oven.

It is also possible to use two methods of retrieval by microwaving the sections first, cooling them to 37°C and then treating them with a protease enzyme.

The choice of retrieval method is largely a matter of personal choice, the method of tissue preparation and the antigen being sought. Some antigens will be demonstrated by heat retrieval but not by enzyme digestion and vice versa. Often there are several different techniques being employed within the same laboratory for different purposes. One beneficial aspect of the use of retrieval methods is that the antibodies can often be used in more dilute solutions with dilution factors in excess of 1/10,000 being cited in some papers.

10.2 LABELLING OF OTHER PROTEINS

Proteins other than antibodies can also be labelled using the same general methods as explained above.

Lectin histochemistry

Lectins are plant, or occasionally animal, proteins that bind to sugar molecules rather than antigens but otherwise the reaction has much in common with antibody binding. They are not immune proteins but occur

Box 10.11 Lectins

Lectins were originally identified by their ability to agglutinate red blood cells. The agglutination can be specific for certain blood groups since the blood group antigens contain sugars and the different blood groups have different terminal sugars. Lectins can be toxic in some cases since, if they are absorbed intact without being digested, they will agglutinate the red cells in blood and cause a haemolytic disorder. Some types of bean contain sufficient lectin concentrations to cause disease in this way if they are eaten uncooked. Not all lectins are dangerous poisons, however, and they are currently being investigated for possible use in drug delivery to specific sites.

endogenously in the tissues of the plant without needing to 'immunize' it. Like antibodies, they can bind more than one sugar (they are polyvalent). Unlike antibodies, many lectins need specific cations to bind effectively and these need to be added, e.g. concanavalin A needs calcium ions to bind effectively. Lectins may be highly toxic (see *Box 10.11*) as they can interfere with sugar interactions.

Only terminal sugars react

The sugars to which the lectins bind can be part of proteins (glycoproteins) or can be complex carbohydrates or in the form of mucins, but in all cases only the terminal sugars can be accessed. Sugars buried inside protein or bound inside polysaccharides are not usually available to the lectins and will not be detected. Lectins can be used as very precise reagents for locating sugars in tissues. *Table 10.1* lists some lectins and their specificities. Lectins sometimes react with other sugars but with a decreased binding strength. The use of lectins in histochemistry has greatly increased in the past few years as the importance of carbohydrates in cell recognition, cell adhesion and metabolic control has been realized.

Table 10.1 **Examples of some lectins and their specificities**

Lectin	Abbreviation	Source	Specificity
Concanavalin A	Con A	*Canavalia ensiformis*	α-Mannose, α-glucose, N-acetylglucosamine (GlcNAc)
Wheat germ agglutinin	WGA	*Triticum vulgare*	GlcNAc-β-1,4-GlcNAc
Horse gram lectin	DBA	*Dolichos biflorus*	GalNAc-α-1,3-GalNAc
Gorse lectin	UAE	*Ulex europaeus*	α-L-Fucose
Horseshoe crab lectin	LPA	*Limulus polyphemus*	N-Acetyl neuraminic acid

Lectins can be located by several different methods

Lectins can be treated simply as an antigen and injected into an animal to raise antibodies against them and used in one of the labelling strategies already explained. Lectins can be applied to tissue sections and, after washing away the excess, any bound lectin can be identified by a standard immunotechnique. Lectins are also available as fluorescent conjugates, biotinylated lectins and enzyme-labelled lectins. These can be employed in a similar fashion to antibodies labelled in these ways.

Finally, lectins can occasionally be demonstrated using carbohydrate-containing enzymes. Glucose oxidase, for example, contains about 18% carbohydrate. The lectin can bind to the sugars present in the enzyme. The glucose oxidase can then be demonstrated simply using an enzyme technique. This greatly simplifies the technique compared with most other labelling methods. This works well for concanavalin A but is less successful with other lectins as the specific sugars they bind to are not always available in the enzyme. HRP can also be used in the same way but suffers slightly from the presence of endogenous peroxidase, whilst human tissue does not contain any glucose oxidase activity so there is no background staining.

Protein A

Protein A is a staphylococcal protein with a highly specific affinity for the Fc part of mammalian IgG. It can be used in the same way as an anti-immunoglobulin. Protein A can be obtained commercially labelled with fluorescent dyes, biotin and enzymes. One benefit of using protein A is that it is not species specific and will detect most mammalian IgGs. This is sometimes useful as it reduces the need to have several different anti-immunoglobulins when using primary antisera from different animal species. Its disadvantage is that it cannot be used in tissues containing endogenous IgG. Anti-human IgG can be used on rat lymph nodes as they will not contain human IgG but protein A cannot be used on any lymph nodes as it will react with all mammalian IgGs.

Specific receptors

Hormones will be bound by their specific receptors within the tissues and this can be used to detect the location of such receptors. This is fairly straightforward if the hormone is a protein and can be labelled in the same way as other proteins.

Some receptors can be detected using exogenous proteins that will bind to the receptor. These techniques using specific binding materials are often unique and, although useful and important, do not have much in common beyond the facts that they bind tightly with a receptor within the tissue and that they can be labelled or conjugated by one of the methods already outlined without altering their binding ability. For example, α-bungarotoxin is found in the venom of a Taiwanese snake and binds to the acetylcholine receptor of the neuromuscular junction and this can be used to locate and identify the receptors. α-Bungarotoxin is available commercially labelled with biotin and fluorescein. The general concept of labelling a protein that binds to the tissue in some specific way applies to all such exogenous binding materials. The source of the binding agent, however, can be quite varied.

There is one final labelling technique that can be applied to many materials and that is autoradiography. This is the subject of the next chapter.

SUGGESTED FURTHER READING

Brooks, S.A., Leatham, A.J.C. and Schumacher, U. (1997) *Lectin Histochemistry*. Oxford: Royal Microscopical Society.

Carlton, S.J. (2002) Immunofluorescent techniques. In *Theory and Practice of Histological Techniques*, 5th edn (eds J.D. Bancroft and M. Gamble). Edinburgh: Churchill Livingstone.

Kiernan, J.A. (2001) *Histological and Histochemical Methods*, 3rd edn. Oxford: Hodder Arnold.

Miller, K.D. (2002) Immunocytochemical techniques. In *Theory and Practice of Histological Techniques*, 5th edn (eds J.D. Bancroft and M. Gamble). Edinburgh: Churchill Livingstone.

SELF-ASSESSMENT QUESTIONS

1. Define the terms antibody and antigen and explain briefly why antibodies are useful as histochemical reagents.
2. Outline how fluorescein is used as an antibody-labelling material.
3. What are the disadvantages of the immunofluorescent technique?
4. What enzymes are used in immunological staining?
5. Outline the steps needed in the PAP (or APAAP) technique.
6. How can the PAP technique be used in electron microscopy?
7. What is meant by antigen retrieval and how can it be achieved?
8. Describe the use of lectins in histochemistry.
9. What is the main use of immunogold labelling?
10. What is the use of avidin in the ABC technique of antibody labelling?

Autoradiography

Learning objectives

After studying this chapter you should confidently be able to:

■ **Outline the principles of autoradiography.**
Autoradiography uses radioisotopes to follow the fate of molecules in the body. The labelled compounds are used in cell cultures or experimental animals and metabolized by the cells. Sections of the tissue can be prepared and the isotopes are located using photographic emulsions. Ionizing radiation released by the isotopes affects the photographic emulsion, which shows blackened areas following development.

■ **Name some radioisotopes commonly used in autoradiography and the nature of their radiations.**
These are ^{3}H (tritium), ^{14}C, ^{32}P and ^{35}S. These are all β-emitters with energies varying from 19 to 1710 keV.

■ **Outline possible problems in autoradiography.**
Incorrect localization may occur due to movement of the emulsion, separation of the emulsion and section or processing causing relocation of the labelled compound. Fogging of the emulsion may cause problems and can be due to light exposure, chemical contamination or mechanical damage.

11.1 THE PROCESS OF AUTORADIOGRAPHY

Autoradiography is a method of accurately following the fate of chemicals in cells and organs using radioisotopes as labels. It is widely used to trace the routes of metabolism of drugs within animals and so this will be used as an example to show how an autoradiographic investigation is planned and carried out. The applications of autoradiography are very widespread and it is one of the most useful techniques in research.

The fate of a drug in the body involves two phenomena:

■ how and where it is distributed within the body; and
■ how it is metabolized and excreted.

Ideally we would like to be able to follow both of these processes. The actual concentrations of most drugs within cells and tissues are generally quite low,

---

Box 11.1 Discovery of autoradiography

The first autoradigraph was done before there was any knowledge of radioactivity and before radioactivity was even suspected. Autoradiography was the first method of identifying radioactivity. Uranium salts were thought to be fluorescent. Antoine Henri Becquerel was testing some salts and left them on top of a paper-covered film in a draw ready to irradiate them with light the following day. They were left unused for a few days, so rather than irradiating them he decided to just develop the film anyway. He was surprised to see blackening since fluorescence should not have occurred in the absence of light. This was the first indication of material producing unknown rays in the absence of heating or absorption of light.

---

so detecting the drug using conventional chemical tests would be difficult or impossible. To overcome this problem, radioactive materials are used, which can allow the detection of just a few molecules of drug.

Steps involved in autoradiography

The first step is to prepare some of the drug but replacing one of the normal stable isotopes with a radioactive isotope. The drug is then administered to an animal or put into a tissue culture medium. The drug is absorbed, distributed in the tissues and may be metabolized. Sections of the animal tissues can then be made. The radioactive isotope will decay and emit radiation, which can be detected using photographic film that reacts to the radiation as it would to light. The exposed film is developed in the same way as for photography and areas that have been exposed to radioactivity will show up as black areas (see *Fig. 11.1*). Only a few atoms decaying radioactively are needed to detect their position in the tissue, so it is extremely sensitive. It is also necessary to be able to locate the film over the original section accurately so that the position of the isotope can be determined. *Colour plate 26* shows an example of microscopic autoradiography.

Autoradiography can also detect metabolic products

Not only can the distribution of the drug be identified but also the way in which it has been modified by the cells. The metabolism of the drug can be followed by autoradiography – as the compound is broken down or changed by the cells or enzymes, the radioactive atoms will be incorporated into the breakdown products. By sampling over a period of time, the fate of the drug can be followed up to its final excretion from the body. Although the body is always full of thousands of different metabolites, only the radioactive drug and its metabolites are actually traced. This is possible since all of the non-labelled compounds are ignored because they lack radioactivity and so do not register on the autoradiogram.

Although autoradiography is relatively simple to do, it requires careful planning to give good results since there are many potential pitfalls in the technique.

1. Prepare a radioactively labelled drug

2. Administer to a laboratory animal

3. Take tissue samples and prepare sections

4. Cover the section with photographic emulsion

5. Leave to allow radioactivity to affect the film. Then develop the emulsion. Blackened areas show the sites of the radiolabelled material.

Figure 11.1
Outline of the steps in autoradiography

11.2 RADIOACTIVE LABELS

Choice of label

Labelling involves making a sample of the drug with one or more radioactive atoms. This is done by synthesizing the drug using a radioactive precursor. Many standard synthetic reagents are available in radioactive form from commercial sources, so it is possible to make almost any compound. However, it is not simple or cheap and should be done by an expert chemist as radioactivity is dangerous and the preparations are usually done on a very small scale since the radioactive starting compounds are so expensive.

It is important to think carefully about the choice of label before getting the radiolabelled drug synthesized.

Box 11.2 Not all important atoms can be radioactively labelled

Some elements have no isotopes that can be used for autoradiography. There are, for example, no useful isotopes of oxygen, nitrogen or chlorine. Thus, labelling cannot be done for every atom in the molecule and the fate of some atoms must be guessed. In some cases, they can be determined by using non-radioactive isotopes and mass spectrometry to determine their fate. This can be done with oxygen, which has a heavy but non-radioactive isotope.

Table 11.1 **Properties of radioactive emissions**

Type of radiation	Nature	Charge	Applications
α	Helium nucleus	+	Good but few α-emitters are interesting biologically
β	Electron	–	Localization poorer than α-particles but many of the atoms found in biological specimens have β-emitting isotopes
γ	Electromagnetic radiation	0	Useless for autoradiography but can be a nuisance since γ-rays are often emitted along with β-particles

Choice of radioisotope

It is not possible to replace every individual element since not all atoms have suitable radioisotopes (see *Box 11.2*). Radioactive decay can produce three forms of radiation, as described in *Table 11.1*.

α-Particles. α-Particles are quite large and heavy. They are able to penetrate only a short distance through tissues or photographic film, so they always affect the film very close to the site of the decaying atom and the accuracy of localization is good. It is made even better because the α-particle causes many electrons to be displaced as it passes through the photographic film so that its track can be seen as a straight line. If the lines all converge on one point (see *Fig. 11.2*), then the position of the isotope can be located very accurately.

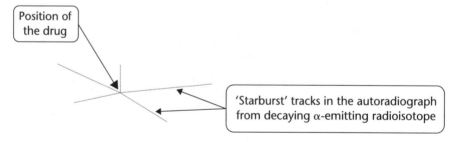

Position of the drug

'Starburst' tracks in the autoradiograph from decaying α-emitting radioisotope

Figure 11.2
Appearance of the effect of α-decay in an autoradiogram. The centre point of the tracks indicates the location of the α-emitting isotope

Unfortunately most of the α-emitting isotopes are not common elements in biological molecules, so although α-emitters would be good for auto-radiography, they are rarely used in biology.

γ-Emitters. γ-Emitters are useless for autoradiography since γ-rays can travel very large distances from their origin. Thus, even if they do cause blacken-

---

Box 11.3 Microradiography

Autoradiography is sometimes confused with microradiography. Microradiography involves placing a small piece of tissue or a tissue section on to a piece of film and then irradiating it with X-rays or γ-rays. This is similar to ordinary radiographic methods used in medicine to visualize bones and teeth and will detect radio-opaque materials in the section. Autoradiography is different in using radioactivity within the tissue and using mainly poorly penetrating β-particles to detect radiolabelled materials.

---

ing of the film it may be several millimeters away from their origin. Since γ-rays are emitted along with β-particles, they can be a cause of background blackening of the film, which is a nuisance.

β-particles. β-Particles are usually used in autoradiography. They are relatively light and have the same negative charge as the electrons in the outer shells of atoms. β-Particles are therefore often deflected by the electron shells of atoms. As a result of these deflections, the electrons do not travel through the tissues or the autoradiographic film in straight lines but tend to wander around. Depending on their energy, they may cause blackening some distance away from the isotope's actual position. They also do not leave linear tracks in the film because they dislodge comparitively few atoms from the radiographic emulsion.

Figure 11.3
The track of β-particles in an autoradiographic emulsion. The left-hand photograph shows the path of the particle, whilst the right-hand one shows the sites of silver grains. Only one or two points on the β-particle's track leave a silver grain. With β-particles, the accuracy of localization is less precise and all that can be assumed is that the radioactivity is somewhere within the circle

If there are many radioactive disintegrations at the same point, then there will be a lot of grains forming a 'cloud' around the site of the radioactivity. The location of the isotope is somewhere within this cloud of dots but its exact position can only be an estimate (see *Fig. 11.3*).

β-Emitting isotopes include useful elements such as carbon, hydrogen and sulphur

There are a lot of very useful β-emitters (see *Table 11.2*). Suitable isotopes include hydrogen (tritium), carbon, sulphur and phosphorus. With β-rays, the localization is affected by the energy of the radiation, which is usually measured in electron volts (eV). Tritium (^3H) is one of the best isotopes for localization as it has a low-energy emission. Tritium can even be used in the electron microscope to localize to the subcellular level; for example, it can determine whether the drug is in the nucleus or the cytoplasm. With very careful technique, it is even possible to estimate whether the isotope is in a mitochondrion or in the cytosol or in the case of the nucleus to which chromosome it is bound.

Table 11.2 Radioisotopes and their properties

	Energy (keV)	Half-life (t½)	Effective resolution (μm)
^3H (tritium)	19	12.3 years	0.5
^{14}C	156	5730 years	2–5
^{32}P	1710	14.3 days	5–10
^{35}S	167	87.4 days	2–5

The effective resolution (*Table 11.2*) indicates how accurately the position of the isotope can be determined. Carbon and sulphur are quite good for light microscopy magnifications and can certainly locate the isotope to individual cells. Phosphorus is less accurate for microscopy but is still useful for macroscopic and electrophoretic uses and can be relied on to locate the isotope to small groups of cells.

The half-life of the isotope is important

As well as the energy of the β-particles from the isotope, it is often important to consider the half-life of the isotope. The half-life is a measure of how quickly the atoms decay. Radioactive decay is a random event, so it is only possible to be specific about the behaviour of many atoms and not individual atoms. We can never tell when an individual atom will decay but we can be quite accurate in saying that, of a thousand atoms, half will have decayed in a set time. That time is the half-life of the isotope. Half-lives vary tremendously. Carbon and tritium have long half-lives (5730 years and 12.3 years) but phosphorus is relatively short-lived (14 days). Isotopes with long half-lives are usually more convenient experimentally as they can be used over long periods, so experiments can last several weeks or years without significant loss of radioactivity. With phosphorus, the experiment needs to be quite brief. If the experiment required a 2 month time scale, then only about 6% of the original isotope would still be radioactive by the end of the experiment.

A second advantage of a long half-life is that the amount of blackening seen in the photographic emulsion can be increased by prolonging the time of exposure of the photographic film. Provided the radioactivity continues undiminished for a long time, the radioactivity will continue to expose the film and increase the density of the image. With a short half-life such as that of phosphorus, doubling the exposure will not increase the blackening effect very much. With an exposure time of 28 days (by no means unusual to detect very low concentrations of drug), three-quarters of all of the radioactivity will have already decayed and leaving the specimen indefinitely would only result in 25% more radioactive decay and 25% more blackening.

The safety also varies with half-life. Isotopes with long half-lives may cause disposal problems as they will remain radioactive long after the experiment has finished. An isotope with a short half-life will lose its radioactivity in simple storage and can be more easily discarded without worrying about the radiation hazard. Storing phosphorus for 1 year will make it effectively non-radioactive.

Safety is important as isotopes may concentrate in the body

The other aspects of safety are concerned with concentration in the body. Tritium is often rapidly diluted in the body because of the large amount of hydrogen present, particularly in water, but phosphorus concentrates in bone. This location does, however, depend on the form of the isotope. If it is incorporated into a molecule, it is not the nature of the isotope but the nature of the molecule that is important. Weaker radiations (e.g. tritium) do not penetrate far and are easily blocked, even by air. Unless the isotopes actually get into the body, they will not cause any damage since the dead cells on the skin will prevent the radiation reaching living cells. If they are ingested, the isotopes will come into direct contact with cells and this is when they are dangerous.

My own choice for a radioactive label would be tritium as it is long-lived, relatively safe and gives the best localization.

Choice of labelling site

The site of labelling must be suitable. Ionizable or exchangeable atoms are of no use since they will not follow the compound. Many hydrogen atoms fall into this category but carbon is more often stable within the compound and will be a better labelling site. For example, take the case of acetic acid. If we were to label it with tritium, it is vital that we choose the right atom. If we synthesize the acetic acid so that the tritium is the acidic hydrogen in the carboxyl group, then when the acetic acid dissociates in water the tritium will be lost into the fluid:

$$CH_3COOH + H_2O = CH_3COO^- + OH^- + 2H^+$$

It will not act as a tracer for the acetic acid. If, however, we synthesize the acetic acid with tritium attached as one of the hydrogens in the methyl group, it will not be displaced so easily and can be used to follow the acetic acid.

Box 11.4 Autoradiography is not a diagnostic technique

Autoradiography can never be a diagnostic tool since it involves administering radioactivity to the subject and usually involves killing the subject to recover the tissues. The results of autoradiography can sometimes be confirmed in humans by using positron-emitting isotopes. The positrons can be detected using detectors outside the body and the fate of compounds can be followed. The positrons are detected using tomography equipment that locates the emission in three dimensions. These investigations are called PET scans (positron emission tomography).

Double labelling is also possible in which two different atoms are replaced. For example, it would be possible to label the acetic acid with ^{14}C replacing the carbon in the carboxyl group and with tritium attached to the methyl carbon. If the acetic acid became split into the carboxyl group and the methyl group, it would be possible to track both fragments separately.

Administration and metabolism of the labelled compound

Once the labelled drug has been synthesized, it can then be administered (see *Box 11.4*). Usually this involves several small animals such as rats or mice being given the drug at the same time so that by examining animals at different times the fate of the drug can be followed. The drug can be given by mouth or injected as appropriate for the drug being tested. The animals are then allowed to metabolize the drug for differing periods before being killed and prepared for histology. How much of the labelled drug to give, how long to leave the animals and how frequently to sample the group of animals are all crucial questions, but it is difficult to give any guidelines since the answers are unique to each experiment. In some cases, it may be necessary to do a pilot study to get an idea of the right answers rather than trying to predict them theoretically.

11.3   HISTOLOGICAL PREPARATION

At the end of the experiment, the fresh tissue obtained from the animal must be sectioned and the processing of the tissue needs to be considered carefully. The main requirement is to ensure that the substance being detected is not lost or redistributed by the processing. Thus, questions need to be asked at every step in the process. Ideally these questions are all answered long before the experiment begins so that there is no delay in knowing how to treat the tissue once the animal is killed.

Choice of fixative

Questions that need to be considered include 'Does the tissue need to be fixed at all?', 'Will using a fixative affect the location of the drug?' and 'Which fixative should be used?'

Aldehyde- and mercury-based fixatives may fog the emulsion since they can react directly with the silver compounds in the film (chemical blackening of photographic film is called **chemography**). Alcohol is probably the safest fixative in this regard but it may dissolve many substances. Fixation in formaldehyde is usually not a problem in autoradiography provided the tissue is paraffin processed, as the formaldehyde will be washed out during processing. Mercury and glutaraldehyde are retained through processing and will cause problems.

Processing

Which technique to use is an important question. Again, this depends on the nature of the labelled compound. Avoiding dissolving or relocating the labelled material is the prime consideration rather than the method that will produce the best sections.

A few examples of experiments may help to explain the concept.

Identification of a labelled steroid

Steroids are lipids and therefore will be dissolved if any lipid solvent is used. Even if the steroid is bound to a receptor, it may be dissolved if any organic solvent is applied. The best method would seem to be to freeze the tissue in liquid nitrogen and cut cryostat sections. These can then be dried quickly to minimize movement of the steroid after cutting. Freeze-drying may not be the best method as it involves using paraffin wax to support the tissue after drying and paraffin wax is a lipid solvent.

Identification of a DNA base or base analogue (e.g. tritiated thymidine)

DNA base analogues can be incorporated into DNA during metabolism and are used as cytotoxic drugs in the treatment of some malignancies. Since the drug is bound into DNA, there is no problem with dissolving it in the usual solvents since DNA is retained in paraffin sections. The tissue can be safely fixed, processed to paraffin wax and sectioned as usual.

Determining whether an antibiotic crosses the blood–brain barrier

Many drugs are excluded from the brain tissue by a physiological barrier. If the drug is injected into an animal and an autoradiograph prepared of the head, it should be possible to see whether the drug has penetrated the neural tissues. In this case, there is no requirement for accurate microscopical location. The question we wish to be answered can be investigated macroscopically. There is no need to fix the tissues since preservation of fine detail is not needed. Processing would be kept to a minimum to prevent relocation of the drug. The simplest method is to freeze the whole head (or indeed the whole rat; *see Colour plate 27*). It can then be sectioned using a heavy-duty microtome. Sections can be relatively thick since again fine detail is not needed. Sections can be supported during cutting by the Sellotape technique (see Chapter 3).

Box 11.5 Autoradiographic emulsions

Photographic emulsions consist of silver halide crystals in a gelatine support. The size of the individual halide grains determines the accuracy of localization. Autoradiographic emulsions have very small grain sizes (fine-grain emulsions) so they can give accurate localization.

When a light ray or β-particle strikes a silver halide grain, it can knock an electron out of the crystal. This results in a silver ion being converted to a silver atom. This one atom then acts as a catalytic site for reduction by photographic developers such as quinol ('hydroquinone'). The whole silver grain turns black giving a visible speck in the autoradiograph. Without that catalytic silver atom, the developers do not cause reduction of the silver grains so they remain as white silver halide crystals.

The unused silver halide crystals must be dissolved out of the autoradiograph before it is examined in the light, otherwise it would slowly blacken in the light. This is done using sodium thiosulphate ('hypo') and is referred to as photographic fixing. This is photographic fixation to remove excess light-sensitive silver salts, not histological fixation in, for example, formaldehyde.

11.4   EXPOSURE TO EMULSION

Once the sections are obtained they need to be placed in contact with the photographic emulsion to detect the radioactivity (see *Box 11.5*). The type of emulsion or film used depends on the accuracy of location required.

For general localization to an organ, such as in the blood–brain barrier example above, this can be done using X-ray film. X-ray film is preferred to simple photographic film as it has a more regular and finer grain structure. The film needs to be held in contact with the specimen for several days and this is most easily done using a 'flower press' type of holder. This consists of two sheets of wood that can have wing nuts at the corners so that the two flat pieces of wood compress and flatten anything sandwiched between them. The film is removed from its wrapper in a dark room (only a faint safelight can be used) and put in contact with the specimen. It is then sandwiched between two or three sheets of thick blotting paper to act as a cushion. It is wrapped in aluminium foil to keep out the light and finally put into the press and the wing nuts are tightened up to hold it in place and prevent movement. It can then be left to expose. If several autoradiographs are being prepared at the same time, it is better to keep them as separate packages. This not only makes it easier to remove just one autoradiograph but also helps to prevent radiation from one sample affecting the film as they are pressed against each other.

Microscopic sections can be prepared by dipping in photographic emulsion

If the tissue is going to be examined microscopically, a more accurate localization is needed. The emulsion needs to be placed in very close contact with the specimen. The dipping technique uses a low melting point photographic emulsion that can be melted at about 40°C and then held as a liquid in a waterbath. Sections of tissue are brought to water, dipped into the liquid emulsion and then drained and cooled to allow the emulsion to harden. They are then stored to allow exposure. All of these preparations must be done in a darkroom lit only with a safelight and the final preparations must be kept dark. The slides are put into a Coplin jar or staining dish with some silica gel to keep them dry. The whole jar is then wrapped in aluminium foil to exclude light and put into a lightproof box to ensure no light affects them. Finally, they are put into a refrigerator until they have been exposed for a sufficient length of time. This dipping technique is quick, economical and simple to do. However, it has the disadvantages that the emulsion thickness is not uniform and the thickness can vary from one sample to the next making quantitation difficult.

Exposure is difficult to calculate

Exposure of the film is a somewhat hit and miss affair (see *Box 11.6*) in most cases, with several specimens being prepared and each one developed after different time to obtain the best results. Once the first one is done, the results give a reasonable idea of how long the total exposure needs to be to get good results. With a high level of radioactivity present, it may only take a few days to get sufficient exposure, but if the levels of radioactivity are low, then exposures can stretch into weeks or months.

Box 11.6 The problem of estimating the exposure time

Knowing how much radioactivity is present within the section is not enough to calculate exposure. The radioactivity might all be concentrated in one small area, so the local concentration might be high but the overall concentration in the section could be low. The best way is trial and error. In some cases, it may need more than one length of exposure. The hot spots of radioactivity will be best seen in short exposures, whilst areas with less radioactivity might need longer to produce sufficient silver grains.

Development is carried out in a high-contrast developer such as an X-ray developer and the emulsion is then fixed.

The section can be stained either before or after application of the emulsion. Staining after autoradiography can lead to the gelatine in the emulsion picking up the stain and becoming coloured. Staining the section before applying the emulsion risks the chemicals in the stains chemically affecting the emulsion and giving a false result. After staining, the stained section and overlying emulsion are examined microscopically. Areas of radioactivity show minute black silver grains surrounding the site of the radioactive decay. The small silver grains are more easily seen using a darkground microscope rather than a brightfield microscope (see Chapter 15).

11.5 PROBLEMS IN AUTORADIOGRAPHY

Although autoradiography is relatively simple to perform, it requires great care and attention to detail to get good results. Some of the potential problems are described below.

Incorrect localization of the radioactive site

This may occur due to movement of emulsion across the specimen resulting in all of the sites of radioactivity being localized at the wrong place.

If there is a gap between the emulsion and the section, then the image of the radioactivity will be spread out and blurred. One common source of such a separation is the trapping of an air bubble under the emulsion. Similar spreading of the radioactivity can occur with thick sections.

Fogging

Fogging of the film occurs when there is darkening of the film even where there is no radioactivity. This is also sometimes called excessive background. Fogging can be due to several causes, most of which are simply lack of due care.

If the emulsion is exposed to chemical agents capable of reducing the emulsion, they will cause similar changes to the radiation. Common sources of such reactive chemicals are fixatives, stains or contamination from fingers. Exposure to light will also affect the emulsion. This can be due to a darkroom that lets in daylight, an unsafe 'safelight' of the wrong type (a Wratten No. 2 safelight is usually recommended) or storage in a container that is not fully lightproof.

Finally, fogging can be due to storage in an area of high radioactivity. This is often done when radiation safety officers try to keep all sources of radiation in one place. The worst place to store an autoradiograph whilst it is being exposed is in a radioactivity laboratory.

Excessive local pressure such as finger pressure (or even more savage fingernail pressure) will also result in strong local blackening of the emulsion.

Quantitation

Quantitation of the amount of radioactivity can be performed by counting the number of silver grains above the area of interest. Although grain counting is quite accurate, it is a little tedious to count all of the grains. Converting from the number of grains to the actual amount of radioactivity requires a number of correction factors. Many things can alter the number of grains seen, such as the sensitivity of the emulsion used, the thickness of the emulsion, the section thickness, absorption of β-particles by the section ('self-absorption') and separation of the emulsion and the section. A simpler way is to incorporate some known standards into the block. These standards are solids with known amounts of radioactivity in them. As they are treated in the same way as the tissue, all of the factors should be the same for both, so the amount of radioactivity can be interpolated between the results that are found in the standards. Standards can be purchased or made in the laboratory by incorporating radioactivity into a sectionable material such as gelatine (which resembles tissue) or Araldite resin, such as that used in the preparation of electron microscopy blocks.

Problems with quantitation can arise from poor technique but there are also some basic physical limitations. β-Particles have a very limited range and will not penetrate through even quite thin sections. If the section thickness is variable, and this is usually the case in histology, it is better to have a thick section than a thin one. The β-particles will only be able to escape and affect the emulsion from the top few micrometres of the block; in the case of tritium this will be about 3 μm. Any β-particle emitted more than 3 μm below the surface will be absorbed by the tissue of the section and will not reach the surface. This means that it does not matter whether the block is 10 μm or 10 mm thick as only the top 3 μm will be measured. This thickness is referred to as the **infinity thickness**. Provided a section is greater than this infinity thickness, then the section thickness is irrelevant.

As a final comment, it can be seen that if you want accurate localization of a radioisotope you need a thin section, but if you want to know how much radioactivity is present you need a thick section. In autoradiography, as in everything else, it is not possible to do everything on a single specimen.

SUGGESTED FURTHER READING

Anon. (1992) *Guide to Autoradiography*. Amersham: Amersham International.
Rogers, A.W. (1979) *Techniques of autoradiography*. Amsterdam: Elsevier.

SELF-ASSESSMENT QUESTIONS

1. How does autoradiography trace chemicals in the body?
2. A new synthetic prostaglandin has been synthesized. Outline how you would plan an autoradiographic experiment. (The drug is hydrophobic with a low solubility in water and is expected to bind to receptors in blood vessel walls.)
3. Name the radioisotope you could use to label the following compounds (a) C_2H_5OH; (b) $HSCH_2CH(NH_2)CO_2H$; (c) H_2O_2 and (d) H_3PO_4. Indicate which atoms would be suitable for stable labelling.
4. What is meant by fogging? Name two possible causes of fogging.

Exfoliative cytology and related techniques

Learning objectives
After studying this chapter you should confidently be able to:

■ **Outline the advantages of exfoliative cytology.**
Collection of material for exfoliative cytology is simpler, quicker and cheaper than surgical collection of biopsy specimens.

■ **Indicate why cytology can be used for screening.**
It is less invasive and can be repeated at regular intervals without undue stress to the patient.

■ **Describe the normal constituents of a cervical smear.**
Normally there will be squamous epithelial cells from different layers of the cervical epithelium (superficial, intermediate and parabasal cells) and endocervical cells from the endocervix. Some blood cells may be present depending on the stage of the cycle (neutrophils, leukocytes, erythrocytes) but large amounts or their presence at certain times may not be fully normal. Some bacteria are normal (lactobacilli) and small amounts of mucin and spermatozoa are not abnormal.

■ **Describe the changes that occur in gynecological smears with age, menstrual cycle and pregnancy and the underlying causes of these changes.**
The appearance of the smear is controlled by the hormones oestrogen and progesterone. Oestrogen increases the number of mature, superficial cells and decreases the amount of mucin and the number of neutrophils seen. Oestrogen effects are seen in sexually mature women during the proliferative stage of the menstrual cycle. Progesterone decreases the maturation so more intermediate and parabasal cells appear, with fewer superficial cells. Progesterone also increases the glycogen content of cells and this may result in an increase in bacteria and as a consequence an increase in the number of leukocytes. Progesterone effects are seen in the secretory phase of the menstrual cycle and also during pregnancy. In the absence of progesterone and oestrogen, there is less growth of the epithelium and more parabasal cells are seen. Lack of both hormones is seen in pre-puberty and post-menopausal smears.

■ **Outline the appearance of a smear showing inflammation and name some common causes of inflammation.**
Neutrophil leukocytes are more common, mucin may be increased and there may be signs of haemorrhage with increased numbers of erythrocytes. The causative organism may be visible. There may be degenerative changes in the cells and altered staining of the cells. Common organisms include *Candida albicans*, *Trichomonas vaginalis* and herpes and human papilloma viruses.

■ **Describe the changes in smears in pre-malignant and malignant states.**
Loss of uniformity is common. Nuclear abnormalities include altered nuclear size and altered nucleocytoplasmic ratio, abnormal chromatin distribution, prominent nucleoli, multinucleation and abnormal staining.

■ **Outline why a smear may be considered inadequate.**
This can be due to too few cells, excessive mucus, pus or erythrocytes that obscure the cells, incorrect sampling technique resulting in air-drying or inadequate fixation artefacts.

One of the major problems with histological diagnosis is the need for a piece of tissue to prepare sections. This means surgery. Surgery is expensive since it needs anaesthetics, sterile conditions and highly trained personnel. It would be much cheaper and simpler if there was no need to cut into the body and cells could be removed without the need for surgery. Exfoliative cytology is just such a method of obtaining cells for diagnosis without having to cut into the body.

Exfoliative cytology relies on cells being shed naturally from a surface (see *Box 12.1*). These cells can be collected without damage to the body so it is simpler and safer. The commonest form of exfoliative cytology is the use of smears from the uterine cervix to recognize the early stages of cancer (malignancy), but it is also useful for diagnosis of other diseases and for monitoring treatment. Although cervical smears are the most common form of smears, they are not the only type and specimens can be obtained from a wide variety of sources.

Box 12.1 The origins of exfoliative cytology

At first the idea of using shed cells was resisted as it seemed unreliable. Since only a sample of surface cells is examined, it was thought that a small or deep tumour would be missed and the accessibility of the cervix for histological biopsy made cytology unnecessary. Cytological diagnosis also relies on different criteria to histological sections since the relationship between cells is lost. It was only the persistence of Dr George Papanicolaou that showed the potential of the method. It still took many years before it became fully accepted. Papanicolaou published his first paper on cancer diagnosis using smears in 1928 but it was not until after the Second World War that it became a recognized clinical method. Cervical screening in the UK began in the late 1940s with an early British pioneer in the field being Stanley Way in Gateshead who set up a screening service in 1948.

12.1   ADVANTAGES AND DISADVANTAGES OF EXFOLIATIVE CYTOLOGY

Advantages

Exfoliative cytology provides a useful alternative to histological examination since it has several advantages when compared with conventional biopsy techniques:

- The collection of specimens is relatively simple and causes very little damage since there is no cutting or incisions. It is considered a non-invasive technique.

- Both specimen collection and processing are quick. Cytology can be used for rapid diagnosis as an alternative to frozen sections. It is easily possible to have a smear ready for diagnosis in a similar time scale to that needed to prepare a frozen section. Speed is not usually the reason for using exfoliative cytology and most smears are processed as non-urgent and routine reports may take several days, but smears can be processed and reported on within an hour if necessary.

- The technique of specimen collection is cheaper since it does not require expensive aseptic surgery or even getting the patient into hospital. In many cases, it can be done during a visit to the GP and it can be carried out by a trained nurse or equivalent trained personnel and does not need a surgeon.

- Exfoliative cytology can be used as a screening method (see *Box 12.2*). Screening involves checking large numbers of apparently normal people for disease in the hope of finding the very early stages of disease in a few of them. It is always easier to treat a disease in the early stages, so early detection is of great benefit to the patient and can be cost-effective by reducing the need for expensive treatment of advanced disease. Screening with cytology is only possible because of the above advantages. It would not be possible to screen patients without symptoms if specimen collection was expensive, involved significant risk to the patient or was very painful.

Box 12.2 Screening

Whether to create a screening programme is a complex decision since it involves ethical, economic and social dimensions. The economic decision is the easiest. The cost of screening is compared with the costs of not screening. The costs of not screening include the extra cost of treating later stages of the disease and the loss of earnings from the disease. The social problems relate to the effects of worry and stress from any false positives or recalls. The ethical problems relate to how much pressure is used to get people to comply with the screening and whether it is morally justifiable *not* to screen for economic reasons. The aim of the Government is to have at least 80% of women between the ages of 25 and 60 screened for cervical disease at least once every 5 years.

Disadvantages

Exfoliative cytology does have some disadvantages when compared with a full histological biopsy:

- A negative result from a smear is less certain than with a histological section since the cells may reflect a poor sampling of the diseased area and not a genuine lack of disease. For this reason, a negative result on a smear should not be allowed to override a clinician's suspicions that there is a genuine disease present. If there is doubt, then the smear should be repeated.

■ Even in a situation where a tumour is detected by the smear, the actual site of the tumour may be uncertain. For example, if a fluid sample is taken, then abnormal cells could have come from anywhere that has come in contact with the fluid.

■ The screening of smears can be very tedious. Most of the cells in most of the samples will be normal and screeners can find it very difficult to maintain the concentration needed to detect the occasional abnormal cell. This is especially true for screening of 'well-women' samples where less than one in a hundred smears may show abnormality and even in the positive cases the majority of cells on a smear may be quite normal.

■ The exact nature of the tumour is less certain than when a biopsy is taken since only isolated cells can be seen and their relationship with adjacent cells is lost in the smearing process. Important characteristics such as tumours invading surrounding tissues cannot be seen directly in smears but only inferred from the appearance of the individual cells.

Because of these disadvantages, many pathologists prefer to confirm a positive cytological diagnosis with a biopsy before planning and applying any treatment.

12.2 GYNAECOLOGICAL SMEARS

The use of smears for the detection of cervical and endometrial malignancy is probably the best known of all the techniques and has been used for many years. When fully applied, it can lead to significant reductions in deaths in the target population. George Papanicolaou pioneered the use of cervical smears as a diagnostic method in the 1940s. He developed the main staining technique for smears and the technique is often referred to as a 'Papanicolaou test' and is often shortened so that the term 'pap smear' is a common designation for the cervical exfoliative cytology test.

Although the actual techniques of preparing the slides may be identical, there are two distinct types of specimen:

1. **Asymptomatic patients.** Samples from asymptomatic patients are collected as part of the cervical cytology screening programme to detect disease before it becomes apparent to either the patient or the clinician. The patients generally appear and feel healthy and the screening is done on a large section of the population. Since most smears are normal, the initial checking of these smears is not done by pathologists but by trained **cytoscreeners** who are mainly trying to separate those smears that are perfectly normal from those that are possibly showing some suspicious signs. The cytoscreeners do not make a final diagnosis although they may indicate the type of abnormality that they find. The positions of all abnormalities are marked on the slide (e.g. by a dot of ink next to the suspicious-looking cell) and the smears are then passed to the pathologist or cytologist for final diagnosis. All abnormalities are

reported and checked, not only malignancy and its early stages. Inflammation and infections are also significant findings and should not be ignored. Improvements in cell-recognition systems have allowed the use of computers for the initial screening. Computers can work continuously, do not tire and are more consistent than human screeners. A £1.3 million trial began in the UK in 2005 to compare manual screening with two automated systems. The results are due to be published in 2010.

2. **Symptomatic patients.** In this case, there is a clinical reason for taking the smear (see *Box 12.3*). The patient may report symptoms or the clinician may detect something during a physical examination. In this case, the purpose of the smear is to diagnose the condition and is not just for screening. The selection of which cases to investigate is done by the clinician, taking into account the symptoms and case history of the patient. The smears may also be used to monitor the effectiveness of treatment. These can often involve more invasive techniques and more frequent sampling since they can be justified by the symptoms. Smears from symptomatic patients should always be seen by the pathologist and not just screened and reported as 'no abnormality seen', since in this case a negative result is not expected and would be considered a significant finding.

Box 12.3 Symptomatic patients

Symptomatic patients will only really be seen if they go to see their GP with a particular problem. Patients will only visit their GP if the problem is one of the following:

- painful or uncomfortable
- worrying
- embarrassing or socially limiting
- disabling

Cervical cancer falls into none of these categories until the disease is well advanced and it is then difficult to treat. In the early stages of the disease, the signs are quite slight and easily missed. This makes cytological screening essential to detect the early and treatable stages of the disease.

The main use of exfoliative cytology is for gynaecological screening

Cancer of the cervix has proved to be a good disease to tackle with such screening. One reason for this is that the earliest signs of malignant change can be seen as simple nuclear changes (dyskaryosis) and alterations in the maturation of cells (dysplasia) in the cervical epithelium. These early changes are not malignant and often subside without progressing to malignancy, but in some cases they can lead to further change resulting in a carcinoma *in situ*. This may then develop into an invasive carcinoma if not treated. *Table 12.1* shows a typical time course of the disease.

Table 12.1   Typical time course of malignant changes in the cervix

	Age at onset (years)	Persistence
Dysplasia	30	10–20 years
Carcinoma *in situ*	40	5–10 years
Invasive carcinoma	60	1–4 years before symptoms become apparent

These times will vary with individual patients and there is evidence that these time scales are changing, even as an average for the population. Some of these changes are now being seen earlier than was previously the case although the reasons for this altered incidence are still disputed.

The pattern, however, remains the same with a significant delay in most cases between the time when the lesion becomes malignant and the time when it begins to invade other tissues. If each woman is checked every 3–5 years, then at least one of the samples should fall in the period between it becoming overtly malignant and the time when it spreads beyond the initial site.

The use of exfoliative cytology for detecting cervical disease has been a success story for screening. The rate of cancer deaths has fallen consistently since the introduction of screening (42% fall in the first 20 years). Mortality rates fell from 8.3 per 100,000 women in 1971 to 3.3 per 100,000 by 2003.

It is estimated that by using screening and early treatment 4500–5000 deaths are prevented in the UK each year. In total, the number of lives saved between 1987 and 2004 is estimated at 100,000.

The degree of protection or confidence that is offered by a negative smear depends on the frequency of testing and the age of the patient. The degree of protection from a single negative smear has been estimated and is shown in *Table 12.2*.

Table 12.2   Degree of protection offered from a single negative smear

	Age of patient (years)		
	20–39	40–54	55–69
3 yearly	41%	69%	73%
5 yearly	30%	63%	73%

The current scheme of testing in the UK is:

Age group	Frequency of screening
25	First invitation
25–49	3 yearly
50–64	5 yearly
65+	Only screened if not screened since 50 or has had a previous abnormal test

These are targets for screening but the frequency of screening is also dependent on how willing women are to be screened (see *Box 12.4*).

The logic of using a variable screening regime depending on the patient's age is that below 25 years of age abnormalities in the smear are common (but most regress) and invasive cancer is very rare so screening has little benefit. Patients over the age of 65 with three clear screens have almost no risk of developing the disease. By reducing the amount of screening the costs are reduced, the system is less overloaded and the psychological/social problems are reduced.

In the USA, screening is based on private medical care rather than a national screening programme and annual smears are carried out from the age of 28 onwards.

Types of gynaecological sample

The cells for cervical smears can be collected in a variety of ways, some of which are largely historical; others are likely to be replaced by the use of liquid-based techniques.

Aspiration of the posterior fornix

This technique collects a fluid sample from the vaginal cavity (see *Fig. 12.1*). This was the original technique used by Papanicolaou but has largely been replaced by direct scraping of the cervix or endometrial brushings. The major disadvantage with this method is that the cells have been shed for several hours (up to 48 h) before being collected and fixed. This long delay between shedding and fixing means that degeneration is more pronounced and this makes diagnosis more difficult and less certain than directly sampling the site.

Cervical scrape

This became the commonest technique when screening became widespread. The method usually used an Ayres spatula (see *Colour plate 28*) or one of its derivatives. The original Ayres spatula is possibly not ideal as it does not have a sufficiently elongated tip to ensure penetration of the external os. The cervix should be viewed whilst taking the smear to ensure

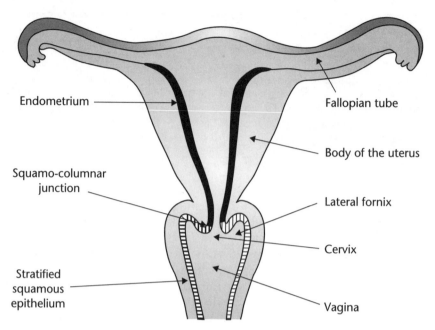

Endometrium

Fallopian tube

Body of the uterus

Squamo-columnar junction

Lateral fornix

Cervix

Stratified squamous epithelium

Vagina

Figure 12.1
Cross-sectional diagram of the vagina and uterus. The posterior fornix is situated behind the cervix and connects with the lateral fornix. The position of the squamo-columnar junction varies so the position in the diagram is an approximation

correct sampling. This requires the use of a speculum but it is best to avoid using lubricating materials as they can contaminate the smear. The spatula is used to lightly scrape the squamo-columnar junction where the columnar epithelium lining the cervical canal changes to the stratified squamous epithelium found in the vagina (see *Fig. 12.1*). The squamo-columnar junction is a very common site of malignant change, so sampling of this precise area is essential in screening. The cells are then smeared on to a slide and fixed. Cervical scrapes are the main method of obtaining cervical smears and are usually performed by clinicians, GPs or nursing staff rather than by cytologists.

Endocervical brushings
The 'brush' can be specially designed or just a cotton wool bud on an applicator. The brush is gently inserted into the endocervical canal and rotated. The cells are then transferred to a slide and fixed. This is less common but will detect endocervical malignancy more reliably and can be used if the squamo-columnar junction is located inside the endocervical canal.

Liquid-based cytology techniques
The problems of efficient cell recovery directly from a spatula or brush has led to the development of a new technique for cervical sampling, which,

although still using the scraping or brushing technique to remove cells from the cervix, uses a fluid to recover the cells. These are replacing the more traditional techniques given above. Several different commercial techniques of liquid-based cytology are available, often using a great deal of automation, which gives a more reproducible result. The cells may be dislodged manually into a transport fluid by simple rinsing into a vial of fluid and the vial containing the cells is then despatched to the laboratory. An alternative is to break off the head of the sampling brush into a vial of fluid and then despatch the vial and the head of the brush to the laboratory where mechanical vortex mixing dislodges the cells.

The cells are separated from the fluid using centrifugation with or without the use of density gradients (e.g. the SurePath system). This results in a cleaner preparation, as mucus and blood cells do not end up on the final slide and obscure the epithelial cells. An alternative is the ThinPrep system, which uses gentle suction through a filter to transfer the cells to a slide.

Both systems were considered by the National Institute for Clinical Excellence in the UK who concluded that the benefits of liquid-based cytology were sufficient for them to be used as replacements for the conventional techniques. The introduction of liquid-based cytology has been accepted and should be completed in 2008.

Liquid-based cytology is hoped to improve the service by reducing the inadequate smear rate (a pilot study showed a reduction from 9% to 1–2%) with no loss (and even possible gains) in detection rates.

Smear fixation

Smears must be fixed immediately whilst still wet. Air-drying results in artefacts (blurring of nuclear detail, for example), especially when the Papanicolaou staining method is to be used, although it is a common method of smear preparation for Romanowsky staining. In addition, the liquid-based cytology techniques often use their own proprietary fixatives and transport fluids. Many fixatives have been tried over the years but two generic fixatives are in common use:

Alcohol (95%, sometimes with the addition of 1–3% acetic acid to improve nuclear preservation). This is the usual fixative but the wet solution is flammable and cannot be sent through the post.

Spray fixatives. These consist of alcohols and polyethylene glycols (PEG or carbowax). The alcohols fix the specimen and then it is coated it with a thin layer of PEG that protects it from drying. The PEG film is easily removed before staining. These are often bought as ready-prepared spray cans or bottles but can be easily made and used from a simple dropper bottle. The advantage of these fixatives is that the PEG acts as a protective coating and stops artefacts caused by drying. The slides can be allowed to 'dry' and this is useful for slides that have to be transported or posted.

Box 12.5 Routine staining

It is a little surprising that in three cellular diagnostic disciplines a single stain has become dominant, yet it is a different stain in each case. In histology, haematoxylin and eosin is dominant, in cytology it is the Papanicolaou stain and in haematology it is the Romanowsky method. The techniques do not transfer effectively across the disciplines. The use of haematoxylin and eosin is non-existent in haematology and minimal in exfoliative cytology. Papanicolaou is not used in routine histology or haematology. The Romanowsky stains do have uses in the other two disciplines but only for very limited applications. This specialization partly reflects genuinely different requirements in the three disciplines but also reflects a historical inertia. Histologists have always used haematoxylin and eosin so they will continue to use it. Papanicolaou has become the most commonly used stain in cytology partly because it was the first stain in the field.

Staining methods

Staining of smears has to bring out both nuclear and cytoplasmic detail and help to differentiate between the different cell types. Although no single method can be perfect for every situation, the Papanicolaou technique has become almost universal in its application for screening of smears (see *Box 12.5*). Other stains are useful for following up abnormalities. Staining needs to be well controlled and reliable since changes in staining are an important feature of diagnosis. Most laboratories use automatic staining machines to ensure a constant staining routine and to cope with the large numbers of smears being stained.

Papanicolaou stain

The Papanicolaou stain was devised in the 1940s and has been the main cytological staining method ever since. To a certain extent, the clarity of this method has been a feature in the acceptance of smears as a diagnostic method. The Papanicolaou method provides good nuclear detail and gives a translucent or transparent cytoplasm that is useful if cells overlap. The ability to see through the cytoplasm of a cell means that it is often possible to diagnose an abnormal cell even if there is another cell overlapping it. The cytoplasmic colour gives some indication of the maturation of the cells and of cellular activity.

The dyes involved are:

- **Haematoxylin.** Harris's or Gill's are the commonest formulae. Harris's requires differentiation, which may result in some unevenness if the smear is thick, but many workers think it gives the sharpest detail when well stained. Gill's is less critical in differentiation and is well suited to automatic staining.
- **OG6.** This is orange G in alcohol with tungstophosphoric acid. This stains the superficial cell cytoplasm a distinct but transparent orange colour.
- **EA (eosin azure).** There are several formulations of this stain and they are designated by numbers EA36–EA65. They all contain eosin, light

green and tungstophosphoric acid and the slightly different formulae vary in the light green concentration and whether or not they contain Bismarck brown and lithium carbonate. The stains do need careful preparation and the commercially available solutions are often used since they give consistent quality.

Haematoxylin and eosin (H&E)

This is the most popular stain for histological preparations and is used by some pathologists as it is a familiar technique and matches more easily with histological appearances. Generally the cytoplasmic differentiation is poorer. It is sometimes considered better for specimens prepared by filtering the cells from fluid samples since it is less likely to give a heavy background colour with the filtered material.

Romanowsky methods

These are more commonly used for blood smears and as special stains in histology and can be used as a stain for cytology specimens. Giemsa, Jenner, May–Grünwald and Leishman are all examples and the formulation used is mainly personal preference. The nuclear detail with the Romanowsky dyes is not as good as with a haematoxylin nuclear stain but differentiation, particularly of non-epithelial cells, is good. Romanowsky smears are usually air-dried and fixed in methanol, rather than the usual wet smear fixation in ethanol.

Shorr's stain

This was the preferred stain for hormone assessment of vaginal smears but is rarely used now as it gives poorer nuclear detail and the cytoplasm is not as transparent as with the Papanicolaou stain. It does, however, distinguish well between the different layers of epithelial cells.

Acridine orange

Acridine orange is a fluorescent stain that differentiates between DNA and RNA in cells. Since malignant cells tend to stain more strongly for RNA than normal epithelial cells, it has been used to detect malignant cells. This method was once proposed as a screening stain for smears and smears can be destained and restained (e.g. by Papanicolaou) to allow confirmation by routine microscopy. The requirement for using a fluorescent microscope made it unpopular for routine use.

Stains for special purposes

There are many other stains that can be used for special purposes, e.g. Feulgen (DNA staining) and methyl green–pyronin (DNA and RNA) are used to distinguish nucleoli, plasma cells and Reed–Sternberg cells. Mucins can be stained with the same methods as in histochemistry. The Perls technique will demonstrate haemosiderin and asbestos bodies. The Gram stain, Ziehl–Neelson and others may be used to detect and identify micro-organisms. Periodic acid–Schiff or Best's carmine are used to detect glycogen.

Normal gynaecological smear constituents

There are many materials and cells that can be found in normal gynaecological smears. Not all of them will be present in every normal smear, so the absence of certain constituents is usually not significant. The presence of some of these constituents is normal only if they are present in small amounts or small numbers but if they are present in larger amounts then it may be abnormal even though the constituent is considered normal for the purposes of this list.

Stratified squamous epithelial cells

These cells arise from the stratified squamous epithelium of the vaginal or ectocervical epithelium. This is the same type of epithelium that is found in skin. The epithelium is quite robust and resistant to abrasion (see *Box 12.6*). The epithelium is multi-layered with the cells being produced in the basal layer, maturing in the middle layers and being shed from the superficial layer (see *Fig. 12.2*). It is this constant renewal from below that makes the epithelium so resistant. At the base of the epithelium, there is a layer of dividing cells. Following mitosis, one of the daughter cells will be separated from the basement membrane and begins to change. The cells become flatter as they mature and they also move gradually upwards through the epithelium as more cells are produced below them. The surface cells are quite flattened and will be lost from the surface with any mild abrasion. It is the upper layers that are sampled in cervical smears and although terms such as 'basal cells' are sometimes used, they do not correspond with the very base of the epithelium where the cells are firmly attached and would not be sampled by the relatively mild abrasion with a spatula.

Skin-type epithelium can become keratinized if the upper layers accumulate large amounts of the protein keratin. Although stratified squamous cells in the cervix do have the potential to become keratinized, this does not

Figure 12.2
Diagram of the layered epithelium of the cervical surface. The cells are produced in the lowest (basal) layer and gradually move upwards

---

Box 12.6 Squamo-columnar junction

The cervix protrudes into the vagina and is lined with columnar epithelium on its outer surface and in the canal leading from the cervix to the uterus (endocervical canal). The junction between the two varies in life. Before puberty (pre-menarche), the squamo-columnar junction is inside the endocervical canal. At puberty, the cervix enlarges and the squamo-columnar junction is now seen in the vaginal region. This results in a gradual, and sometimes patchy, replacement of the columnar epithelium with stratified squamous epithelium. The stratified squamous epithelium is a more resistant epithelium and is better suited to the vaginal environment. This replacement of the columnar epithelium is called **squamous metaplasia**. The appearance of the squamo-columnar junction in the vaginal region has been referred to by various terms including **ectopy, ectopion, erosion** and **cervical discontinuity**. This is not a disease but a normal phenomenon.

---

usually happen in humans, although it does in other animals. The distinctions between cells and layers are not rigid since cells gradually change as they mature and the classes of cell are only convenient labels for identifying the stages in cell maturation. Every superficial cell has passed through all of the stages and the cells do not suddenly alter but change gradually so that some cells are in between categories. Some workers include extra types of cell (e.g. pre-cornified) but these are not included in this list.

Superficial cells. These are large (50–60 µm) cells. They have a very small central nucleus that stains very darkly. This condensed nuclear appearance is called **pyknosis** so the nucleus is called a **pyknotic nucleus**. Superficial cells also have an acidophilic translucent cytoplasm (pink or orange with the Papanicolaou stain), which is often angular or 'squared'. This is the most common type of cell in most smears (see *Colour plate 29*).

Intermediate cells. These are smaller (40–50 µm) cells. They have a larger central nucleus with finely granular chromatin. The cytoplasm is pale green with the Papanicolaou stain and the overall cell shape is angular or 'squared'. These are quite a common type of cell in many smears (see *Colour plate 30*).

Parabasal cells. These are even smaller (20–30 µm) cells. They have a larger central vesicular nucleus with a coarser granular chromatin. The cytoplasm is a denser green with the Papanicolaou stain and the whole cell is rounded or ovoid. This is a less common type of cell in most smears (see *Colour plate 31*).

Basal cells. These are similar to the parabasal cells in most respects. They are even smaller (15–20 µm) cells but have a larger nucleus with a coarser granular chromatin, which may be central or slightly eccentric. The cytoplasm is a dense green with the Papanicolaou stain and is rounded or ovoid. This is an uncommon type of cell in most smears since it is not normally shed from the surface.

Uterine columnar cells

Endocervical cells. These cells come from the endocervical canal, which is lined with ciliated columnar epithelium. Endocervical cells in smears often vary in how well they are preserved. Cells that are poorly preserved may cause confusion and difficulties in identification, especially for less experienced workers. They are smaller than the squamous cells (15–20 μm). The nucleus of these cells varies quite considerably in size, even in normal cells, so variation in nuclear size on its own should not be taken to indicate malignant change. The nucleus is often eccentric, usually at the base of the cell. The cytoplasm stains a green/grey colour with the Papanicolaou stain and may contain droplets of mucin in the upper part of the cytoplasm.

The top border of the cells may be ciliated. The cilia themselves can be seen in well-preserved cells but more often only the terminal plate below the ciliated surface is seen. These cells may occur in clumps. In side view, the clumps appear as a palisade of cells but in vertical view they appear as a honeycomb pattern. Degenerated cells may appear as little more than bare isolated nuclei.

Endometrial cells. These arise in the endometrial lining and are columnar cells but are usually degenerating since they cannot be sampled directly in a simple cervical scrape and may have been shed several days before and then travelled slowly down to the cervix before being collected and smeared. Endometrial cells are small (10–12 μm). The nucleus is quite large and is usually eccentric with a well-defined nuclear border; often one or two large chromatin clumps are seen. There is very little cytoplasm and this usually stains a green/grey colour with the Papanicolaou stain but may occasionally be pink. The cells may overlap or be bunched together. Endometrial cells are only considered as a normal constituent of cervical scrapes around menstruation; significant numbers at other times in the menstrual cycle should be noted and investigated. Endometrial cells may be more common in women fitted with a coil or other intrauterine device.

Blood cells (see Box 12.7)

Erythrocytes. These are easily recognized, as they are strongly eosinophilic small cells (7–8 μm) without any nucleus. Erythrocytes are common around menstruation but may indicate bleeding if seen at other times.

Neutrophils or polymorphs. The full name of these cells is polymorphonuclear neutrophil leukocytes but this is usually abbreviated to neutrophils, polymorphs or even just polys. The name indicates their multiple-lobed nucleus (*poly* = many, *morph* = shape), which may have between two and four lobes. They are very easy to recognize by their small size and strongly basophilic lobed nuclei. Polymorphs are about 9–15 μm in diameter with a pale green/blue cytoplasm. Small numbers are normal but larger numbers are usually associated with inflammation (see *Colour plate 32*).

Box 12.7

The blood cells are complex since they can represent menstruation, which is a normal condition. They can, however, also represent disease states such as inflammation and bleeding. Deciding which it is can be difficult and so smears from around the menstrual period should not be used for diagnosis.

Macrophages (histiocytes). Macrophages are motile cells so they can be very variable in shape and this makes them difficult to identify. Macrophages are larger than other leukocytes (16–20 µm) with a large lightly stained eccentric nucleus. The colour of their cytoplasmic staining depends on how active they are and in particular whether they are actively phagocytosing material and the nature of any phagocytosed material. The most common cytoplasmic colour is a light green. The cytoplasm is often vacuolated and may appear foamy if there are large numbers of vacuoles. The vacuoles may contain debris (bacteria, degenerating cells, etc.) left over from phagocytosed material. Usually only a few macrophages are present in a normal smear and large numbers are associated with inflammation.

Lymphocytes. Lymphocytes are smaller cells (8–12 µm) with a large round basophilic nucleus that occupies most of the cell. They have only a small amount of cytoplasm, which is basophilic. They are rare in normal smears and if found in large numbers indicate chronic inflammation. **Plasma cells** are produced from lymphocytes after they have been stimulated by antigen. Plasma cells have a larger amount of basophilic cytoplasm and an eccentric nucleus with prominent chromatin granules scattered around the nuclear border. This may be referred to as a 'clock-face nucleus' (see *Colour plate 32*).

Other constituents

As well as the cells coming from the epithelia and blood of the woman, there are a number of other materials and contaminants that can occur.

Mucus. Mucus is secreted to keep the epithelium moist and prevent the cells becoming desiccated. Mucins appear as translucent strands when stained with the Papanicolaou technique but may stain more strongly with other stains. Only small amounts are usually found in smears and because the small deposits and thin films are translucent the presence of mucin does not interfere with cell recognition. If larger amounts of densely staining mucus occur, it will stain more darkly and may obscure some cells making diagnosis difficult. Large amounts of mucus may occur if there is inflammation present.

Fibrin. Fibrin is an insoluble fibrous protein and is produced from the soluble plasma protein fibrinogen by the coagulation cascade. Fibrin appears as pink strands with the Papanicolaou stain and is usually associated with bleeding. It is normal around menstruation; at other times it usually indicates a haemorrhage but it can also indicate an inflammatory exudate.

Doederlein (Döderlein) bacilli. These are lactobacilli and are a common commensal organism in the female genital tract. They break down the glycogen that occurs in epithelial cells and release lactic acid as a product of their metabolism. If bacteria are present in large numbers, they can cause cytolysis of intermediate cells, which therefore appear irregular or 'ragged'. The lactic acid produced by these bacilli lowers the vaginal pH to around pH 4–4.5 and this helps to inhibit the growth of pathogenic organisms (see *Box 12.8*).

Box 12.8 Lactobacilli in the vagina

The term commensal means that the organism is not causing disease. The presence of these bacteria is often beneficial in this case, so it is almost a symbiotic relationship. The loss of this **normal flora** may have serious consequences. If the woman is treated with a broad-spectrum antibiotic, it may kill off all of the lactobacilli and result in the growth of more-pathogenic organisms such as *Candida albicans*. This fungus causes the disease thrush and one treatment for thrush is to use a living culture of lactobacilli to re-establish a healthy and acidic environment. One such culture is live yoghurt, so yoghurt can be used to treat thrush. It must of course be a live yoghurt and not a pasteurized one. Although this 'organic' treatment can help, it is always wise for the patient to consult their doctor and not self-treat in isolation.

Lactobacilli appear as small rod-shaped organisms (1–2 µm long), which may form chains. They stain pale blue with the Papanicolaou stain and are Gram-positive. Lactobacilli are common during secretory-phase smears and in pregnancy when glycogen is abundant in the intermediate smears.

Spermatozoa. These are simple to recognize as they have a dark-staining head with a pale cap (acrosome); the tail fibres are not always easy to distinguish. The presence of large numbers may make a smear unsatisfactory for diagnosis.

Normal changes in gynaecological smears

The appearance of cervical smears alters with time and with the physiological state of the woman. The main controlling feature of the changes is the levels of the hormones oestrogen and progesterone (see *Box 12.9*).

Oestrogen and progesterone levels in the blood vary on two time scales:

■ **Short-term changes.** These occur in normal menstruating women with roughly a monthly cyclic change. Although the menstrual cycle is nominally a 28 day cycle, it can vary considerably in some women.

■ **Long-term changes.** Lifetime changes are associated with the onset of puberty (menarche) and the menopause, whilst a pregnancy interrupts the normal menstrual cycle for 9 months.

Box 12.9 Therapeutic hormones

The effects of hormones are not limited to the natural hormones and will be mimicked by artificial hormones such as those in the contraceptive pill and hormone-replacement therapy. The normal menstrual cycle is only nominally 28 days in women and can vary depending on conditions. The use of the contraceptive pill usually results in a regular 28 day cycle because of the exogenous hormones so the cycle becomes constrained. Pheromones are scents that can control aspects of physiology and behaviour in another animal. Women sharing a flat as students often become entrained and will menstruate at the same time and this is believed to be due to pheromone influences. To get into step with each other, the length of the cycles must change.

Cytology of the menstrual cycle

There are four main phases and two intermediate phases that can be identified:

1. Proliferative (oestrogenic) phase.
2. Ovulatory phase.
3. Secretory (progestagenic) phase.
4. Menstrual phase.

Menstruation is classed clinically as the beginning of the menstrual cycle since the onset of bleeding is the easiest point in the cycle to recognize. Menstruation is, however, really the last phase of the cycle when the body is removing the unwanted remains of the previous cycle and preparing the uterus for regrowth of the epithelium. The start of epithelial growth is a more logical start to the menstrual cycle but the simplicity and reliability of the menstrual blood flow as a marker makes timing and counting the days from this occurrence the best method for clinical purposes. Thus, the first signs of menstrual blood flow are counted as the first day.

Proliferative phase

The proliferative phase occurs from the 9th to the 14th day of the menstrual cycle. It is a period of increasing oestrogen levels in the blood and the oestrogen stimulates the epithelium of the cervix and uterus to grow and thicken. The stratified squamous epithelium includes more mature cells. A smear from this phase shows predominantly superficial cells (60% or more in the later stages) and there is a low number of polymorphs and histiocytes. The squamous cells separate well and so appear isolated and they usually lie flat on the slide with very little wrinkling or folding of the cells. This type of smear or the next type (ovulatory) is preferred for diagnosis as they are easier to screen because of the 'clean' smears produced.

Ovulatory phase

The ovulatory phase occurs around days 15 and 16 of the cycle and smears taken at this stage consist almost exclusively of superficial cells. Polymorphs and other background materials are mostly absent giving a very clean smear. This appearance indicates a high level of oestrogen in the blood but, although referred to as ovulatory, it cannot be taken to mean that ovulation has actually occurred.

Secretory phase

Following ovulation, oestrogen concentration in the blood declines and progesterone becomes the dominant influence from day 17 through to about day 24. The effect of this progesterone on the cells in smears is to decrease the number of superficial cells and increase the number of intermediate cells in the sample. The intermediate cells have more glycogen and are more likely to be folded and wrinkled than superficial cells. The epithelial cells often occur in clumps rather than being well separated. Lactobacilli become more noticeable both in numbers and in their cytolytic effect on the cells. Secretory phase smears also have more polymorphs, possibly due to the increased numbers of bacteria. The later stages of the secretory phase, from day 25 until the onset of bleeding on day 28, form one of the minor phases termed the pre-menstrual phase. The progesterone levels are beginning to fall. The appearance of smears is similar to those in the rest of the secretory phase although possibly more pronounced. In the last stages, some superficial cells may begin to reappear if the falling concentration of progesterone is accompanied by an early increase in oestrogen secretion from a developing Graafian follicle.

Menstrual phase

This covers days 0 to 5 of the menstrual cycle and is characterized by bleeding and sloughing of the epithelium of the uterus. During the menstrual phase, the appearance of the smear is dominated by red blood cells and white cells from the menstrual blood flow. Also carried with the blood are endometrial cells and mucus from the sloughed endometrium. Diagnostic examination of these smears is difficult as the cells are clumped, degenerating and obscured by the high numbers of red cells. Generally they are unreliable for diagnosis and a repeat smear should be done.

The 5th to 8th days of the cycle are sometimes distinguished as the post-menstrual phase where the numbers of red cells diminishes, although white cells are still present in quite high numbers. Endometrial cells are more common in this late menstrual phase than in most other phases and the predominant squamous epithelial cells are intermediate cells.

Hormonal assessment of smears

Since the types of cell vary with the hormone content, it is possible to assess the levels of circulating hormone from the pattern of cells seen in the smear. The relative amount of hormone present can be assessed by counting the number of each cell type. Although modern biochemical tests can give a more accurate measure of the actual concentration of hormones, counting of cells can still be useful in correlating with hormone levels and may detect cases where, although there is a high concentration of oestrogen, the cells are not responding to the oestrogen. This may occur if the hormone receptors are defective in some way.

Three indexes have been used in hormone assessment, as outlined below.

Maturation index

The parabasal, intermediate and superficial cells are counted and reported as a percentage of the total, e.g.:

Parabasal	Intermediate	Superficial	
4	27	69	= oestrogen effect
45	42	13	= low oestrogen

Eosinophilic index

This counts the number of eosinophilic cells, i.e. superficial cells. This measure is only accurate in the absence of inflammation and is very dependent on predictable and reliable staining of cells. In the example above, the eosinophilic index would be 69% and 13%.

Karyopyknotic index

The karyopyknotic index uses nuclear morphology to count superficial cells rather than their staining characteristics. The nuclei counted should be dark, homogeneous and less than 6 μm in diameter. This is also reported as a percentage.

Lifetime alterations

Pre-menarche

The onset of menstruation at puberty is referred to as the **menarche** so **pre-menarche** smears refer to smears taken from sexually immature patients. Children are not randomly screened so pre-menarche smears are only taken as diagnostic smears and only when the clinician believes there is a good reason for the investigation. Girls have very little sex hormone secretion before the menarche, so there is little stimulation of the epithelium and the lack of growth is termed atrophic. The appearance of an **atrophic** smear is one in which parabasal cells are the most common epithelial cell type, although leukocytes and commensal bacteria may also occur in the smears. This pattern persists until the onset of the menstrual cycle when intermediate and superficial cells begin to appear. The full regular cyclic activity may not appear, however, for a year or more following the menarche and the appearances of the smears may temporarily revert to a more atrophic state if a particular cycle is missed.

In the newborn during the first few weeks of life, the appearance of smears may be quite different due to hormones coming from the mother and placenta acting on the foetal epithelium whilst the child is in the uterus. This effect will disappear rapidly as the hormone levels fall in the first couple of weeks of post-natal life. The taking of smears from such young babies is extremely rare.

Pregnancy

The predominant hormone is progesterone so the pattern of cells seen in a smear resembles a late secretory phase smear but these appearances are more prolonged and the pattern becomes more established. The cells in the smear are often clumped and folded, with intermediate cells as the predominant type of cell present. The cells may show a **navicular** form. This refers to elongation of the cells with curling edges giving a boat-shaped cell with an eccentric nucleus.

Some superficial cells may be present, depending on the amount of oestrogen being secreted, but the numbers of superficial cells should be low in a normal pregnancy. If more than a third of the cells that are seen in a smear taken in the first trimester (the first third of the pregnancy) are super-ficial cells, then this is significant and should be reported to the clinician as it may indicate an early sign of abortion (miscarriage). This is most likely to occur when the production of progesterone switches from the corpus luteum to the placenta around weeks 10–12 of pregnancy. In the second and third trimester, the critical number is only 10–15% superficial cells and if a larger proportion of cells is seen, then it should be reported quickly.

Many of the intermediate cells in pregnancy have a high glycogen content and this encourages the growth of lactobacilli, which are therefore common in such smears. This may lead to large amounts of cellular degradation (cytolysis). Parabasal cells are uncommon in smears taken during pregnancy except in cases where there is inflammation. Trophoblastic cells from the placenta may sometimes occur in smears and are another possible indica-tor of the risk of a miscarriage.

Post-natal smears

Smears taken from a mother during the first week or so following delivery show the presence of erythrocytes, leukocytes and groups of **decidual** cells shed from the remains of the placenta. Parabasal cells are more common than the intermediate cells characteristic of pregnancy. A couple of weeks after the end of pregnancy, the appearance of the smear reverts to the more usual patterns and, depending on the hormones present, the appearance may vary from a secretory pattern to a late proliferative one.

Post-menopausal smears

The menopause is when the usual monthly menstrual periods stop. During this period, there is a gradual cessation of hormone secretion by the ovary but this decline may take months or years. The pattern of cells in the smear varies from a typical proliferative pattern to an atrophic pattern. Most smears will show a more transitional state with many intermediate cells. If a strong progesterone pattern is seen in a reportedly post-menopausal smear, the possibility of pregnancy should be considered.

The atrophic pattern developing shortly after the menopause is often associated with vaginal discomfort and the patient may need hormonal

---

Box 12.10 Therapy can alter the appearance of smears from post-menopausal women

Hormones are also capable of acting on cells elsewhere in the body. The epithelial cells in the mouth and trachea also react in the same way as the vaginal and cervical cells but to a lesser extent. The loss of hormones during the menopause can occasionally cause severe problems with thinning of skin and drying of the mucosa and the person may need to have hormone-replacement therapy. The patient can be returned to the same condition as a pre-menopausal woman although the lack of ova prevents natural pregnancy. Women can become pregnant, however, by *in vitro* fertilization. Women into their sixties have become pregnant in this way. This use of hormones and other treat-ments can complicate the interpretation of smears from older women.

treatment to produce a thicker epithelium that is more resistant and less easily irritated.

Post-menopausal hormone treatment will of course alter the cellular pattern (see *Box 12.10*) so any hormone treatment needs to be known. Highly oestrogenic smears after the menopause in the absence of hormone treatment should always be investigated further.

Inflammatory changes in smears

Inflammatory changes occur in a wide variety of conditions and diseases (see *Box 12.11*). The inflammation may vary in intensity from mild to severe and can be either short-lived (acute inflammation) or long-lived (chronic inflammation). Sometimes the cause of the inflammation may be directly visible and identifiable in the smear or there may simply be an unidentifiable inflammation present, in which case it would be reported as non-specific inflammation. The classical changes associated with inflammation in tissues are pain, redness, heat and swelling, but these are not, of course, visible in smears so inflammation is recognized by changes in the cells of the smear.

The changes that occur in smears can be considered as either destructive changes or reactive changes.

Box 12.11 Inflammation is not a disease

Inflammation is one of those areas of physiology and pathology where it is not possible to decide completely what sort of process it is. Normally we would consider a process in the body to be either normal (often called physiological) or the result of disease (pathological). Inflammation is normal in the sense that it occurs as a method of maintaining the body in a healthy state. It is a normal body response to an abnormal situation, such as infection or trauma. However, the presence of inflammation always indicates that a pathological situation exists and the body needs to repair or resist the change, so inflammation is always associated with pathology.

Destructive or degenerative changes

These occur when the causative agent of the inflammation induces degradation in the cells of the tissues.

Cytoplasmic degradation. The destruction can be directly due to the bacteria or fungi causing inflammation, with the cells showing direct cytolytic effects; there may be loss of the cellular border giving a ragged edge to the cell (sometimes described as looking 'moth-eaten'). The cytoplasm may contain vacuoles and if there is perinuclear vacuolation it will give the appearance of a pale halo around the nucleus. In extreme cases, degradation may lead to all of the cytoplasm being lost, leaving bare nuclei free in the smear.

Cytoplasmic staining is often altered, with cells that would normally stain as basophilic now showing eosinophilia (e.g. parabasal cells may be red/brown). This eosinophilia is the most likely finding, although other altered staining can occur.

Phagocytosis may occur with the appearance of the engulfed material inside the cells.

Nuclear degradation. There may be pyknosis or the nucleus may fragment into small dense particles of chromatin (a process called karyorrhexis).

Reactive changes

Reactive changes are due to the inflammatory reaction in the tissue, rather than the direct effect of the bacteria. The most important reactive change is the production of inflammatory exudate. In inflammation, there is an increase in the permeability of blood vessels in the inflamed area. The increase in permeability to allows protein-rich fluid to pass out of the blood vessel. This is the cause of the swelling (oedema) that is found in acute inflammation. The constituents of the exudate can vary. The most frequent finding is an excess of leukocytes, particularly neutrophils and macrophages (see *Colour plate 32*). If there is bleeding as well as exudation, then erythrocytes will be seen even in non-menstrual smears. Fibrin strands may be present either from haemorrhage or from a protein-rich exudate.

Chronic inflammation differs slightly in that it is a much longer lasting change. The fluid exudate is usually much less than in acute inflammation and the cells will be mainly lymphocytes, plasma cells and macrophages. The macrophages may form large multinucleated phagocytic cells called giant cells.

In addition to the exudate, there may be reactive changes in the epithelium resulting in altered cell maturation and desquamation (shedding of cells). The normally non-keratinized epithelium may become hyperkeratotic (increased keratin) in response to continued irritation and this can result in white patches on the surface (leukoplakia). In hyperkeratosis, the cells appear as large flat cells without a nucleus although they may have a clear area in the centre of the cell where the nucleus has lysed. The cells are polygonal in shape and the cytoplasm is acidophilic and stains orange with the Papanicolaou method.

The agent causing the irritating can be physical, chemical or may be one of several infective agents (see below). The infection may be protozoan, fungal, viral or bacterial in origin. Many of these infections are considered to be sexually transmitted diseases, although this is not necessarily the only method of transmission (see *Box 12.12*).

Infective agents

Trichomonas vaginalis ('Trikes' or TV) is a unicellular flagellate that is found in up to 20% of females. In infections, it is associated with a yellow/green discharge that can be frothy and has an unpleasant odour. TV can be trans-

Box 12.12 Sexual transmission

Many of the diseases of the female genital tract can be transmitted by sexual intercourse. Such diseases were called venereal diseases but the term sexually transmitted disease (STD) is now preferred. Although a disease can be transmitted sexually, this may not be the only route of infection. Infection from inanimate objects such as towels, toilet seats, etc. is possible in some cases. Contaminated inanimate objects that can transmit disease are sometimes called **fomites**. Other infections are almost totally restricted to direct sexual transmission and cannot be caught from inanimate objects, as the organisms are unable to exist away from the human body. An example of this is syphilis, which is almost impossible to catch except by direct, usually sexual, contact. It requires tact to tell someone or their partner that they have a disease that can be sexually transmitted as there can be the hidden suggestion that one or other partner has been involved sexually with a third party. This can lead to emotional problems for the people involved. It is essential that the possibility of non-sexual transmission is explained.

mitted as an STD but infection from inanimate objects such as toilet seats is also possible. It can also occur in males so if an infection is found then both partners need to be treated. There is no longer thought to be a strong correlation between TV infections and a higher risk of cervical malignancy. Early reports of such a link were probably due to confusing factors such as promiscuity (which increases the risk of both TV and cervical malignancy).

TV stains rather poorly with the Papanicolaou stain and the flagellae are rarely visible. They appear as pear-shaped faint grey/green structures (8–20 μm) with an eccentric nucleus ('Mongols eye'). They can be seen more easily in wet preparations using phase-contrast microscopy where they can be seen to be motile. The organism can also be cultured to confirm its presence if necessary.

The presence of TV can often be inferred even when the organism itself is not seen, since it usually causes a characteristic red staining of the cytoplasm of the epithelial cells. Vacuolation and perinuclear haloes are also common. The inflammatory changes in the smear are often severe. Some cytopathologists have reported the reactive changes as 'appearances suggestive of *Trichomonas* infection'.

The changes seen with TV may mimic some of the signs of early malignant change so the patient should be treated to get rid of the infection and a repeat smear taken so that dyskaryotic changes are not missed.

Candida albicans (monilia, thrush) is an eosinophilic yeast that may appear as long eosinophilic threads ('pseudohyphae'). Squamous cells often appear to cluster around these pseudohyphae in smears. *Candida* is a common finding in smears and may behave as a commensal or a pathogen depending on the conditions. In heavy infections, there should be treatment of both the female and any male partners. It occurs mainly in reproductive life, more frequently in pregnancy and following antibiotic therapy. It does not seem to be associated with the modern low-oestrogen pill formulations but high-progesterone pills may increase the risk of infection.

Herpes simplex virus is a virus that infects humans and has several variants. Herpes simplex virus 1 (HSV-1) is usually associated with oral infections (cold sores or fever blisters), whilst HSV-2 is more common in genital infections and is considered an STD. It causes ulceration of the cervix. If infection occurs during pregnancy, it can be transmitted to the foetus with fatal results (foetal malformation and miscarriage). This usually only applies to women acquiring the infection during pregnancy; once infected, the antibodies in the maternal blood usually protect the foetus. There is a higher incidence of anti-herpes antibodies in women who develop cervical malignancy than there is in the general population. There is no direct evidence that herpes virus is actively involved in malignant change and there is often no sign of herpes DNA or any viral antigen in the malignant cells.

Smears show characteristic changes during the active phase of a herpes infection but simple morphology is not as reliable as cultures. The most characteristic cell seen during an active infection is a large multinucleated (up to 30 nuclei) giant cell (50–200 µm). The chromatin is often most prominent around the margins of the nucleus, which makes the nuclei well defined and results in a 'ballooned' appearance with the empty centre of the nucleus having a ground glass appearance. The virus may cause eosinophilic viral inclusion bodies in the nucleus but this depends on the stage of infection and is not always present. Confusion with malignant change is possible, so accurate recognition of the changes caused by herpes virus is important. Immunological techniques using anti-HSV antibodies may be useful in some cases.

Human papilloma virus (HPV) is the cause of genital warts and is also passed on through sexual intercourse. There are many variants of HPV (more than 50 have been recognized), with each type having a characteristic pathological condition. Fifteen types have been found in the vaginal environment and some may pre-dispose the person to cervical malignancy. Two forms have been identified with a high risk of cervical cancer (HPV-16 and HPV-18), whilst some others are less strongly linked but still possible factors (e.g. HPV-31 and HPV-33).

HPV infections usually disappear after 6–9 months but 10–20% of infected women remain infected. It is the persistent infection that is linked to malignancy. Thus, a single positive test is not significant in itself but is cause for an earlier recall. Persistent HPV infections have been found in >90% of cervical cancers. In the absence of infection, disease rates are very low. Research is therefore being carried out into the possible use of vaccination against HPV to protect women from the virus and thus prevent cervical cancer.

The possibility of using HPV testing either as well as or instead of the standard morphology is also being considered. An NHS study started in 2001 and is due to report in 2008. Currently the suggestion by the Health Technology Assessment review of the current evidence is that it should be used selectively. It is being used in pilot studies to triage women for high risk. In the pilot studies, women who show abnormal morphology are tested for HPV. If a woman is HPV-positive, she can be referred for immediate colposcopy. (In some trials only those over 35 are immediately referred.) If the patients are HPV-negative, they can be recalled in 6 months. If the second test shows persistence of dyskaryosis or is HPV-positive, they are then referred for colposcopy. If the disease has regressed and the HPV test is still negative, the woman is simply returned to the normal screening programme.

Early pilot studies suggest that HPV testing may be more reliable than morphology alone. The sensitivity of HPV tests may be as high as 95% (current morphology targets are 85% sensitivity) and the negative predictive value is >90%. In a sample of 11,000 women, HPV testing picked up 97% of anomalies, whilst standard cytology detected only 76%. Combined negative predictive values for morphology and HPV testing approached 100%. Both the standard morphological testing and the HPV screening can be done from same liquid-based cytology sample, making the process simpler and less stressful for the patients.

The most characteristic feature of HPV infections is the presence of **koilocytes**, which have a distinct perinuclear halo. There is usually some abnormal keratinization associated with the infection. Following a diagnosis of HPV warts, it is probably wise for the patient to have annual cervical smears because of the increased risk of cervical malignancy. Again, like HSV, the use of antibody techniques and in some cases nucleic acid hybridization methods may be useful.

Many other infections may occur from bacteria (*Leptothrix, Gardnerella, Neisseria, Treponema* and *Mycobacteria*) and other infectious agents including actinomycetes and chlamydia.

Malignancy

The diagnosis of malignancy (see *Box 12.13*) has two related aspects. One is the recognition that the cells have changed from their normal growth pattern and become malignant. This change is often called transformation. The other diagnostic task is to recognize exactly which type of malignancy is present. The cytological recognition of malignant transformation is most obvious in the nuclear abnormalities of the transformed cells. Cytoplasmic changes are frequently present in malignant cells but are less useful in recognizing that malignant change has occurred. The appearance of the cytoplasm is more important in determining which type of malignancy is present in the smear.

One outstanding feature of malignancy is the loss of regularity and uniformity of the cells. The malignant cells show a much greater range of size, shape and structure than normal tissue.

There is no single change that is pathognomonic, i.e. totally and solely characteristic of malignancy, so the diagnosis depends on several of the following list of features being present. The more features that are present

---

Box 12.13 Cancer

Malignancy is often referred to by the general public as cancer. It is a very emotive disease and a diagnosis of cancer is often regarded as indicating almost certain death from the disease. Malignancy can certainly be dangerous if left untreated but most malignant diseases can be treated effectively if caught early. The danger with many malignancy is that if left untreated it will gradually get worse and can spread. This increase in the aggressive growth of the tumour is called **progression**. Cancers can spread by invasion or metastasis. **Invasion** is where cells move into adjacent tissues by direct connection, whilst **metastasis** is when cells are spread by transport in blood, lymph or other body fluids. Both make treatment much more difficult as there will be more malignant cells and more widespread growth. Surgery is difficult once metastatic spreading has occurred. Surgery is usually the most effective cure, so metastasis usually means a much worse prognosis. The success of early treatment is, of course, the reason for using cytological screening.

---

within the cells, the greater the likelihood that malignant change has occurred. If only one or two features are present, then full malignant transformation is less likely. There may still be a suspicion of early malignant change, so the result is still important. Some changes are more significant than others, e.g. disturbed chromatin patterns are much more significant than simple nuclear enlargement, which can be found in a number of non-malignant conditions.

Nuclear changes (see Colour plate 33)

Disturbed chromatin distribution. The pattern of dark heterochromatin and pale euchromatin is usually regular and distinctive. Malignant cells usually have a less regular and coarser chromatin pattern in the nucleus. This finding is one of the more significant findings and would be expected in most malignant cells.

Alterations in size. Nuclear enlargement is common but some tumours with small malignant nuclei do occur. Simple alteration in size can be difficult to spot but it is often easier to see the change in the relative proportions of the nucleus and the cytoplasm, so the altered size is often referred to as an increased nucleocytoplasmic ratio. Humans are much better at recognizing relative changes than identifying absolute size changes.

Increased DNA content in the nucleus. The increased amount of nuclear material (chromatin) may not always be apparent if the nucleus is greatly enlarged. The enlargement of the nucleus means that the chromatin is more spread out giving a large pale nucleus. The increased DNA content comes from two sources. One is that malignant cells are usually actively dividing and, as part of the mitotic activity, the DNA in the cell must be duplicated before the cell divides. Thus, many of the cells will be synthesizing new DNA prior to division and as a consequence they may have twice as much DNA as other cells. The malignant cells may also have extra chromosomes present over and above the normal diploid 46.

Prominent nucleoli. Although abnormal and not always present in malignant cells, they are quite significant. The nucleoli may be enlarged or irregular in shape and there may be more than one present in a single cell. The nucleoli are indicative of the increased protein production characteristic of cell proliferation.

Abnormal nuclear outline. The nuclear border in malignant cells is often quite irregular and may be less well defined than in normal cells. With a pale nucleus, an irregular and an ill-defined border, the nucleus may appear to merge with the cytoplasm rather than being distinctly separated from it.

Multinucleation. The presence of more than one nucleus in a cell is a significant finding but they must be distinguished from non-malignant cells that can be multinucleate such as giant cells.

Mitosis. Cell division is usually more frequent in malignant tumours than it is in normal tissues and mitosis may occur in superficial cell layers that are normally non-mitotic. This may mean that cells in mitosis may appear in the smear. If an irregular mitosis is seen, e.g. a tripolar mitotic figure, this is even more significant.

Abnormal staining. The malignant cells often have quite odd colours. The cells may be darker than normal (hyperchromatic), paler than normal (hypochromatic) or stain in different colours to normal (polychromatic).

Cytoplasmic changes

Cytoplasmic changes are less important in recognizing malignancy but the sorts of change that occur include variation in the total cell size, variation in shape of the cell, abnormal cytoplasmic vacuolation and abnormal cytoplasmic staining. Malignant cells may also lose the characteristic features that make them identifiable as a particular cell type. This loss of differentiation is an important feature. The less well differentiated the cells are, the more likely it is that the tumour is an aggressive tumour and is spreading.

Different descriptive terms used to describe the changes

The recognition and reporting of malignant changes is complicated by various factors and varies from centre to centre (see *Box 12.14*). There is no absolute test of the degree of malignancy and the diagnosis is made on the basis of experience.

Malignancy does not happen as a single change but as a gradual development. There is a continuous spectrum of changes from mild changes (which may never progress to a full malignancy) to invasive tumours (which are life-threatening). There are no sharp breaks in this spectrum of changes, so deciding into which category a particular smear should be classed can be difficult.

The reporting phrases also differ even though they refer to the same condition and this may be confusing. The main categories of description are:

Box 12.14 Problems with missed diagnoses

The missing of abnormal cells is a serious problem. The target rate for detecting abnormalities with conventional smears was set at between 85 and 95%. In 1996, there was a case (The Times, 6 Feb 1996) where one laboratory fell below this expected standard, resulting in the rescreening of 70,000 smears at a cost of £140,000. It was expected that 350 previously undiagnosed abnormalities would be detected although none of these was expected to be full malignancy. However, the scale of the problem at that laboratory may have been underestimated. There are reports of five invasive carcinomas, 15 hysterectomies and five deaths in women involved in the screening programme. Many of these women are now involved in litigation against the hospital and the hospital is no longer screening smears.

In 1997 (The Times, 6 Feb 1997), a woman was awarded £60,000 following a missed diagnosis that resulted in her losing a child when she became pregnant.

- **CIN.** This stands for cervical intraepithelial neoplasia and the degree of severity is indicated by numbers CIN1 to CIN3 (with three being the most severe). The only way to be sure it is intraepithelial is to examine a histological section, so this is a histological description rather than a cytological one.
- **Dysplasia.** This is also a histological description and relates to the changes in cell maturation within the epithelium. Severity is usually indicated by words (mild, moderate and severe).
- **Dyskaryosis** (originally introduced by Papanicolaou). This is a cytological description of the nuclear changes and indicates severity either using the same phrases as dysplasia (mild, moderate and severe) or by relating it to the cytoplasmic appearance of the cells (superficial cell dyskaryosis, intermediate cell dyskaryosis and parabasal cell dyskaryosis). In addition, smears may be classified as negative, borderline, ?glandular or ?invasive. This is the classification favoured by the British Society for Clinical Cytologists (BSCC).

In the USA, the Bethesda system 2001 is used to classify the changes into only two categories: low-grade squamous intraepithelial lesions (LSIL) or high-grade squamous intraepithelial lesions (HSIL). The classification also includes negative and atypical squamous cells (ASC), which may be qualified as 'atypical squamous cells of undetermined significance' (ASC-US) or 'cannot exclude HSIL' (ASC-H).

Within the limits already mentioned, the use of CIN, dysplasia and dyskaryosis correspond reasonably as follows:

CIN1	Mild dysplasia	Mild dyskaryosis
CIN2	Moderate dysplasia	Moderate dyskaryosis
CIN3	Severe dysplasia	Severe dyskaryosis (and carcinoma *in situ*)

The Bethesda 2001 classification is less directly comparable to the system above. The LSIL classification covers HPV cytopathic changes and the CIN1/mild dysplasia category, whilst HSIL covers the CIN2 and CIN3 and carcinoma *in situ* categories.

The cytological changes corresponding to the three categories are outlined below (also see *Colour plate 33*).

Mild dyskaryosis. Cells resemble superficial or intermediate cells by having abundant cytoplasm with angular outlines. The nucleus may show slight irregularities but occupies less than half of the cell.

Moderate dyskaryosis. The nucleus is more enlarged and may stain irregularly and the nuclear border may be less distinct and irregular. The enlarged nucleus occupies one-half to two-thirds of the cell.

Severe dyskaryosis. Only a thin rim of cytoplasm is usually present. The cell is largely occupied by an irregular nucleus. Sometimes the cytoplasm is larger but there is extra cytoplasm present. The appearance can resemble the nucleocytoplasmic ratio in mild dyskaryosis but the nucleus in severe dyskaryosis is actually much larger than in mild dyskaryosis.

The severity of the disease is judged purely on morphological grounds. The number of cells is not significant. A single cell is just as significant as hundreds, provided the cytological changes are the same. The number of cells seen to be abnormal is as much an indication of the sampling as of the severity of the disease.

The term **carcinoma *in situ*** refers to the stage when the cells are showing all of the cytological signs of full malignancy but have not yet begun to invade or metastasize. This is a histological diagnosis since it is not possible to tell whether invasion has occurred from isolated cells.

The final stage of the diagnostic spectrum is **invasive carcinoma** where the cells have begun to spread beyond the epithelium and into other tissues. This again is a histological diagnosis but a smear will often have cells that indicate that invasion is occurring, so the smear can be reported as 'suspected invasive carcinoma'. The change from the pre-malignant state to the frankly invasive malignancy is usually marked by the appearance in the smear of bizarre cell shapes of which the **tadpole** and **fibre cells** are the most distinctive. Tadpole cells are named from their shape and have a malignant nucleus in the 'head' of the tadpole. Fibre cells are excessively elongated and often have an elongated hyperchromatic nucleus. The cytoplasmic staining is irregular in both cell types.

Other types of malignancy apart from squamous cell carcinoma may also occur (e.g. adenocarcinoma) but their appearance will not be dealt with in this account.

The other report that can be made is for an 'inadequate' or 'unsuitable' smear. An inadequate smear is one that cannot be satisfactorily diagnosed. The inadequacy may be due to one or more of the following:

- Too few cells in the smear to be reliably diagnosed as negative.
- The presence of red cells that are obscuring detail.
- The presence of pus that is obscuring detail.
- Air-drying or inadequate fixation. If the cells have been badly treated during preparation, a reliable diagnosis is not possible.

Assessment of the suitability or otherwise of a smear is subjective and again varies with the laboratory. If the smear is unsatisfactory, then the reason why it is unsatisfactory should be reported back to the requesting doctor and a repeat smear obtained as soon as possible. It is hoped that the introduction of the liquid-based cytology systems will result in a much lower rate of inadequate smears.

12.3   OTHER CELL PREPARATION TECHNIQUES

As well as the direct scraping technique used in cervical smears and buccal smears, there are a variety of other samples, mainly non-gynaecological, that can be made into cytology smears. These are derived from fluid samples.

Fluid samples

Many body fluids contain exfoliated cells and can used to prepare smears. They can be collected by inserting a fine needle into a fluid-filled area (see *Box 12.15*). Fluid samples include pleural and peritoneal aspirates, urine, cerebrospinal fluid, amniotic fluid, breast cyst fluids and breast (nipple) discharges. They vary in volume from about 1 ml to more than 1 litre in volume. They can vary in consistency from watery urine to more viscous discharges and they vary in their cell content from very sparse to heavily cellular. Not surprisingly, then, there are several different ways of preparing smears from fluid samples.

Heavily cellular specimens can be directly smeared but most fluids require some method of concentrating the cells. Concentration of fluids can be achieved by centrifugation or filtering.

Box 12.15 Fine needle aspirates

Fine needle aspirates are not really 'exfoliative' cytology since they involve introduction of a needle into tissue under local anaesthetic to withdraw cell samples from small nodules that have been detected by palpation or some form of imaging (X-ray, ultrasound or magnetic resonance imaging). The needle can be guided by ultrasound into the lesion. The use of fine needle aspirates is increasing and is a great advance in the management of breast tumours but is also used for thyroid and lymph node lesions. The cells recovered by these techniques can be examined by the same methods that are used for other smears, so the specimens are examined by cytologists along with the more conventional exfoliated cell smears.

Centrifugation

Centrifugation may be done in one of two ways:

Simple centrifugation. This involves putting the fluid sample into tubes and then centrifuging them (e.g. 2500 r.p.m. for 5 min). Centrifuge tubes can be quite large so reasonably large quantities can be concentrated in this way. Following centrifugation, the supernatant is carefully decanted off leaving

Slide

Funnel for fluid

Absorbent pad

Figure 12.3
Cytocentrifuge chamber. The centrifugal force would be from left to right forcing fluid out of the funnel on to the slide

the deposited cells in the bottom of the tube. The tubes are drained and the cells resuspended in a few drops of fluid. The concentrated suspension can then be smeared using a wire loop or a pipette and the smears are fixed in the usual way. Very watery fluids may not have sufficient protein to allow the cells to adhere and may need the addition of protein such as serum or albumen to aid adhesion of the cells.

Cytocentrifugation. This involves a special centrifuge that spins small (about 0.5 ml) samples of fluid directly on to the slide (see *Fig. 12.3*). This has proved very effective although early techniques did not always give good cell yields as cells were lost before being spun. The very discrete pellet of cells produced by the cytocentrifuge makes screening easy and cell yields are now usually very good. Again, watery fluids may need additional protein to aid adhesion. With the cytocentrifuge, it is critical to have the correct number of cells in the fluid sample. If there are too many cells in the sample, they will produce several layers of cells instead of a monolayer, whilst if there are too few cells in the small volumes used in the cytocentrifuge, then the smear will be very sparse. The samples may need to be diluted or concentrated before use. Concentration is normally be done by simply centrifuging a larger sample as outlined above.

Filtering

This involves using a specialized plastic membrane filter (such as Millipore or Nuclepore filters), which can be made translucent if immersed in xylene. The fluid containing cells is placed in a funnel with a filter and the fluid is gently sucked through the membrane using reduced pressure. Filtration is suitable for concentrating large volumes of fluid containing very few cells as all of the cells are trapped on top of the filter.

The cells can be stained whilst still on the filter, which becomes reasonably transparent in the mounting process. Staining and processing of the filters is comparatively simple and the filters are mounted on a slide under

Figure 12.4
Filter with a cell trapped on the upper surface

a coverslip. The filter does obscure the cells slightly and cells may be distorted by the filter, especially if too much pressure is applied (see *Fig. 12.4*).

This gives very high recovery rates for cells and can be carried out with fixed cells. This is useful if specimens need to travel some distance to the laboratory since the specimen can be stabilized and rendered less of a health hazard by adding fixative to the fluid sample before despatch. The filters effectively trap epithelial cells but smaller cells such as bacteria and blood cells may pass through the small pores in the filter. The filters are not suitable for Romanowsky staining methods that tend to stain the background. The filters are not suitable if there are many cells since with a high cell content the filters will quickly become clogged. The method is not generally popular and has largely been replaced by the cytocentrifuge, but it does have some advantages so most laboratories have the capability to filter specimens, even if they usually prefer to use other methods. Filtration is an essential part of some liquid-based cytology methods, which are replacing traditional gynaecological scrapes.

Thick fluid samples

If a fluid sample is very thick, it may be thinned to allow easy separation of cells. Thinning can be done by enzyme digestion, the use of HCl (8%) or ultrasonic treatment.

Specimens that are heavily contaminated with blood may be similarly cleaned up using acetic acid to lyse the red blood cells or enzymes such as streptolysin, but separation by careful centrifugation is probably better as it produces fewer problems with staining and later cell identification. The red blood cells are denser than other cells and so get pushed to the bottom of the tube with a thin layer of other cells on top ('buffy layer') allowing separation of the red blood cells from the other cells. The separation can be enhanced by using a flotation material such as Histopaque. The flotation material is prepared to have a density between that of red blood cells and the epithelial cells. When it is used in a centrifuge, the red cells, being denser than the medium, go to the bottom of the tube but the other cells are less dense and float in the medium instead of being deposited along with the red cells.

Exfoliative cytology samples and potential infection

In all smearing techniques it is important to take full precautions against infection since the samples are usually unfixed when they arrive and so may be contaminated with pathogenic (disease-causing) organisms. This is most likely in specimens from ill patients. Bacteria may even be able to multiply in some samples, making the bacterial count even higher if the samples are delayed or stored inappropriately.

SUGGESTED FURTHER READING

Coleman, D.V. and Chapman, P.A. (1989) *Clinical Cytotechnology*. London: Butterworths.

Hopwood, J. (1995) *Background to Cervical Cytology Reports*. Burgess Hill: Schering Health Care Ltd.

Kiernan, J.A. (2001) *Histological and Histochemical Methods*, 3rd edn. Oxford: Hodder Arnold.

Kocjan, G., Priollet, B.C., Desai, M. *et al.* (2005) BSCC, Bethesda or other? Terminology in cervical cytology. *Cytopathology* **16**, 113–119.

Morse, A. (2002) Diagnostic cytopathology: cell appearances. In *Theory and Practice of Histological Techniques*, 5th edn (eds J.D. Bancroft and M. Gamble). Edinburgh: Churchill Livingstone.

Morse, A. (2002) Diagnostic cytopathology: specimen collection and preparation. In *Theory and Practice of Histological Techniques*, 5th edn (eds J.D. Bancroft and M. Gamble). Edinburgh: Churchill Livingstone.

National Institute for Clinical Excellence (2003) *Guidance on the Use of Liquid-based Cytology for Cervical Screening*. Available at http://www.nice.org.uk/pdf/TA69_LBC_review_FullGuidance.pdf

SELF-ASSESSMENT QUESTIONS

1. What are the characteristics needed for a screening method? Outline the properties of exfoliative cytology that make it useful for screening.
2. What staining method is used for gynaecological smears? Why is this method preferred to other staining methods?
3. Which of the following are normal smear constituents, which are abnormal constituents and which are normal but only under specific circumstances? (a) Superficial cells; (b) parabasal cells; (c) *Trichomonas vaginalis*; (d) dyskaryotic cells; (e) koilocytes; (f) erythrocytes; (g) plasma cells.
4. What is meant by a navicular cell and when would you expect to see them in smears?
5. Which stage(s) of the menstrual cycle are best for taking smears and which are not suitable?
6. What effect does acute inflammation have on a vaginal smear? How does this differ from chronic inflammation?
7. Name four common infectious organisms that can cause inflammation.
8. What do the initials CIN stand for?
9. List the characteristics that would make a smear unsuitable for diagnosis.

Cytogenetics and molecular genetics

Learning objectives

After studying this chapter you should confidently be able to:

■ **Outline the diagnostic applications of cytogenetics.**
Cytogenetics can be used to diagnose genetic disease caused by alterations in chromosome number and structure. This can be either pre-natal or post-natal diagnosis. It can also be used in some acquired conditions such as leukaemia where there may be a change in the chromosomes.

■ **Describe how chromosomes are prepared for examination and describe a normal human chromosome complement.**
Chromosome examination requires cells to be grown in culture to ensure they are in mitosis, which is the only time when chromosomes are visible. Chromosomes need to be spread using hypotonic treatment of cells. Fixed smears can then be stained to show the bands and this allows recognition of altered number or structure. A normal human cell contains 46 chromosomes including 22 paired chromosomes (autosomes) and two sex chromosomes, which differ between the sexes (two X chromosomes for females and one X and one Y chromosome for males).

■ **Describe the effects of alterations in chromosome number on spontaneous abortions and live births.**
Spontaneous abortions are more common in chromosomally abnormal pregnancies. Chromosomal abnormalities are the commonest cause of spontaneous abortions.

■ **Briefly discuss and name the syndromes that occur in humans from altered chromosome number.**
Chromosomes may be altered either in complete sets of the 23 human chromosomes (euploid variations), giving an embryo or fetus with 23 or 69 chromosomes, or the change may only affect one chromosome (aneuploid variations). All euploid variations are inviable. Most autosomal aneuploid variations are also inviable with only Down's syndrome surviving to birth in significant numbers. Aneuploid variations in the sex chromosomes are less vulnerable and several syndromes occur, notably Klinefelter's, Turner's, supernumerary X and double Y syndromes.

■ **Outline the effects of alterations in chromosome structure.**
Chromosome structure changes can result in less-severe forms of genetic disease than loss or gain of complete chromosomes. Deletions act as incomplete monosomy, whilst insertions act as incomplete trisomy. Translocations may not cause problems if there is no loss or gain, only simply rearrangement of genetic material (balanced translocation).

However, translocations may cause problems to the offspring of carriers as the meiotic rearrangement of genetic material can result in an unbalanced chromosome structure. Inversions may also cause problems during gamete formation but by a different mechanism.

- **Interpret an abbreviated karyotype.**
- **Briefly describe the role of *in situ* hybridization.**
  In situ hybridization allows changes in the DNA sequence to be identified and localized. This can be used to identify mutations in individual cells as well as whole-body changes.

Genetics is the study of inheritance and encompasses three areas of study, two of which involve aspects of cellular pathology and histology:

- Classical genetics is the study of pedigrees and the pattern of inheritance from one generation to the next. The basis for classical genetics was laid in the nineteenth century by the Austrian monk Gregor Mendel whose name is associated with this type of study as Mendelian inheritance.
- Cytogenetics is the part of genetics involved in the study of genetic changes that occur in cells and can be seen down the microscope. These include changes in chromosome number or structure. The chromosomes can be stained so that they show **banding**. The banding is unique to each chromosome and individual chromosomes can be recognized. By sorting the chromosomes into order, a person's **karyotype** can be determined. The karyotype shows whether any chromosomal abnormalities are present. It is even possible to recognize changes within an individual chromosome such as loss of certain bands. The techniques involved include smear preparation and staining and are quite closely allied to histology and cytology.
- Molecular genetics studies the changes in the sequence of DNA bases. These changes can be visualized in sections or smears by using molecular biological techniques and the role of these techniques is rapidly increasing, including their use in histology.

Only cytogenetics and molecular genetics will be considered in this chapter.

13.1 CYTOGENETICS AND CHROMOSOME STUDIES

Chromosomes are the structures that contain the DNA of the cell and normal humans have 46 chromosomes. Abnormalities in the number and structure of these chromosomes are important in many fields of medicine.

Chromosomal abnormalities

Chromosomal abnormalities are a common cause of abortion

Abnormalities of chromosomes are often present from the instant of fertilization and remain until the death of that individual since there are no cures

Box 13.1 Abortion and miscarriage

The term abortion is often misused by the general population. In medical terms, an abortion is any premature termination of pregnancy before the foetus is viable.

There are several different forms of abortion. **Spontaneous abortions** are where the pregnancy terminates because of physiological reasons without any intervention or traumatic cause. **Induced** or **artificial abortions** are where the pregnancy is terminated medically and a **criminal abortion** is an induced abortion carried out by someone other than trained, licensed medical personnel. **Therapeutic abortions** are induced abortions performed to save the life of the mother.

To many people, the term abortion means an induced abortion and they would use the term **miscarriage** for a spontaneous abortion. The term miscarriage in medicine strictly only applies to spontaneous abortions in the second trimester of pregnancy. Pregnancy is divided into three trimesters, each lasting 3 months, so the second trimester refers to the 4th, 5th and 6th months of a pregnancy.

for chromosomal abnormalities. Many chromosomal abnormalities will spontaneously abort and only become apparent as miscarriages in the pregnancy (see *Box 13.1*). Although diagnosis of a miscarried foetus may seem like a low priority in medicine, it can be important to the parents by indicating that the dead foetus would never have been able to have had a full and normal life. Knowing this often helps parents come to terms with their grief.

Diagnosis of the cause of foetal death may also be important to rule out other causes of abortion. Some unfortunate couples suffer repeated abortions and recognition of the cause of the miscarriage is often a necessary first step in helping to overcome the problems.

A somewhat similar argument also applies to children and adults who are born with chromosomal abnormalities. Although at present little can be done to help people with these conditions except for treating individual symptoms or aspects of the syndrome, it can be helpful if the parents and the individual understand the nature of their abnormality. Knowing the cause of a problem can also eliminate the need to search further for a diagnosis.

Pre-natal diagnosis may allow termination of the pregnancy

Diagnosis of chromosomal abnormalities in the foetus during the early part of pregnancy allows more active intervention. This may involve a medical termination or abortion of the pregnancy if the defect is severe and the prospective parents do not wish to have a severely affected child. Pre-natal diagnosis is controversial because of this link with induced abortions.

Diagnosis of the sex of the foetus can also be used as a method of preventing certain diseases, even though the presence of the disease itself cannot be identified directly. Diseases that can be controlled in this way are those carried on the X chromosome. Such X-linked or sex-linked disorders only affect males. Females can carry the recessive aberrant gene but are not affected. Sex-linked abnormalities include Duchenne-type muscular dystrophy, adrenoleukodystrophy and haemophilia. Although these diseases cannot currently be recognized in the foetus, it is possible to prevent the birth of affected children by only allowing female foetuses to go to full term and be born. Females are not affected so this will effectively prevent the disease occurring in these individuals, although they may still be carriers. It does mean, however, that all male foetuses need to be aborted. Half of these male foetuses would be expected to be normal. This again is ethically controversial.

It may be possible to diagnose abnormalities before pregnancy begins

The increasing use of *in vitro* fertilization also allows the early diagnosis of abnormalities. The prospective mother is stimulated with fertility drugs causing her to hyperovulate and produce several viable ova instead of the usual single ovum produced in a normal ovarian cycle. The fertile eggs are collected by a minor surgical procedure using ultrasound to detect and aspirate mature Graafian follicles that contain eggs. The eggs are then mixed with the father's sperm in the laboratory and grown in culture until they form a small ball of cells (called a **morula**). At this stage, every cell is identical and indeed each cell is capable of forming a whole human being and it is separation of the cells at this stage that leads to identical twins. Removal of a single cell from the morula will not affect the foetus or its development adversely. The removed cell can then be used to produce a diagnosis. Normal embryos can be used for implantation and abnormal embryos would be discarded. By diagnosing before conception, the problems of abortion can be avoided. This technique is being used on a trial basis but is not yet routinely available.

Chromosomal abnormalities arising after birth may be a cause of malignant transformation

There is another use for cytogenetic investigation and this is in the study of chromosomal abnormalities that have arisen after birth in one or a few cells. The majority of the body's cells will be quite normal but the altered cells may cause disease. The commonest disease involving altered chromosomes is malignancy. Alteration of the normal chromosome complement is frequent in malignant tumours and some abnormalities are characteristic of certain diseases. In chronic myeloid leukaemia (CML) there is a large abnormal chromosome called the Philadelphia chromosome formed from a translocation between chromosomes 9 and 22. About 90% of CML cases have this abnormal chromosome and only 10% do not. The presence of the chromosome gives a better prognosis (median survival of about 4 years) compared with those without (median survival of about 1 year).

Preparation of chromosomes for karyotyping

Chromosomes are only visible during cell division

In order to recognize chromosomal abnormalities microscopically, the chromosomes must be visible. The chromosomes are not normally visible within the cell since the DNA is, for most of the time, in the form of euchromatin, which is very spread out in the nucleus. The chromosomes are only visible at mitosis and meiosis when the DNA becomes highly compacted by coiling and supercoiling into relatively short rods. In humans, meiotic divisions only occur in the gonads and are not used in normal cytogenetic investigations. Mitosis occurs in a large number of cells and tissues during normal cell division and is much more easily investigated and so forms the main target of cytogenetic investigations.

Chromosomes can be studied during prophase and metaphase

The chromosomes begin to appear during the first stage of mitosis (**prophase**) as long tangled threads and become shorter and less tangled as prophase progresses into **metaphase** where the chromosomes line up along the central plane of the cell and attach to the microtubules of the mitotic spindle. It is at metaphase that the chromosomes are at their shortest and thickest. The spindle fibres then pull the chromosomes apart at **anaphase** and the chromosomes begin to lengthen again. The two new nuclei develop a membrane and the cytoplasm divides during **telophase** and **cytokinesis**. Thus, the only time that chromosomes can be seen is in these stages. To ensure seeing cells in mitosis, it is necessary to grow them in culture and even then they need treating to make the chromosomes separate and allow them to be easily visualized.

The technique of chromosome preparation can be divided into three stages: (i) collection of the cells; (ii) growth of the cells in culture; and (iii) the preparation of stained smears.

Collection of cells

The cells must be capable of mitosis so not all samples are equally useful. The most common cell samples in the adult are blood lymphocytes, which can be stimulated into mitosis, small skin biopsies from which fibroblasts can be grown and bone marrow cells. Naturally exfoliating cells are not suitable as they are usually dead or at least non-mitotic.

In pre-natal testing of the foetus, the samples are usually taken either from amniotic cells floating in the amniotic fluid, which can be sampled by amniocentesis, or from chorionic villus cells (see *Box 13.2*). Foetal blood samples can be used to produce mitotic samples but are less common.

Several different sites may need to be sampled if the disease is believed to be a **mosaic** where not all of the cells of the body are affected (see section on Mosaicism in this chapter).

Growth of cells in culture

Growing cell and tissue cultures is a difficult and painstaking procedure. Cells in the human body are supplied with fresh nutrients, oxygen, hormones and other signalling molecules by the bloodstream. The same

---

Box 13.2 Pre-natal collection of cells

Amniocentesis is the collection of amniotic cells from the amniotic sac. It is carried out by inserting a needle through the abdominal wall into the uterus and through the membranes surrounding the foetus and drawing off some fluid and cells. This is a fairly safe procedure and rarely (less than 1%) causes an abortion. Amniocentesis can only be done after about week 16 of pregnancy. The cells grow rather slowly so it may take 2–3 weeks to get a diagnosis. This makes it quite late in pregnancy before the results are known and a decision on termination taken.

Chorionic villus sampling is usually done through the cervix and can be performed as early as 8 weeks. The cells grow more quickly so the results can be determined much earlier. Chorionic villus sampling has a higher risk of inducing an abortion than amniocentesis. If it is performed very early (before 10 weeks) there is also the risk of some foetal deformations being caused.

---

vascular system then removes carbon dioxide and other waste products. The vascular system is dynamic and modifies its pattern of blood flow in response to signals from the cells, e.g. if oxygen levels become low. This ideal situation cannot be reproduced exactly in culture and instead the cells are grown in a static fluid that is only occasionally renewed. Nevertheless, some cells can be cultured successfully, provided they are given certain requirements. The method of culture varies depending on the type of cell sample available and the reason for culturing the cells.

Cell cultures are grown from cell suspensions

Cell cultures are where the cells are separated into individual cells before being grown. The cells are prepared as a suspension and can be handled easily using pipettes. This type of culture is easy when the original samples are already suspensions of cells, as would be the case with blood samples and samples of amniotic fluid. It is slightly more complex when the cells are firmly attached to each other, as they would be in a skin sample or a chorionic villus biopsy. The cells must first be separated by treatment with chemicals or enzymes. Trypsin, a proteolytic enzyme, and ethylene diamine tetra-acetic acid (EDTA), which is a calcium-chelating agent, are useful in disrupting tissues without killing or lysing cells. Mechanical disruptions with pipettes or dissecting instruments also help. The cells are then seeded into a plastic culture bottle (see *Colour plate 34*), which has a large flat base on which the cells can settle and grow.

Human cells will not grow whilst in suspension and must attach to a surface of some sort before they will settle down and divide. The density of seeding is important. If too many cells are added, the cells will be crowded and not grow. If too few cells are added, then they may find that they cannot adapt to the culture medium and will fail to thrive.

Tissue culture involves growing cells from a small piece of tissue

Tissue culture involves placing a small intact piece of tissue into a culture flask. The cells can then grow and spread from this explanted piece of tissue to form a layer of cells covering the bottom surface of the flask. Small

---

Box 13.3 Organ culture

Although not relevant to chromosome studies, organ culture is a method of culturing cells in which more than one cell type is cultured in the same flask. Various tricks are used to encourage the cells to interact and produce small clusters of cells arranged in the same way as tissues in the body. This is a research method for investigating how cells interact rather than a method of providing a source of cells for diagnosis. The long-term goal of such research is to be able to grow whole organs from a small sample of cells. The growth of small amounts of simple tissue such as skin and bladder has been achieved and used clinically, but the growth of complex organs such as kidney is still not possible. Organ culture would be a valuable way of producing new organs to replace organs that are failing in a patient. Cells taken from a patient in renal failure could be used to produce a new kidney, which would then be transplanted back into the patient. The use of an organ grown from the patient's own cells would avoid the problem of organ rejection. Although currently in the realms of science fiction for complex organs, such a technique may one day be possible.

'punch' biopsies of skin can be grown in this way and fibroblasts will readily spread from the connective tissue layers of skin. Fibroblasts are one of the easier cell types to grow, so this is a good method for obtaining cells. The advantage of this technique is that there is no need to use enzymes or chemicals that may damage the cells.

A further type of culture, organ culture, is described in *Box 13.3*.

Primary cultures are taken directly from tissues

Along with the way cells are obtained, there is also a difference between the cultures depending on how long they have been cultured. Cells grown directly from the body are termed **primary cultures** and are the most reliable in genetics since they represent cells that have been in artificial culture for only a few divisions. When cells are grown for long periods, they need to be subcultured periodically to keep them growing.

Subculturing cells helps to keep them growing

Subculturing is needed not only to replace the nutrients by replacing the culture medium but also to separate the cells. When cells divide in culture, they spread across the surface and will eventually form a complete layer of cells. The cells then stop growing. This stoppage is called **contact inhibition** and can be overcome by gently stripping the cells off the plastic using trypsin or chelating agents and then dividing them into several new flasks. Subculturing ensures that the cells have more room to grow and keeps the cells dividing rapidly. Once cells have been subcultured in this way they are known as **primary cell lines**. Primary cell lines are still useful as the cells should still be identical to the original cells. Normally, primary cell lines will stop growing after a few subcultures as they become senescent and die. Human cells can divide between 10 and 50 times before this senescence occurs. The limited number of divisions is called the Hayflick limit and is believed to be a property of the cells in the body and not an artefact of the culturing technique.

Box 13.4 Transformation

Transformation to form established cell lines is believed to be due to mutation within the cell, possibly caused by viruses, radiation or chemicals. Transformation is very similar to the alterations seen in malignant change in the body and primary cultures from malignant tumours often grow immediately in the same way as established cell lines. This has made the process of transformation an important tool in investigating carcinogenesis. The most famous of the tumour-derived established cell lines is the HeLa cell line (the name HeLa come from the initials of the patient with the original tumour) derived from a cervical cancer in an American woman in the 1950s. This cell line is still rapidly dividing today and is one of the easiest cell types to culture. The cells grow so readily they have been able to spread to other cultures and many cell lines have become infected by this aggressively growing cell.

Established cell lines

When cells are grown through several subcultures, sometimes a few of the cells may change. This is called transformation (see *Box 13.4*). The transformed cells have quite different growth characteristics and their genetic make-up alters so they are not suitable for genetic analysis. These transformed cells can divide without limitation and are called **established cell lines**. Established cell lines can be important in biological and medical research but not for cytogenetic diagnosis of the original donor.

Requirements for cell growth

Cells require several critical factors for their active growth. These factors are now largely understood and we know the specific growth requirements for many cells, including those used in chromosome studies. The growth media are usually made from many individual components and can be quite complex.

Nutrients

This is the most obvious requirement since nutrients provide the energy needed for metabolism and the building materials needed to synthesize new proteins and other cell constituents. Unlike bacteria and plants, most human cells require a complex mixture of nutrients and cannot synthesize many of the basic building blocks of proteins. Cells require a variety of nutrients to be supplied including (see *Box 13.5* for a formulation of Medium 199):

- **Carbohydrates.** All cells need a supply of energy and carbohydrate is the most readily used energy source. Human cells do not usually need any specific sugars and most media simply use glucose as the energy source.
- **Amino acids.** These are the basic building blocks of protein and a wide variety of amino acids needs to be supplied.
- **Vitamins.** Again, human cells cannot synthesize many vitamins that are often essential enzyme cofactors. Individual cells do not necessarily require the full range of vitamins that a complete human being would, e.g. vitamin K is not essential in culturing cells as it is needed for the production of blood clotting factors rather than cellular materials.

Box 13.5 Constituents of culture medium

The complexity of a cell growth medium can be seen from the following formula for 1 litre of Medium 199.

Amino acids:
L-Alanine 25 mg
L-Arginine HCl 70 mg
L-Aspartic acid 30 mg
L-Cysteine HCl 0.1 mg
L-Cystine 20 mg
L-Glutamic acid 75 mg
L-Glutamine 100 mg
Glutathione 0.05 mg
Glycine 50 mg
L-Histidine HCl 20 mg
L-Hydroxyproline 10 mg
L-Isoleucine 20 mg
L-Leucine 60 mg
L-Lysine HCl 70 mg
L-Methionine 15 mg
L-Phenylalanine 25 mg
L-Proline 40 mg
L-Serine 25 mg
L-Threonine 30 mg
L-Tryptophan 10 mg
L-Tyrosine 40 mg
L-Valine 25 mg

Vitamins
Ascorbic acid 0.05 mg
Biotin 0.01 mg
Calciferol 0.1 mg
D-Calcium pantothenate 0.01 mg
Choline chloride 0.5 mg
Folic acid 0.01 mg
Inositol 0.05 mg
Menadione 0.01 mg
Niacin 0.025 mg
Nicotinamide 0.025 mg

p-Aminobenzoic acid 0.05 mg
Pyroxidol HCl 0.025 mg
Pyridoxine HCl 0.025 mg
Riboflavin 0.01 mg
DL-α-Tocopherol phosphate 0.01 mg
Thiamine HCl 0.01 mg
Vitamin A 0.1 mg

Other components:
Sodium acetate 50 mg
D-Ribose 0.05 mg
2-Deoxy-D-ribose 0.5 mg
Adenylic acid 0.2 mg
Adenine 10 mg
Guanine HCl 0.3 mg
Hypoxanthine 0.3 mg
Thymine 0.3 mg
Uracil 0.3 mg
Xanthine 0.3 mg
ATP 10 mg
Cholesterol 0.2 mg
Tween 80 5 mg
$Fe(NO_3)_3.9H_2O$ 0.72 mg

Hanks' salts:
$CaCl_2.2H_2O$ 185 mg
Glucose 1000 mg
KCl 400 mg
KH_2PO_4 60 mg
$MgSO_4.7H_2O$ 200 mg
NaCl 8000 mg
$NaHCO_3$ 350 mg
Na_2HPO_4 (anhyd.) 47.5 mg
Phenol red 17 mg

■ **Minerals, trace elements and anions.** These are sometimes needed both as nutrients to be included in structural or enzymic proteins and as part of the osmotic and buffering system of the culture medium.

Gases

It is usually appreciated that cells need oxygen since this is the driving force of energy production in the cell but it is less obvious that carbon dioxide is also needed. Human cells produce carbon dioxide as part of their metabolism and it is thought of as a waste product, but of course in the immediate environment of the cells, the concentration of carbon dioxide is much higher than in the atmosphere as a result of the build-up from metabolism. The cells are adapted to this level of carbon dioxide and use it as part of their buffering system. Carbon dioxide levels therefore need to be maintained in the medium. Sometimes the medium is formulated to include carbon dioxide as bicarbonate ions and the medium can then be used in ordinary air, but some media require the atmosphere in contact with the medium to contain 5% carbon dioxide and cells grown in such media require a special atmosphere of gases.

pH

Cells are very sensitive to pH. They must be kept very close to neutrality and will only grow at about pH 6.8–7.4. The pH in the medium gradually changes as nutrients are used and waste products such as lactic acid accumulate. The growth medium is always buffered to minimize these changes using phosphate and bicarbonate buffers, but the pH will still fall slowly. In order to show the changes in pH, the growth medium usually includes phenol red as a pH indicator. Phenol red changes from red (at pH 7.4) to orange and then yellow. Thus, tissue culture media are red at the beginning of the culture and then gradually change colour. Once the orange/yellow colour develops, the medium is exhausted and must be replaced (see *Colour plate 35*).

Osmotic pressure

Osmotic pressure (sometimes called tonicity) again alters during the culturing of cells mainly due to the gradual loss of glucose and other nutrients. The original osmotic pressure is calculated to include these materials so as they are broken down or incorporated into proteins the osmotic pressure gradually falls. Changes in osmotic pressure of the medium are rarely a problem in practice since the medium needs to be changed more quickly for pH changes than osmotic pressure changes. Thus, provided the pH is acceptable, the tonicity will also be acceptable. Osmotic pressure is usually kept in the range of 280–320 mOsm.

Complex molecules

In addition to the direct nutrients needed for growth, human cells also need hormones, growth factors and other complex molecules to grow properly. These play no structural role in growth but act as stimulants for the cells. Without such stimulation, most cells are not mitotic and will not divide or grow. These complex molecules can be added in pure form but it is more common to add a natural source of these as serum (e.g. foetal calf serum) or embryo extracts (made from fertile hen's eggs), which are rich sources of these growth-stimulating substances.

Even then, some cells will not grow adequately and will need further stimulation. Adult human lymphocytes will not enter mitosis unless they are first stimulated by one or more special mitogens. The mitogens used include the lectins phytohaemagglutinin and pokeweed mitogen, which can be added to the culture medium and will stimulate cell division.

Temperature

Cells are very sensitive to slight rises in temperature and are easily killed at even a few degrees above normal body temperature. Lower temperatures than normal are better tolerated by cells but will greatly slow growth. It is quite usual to handle cells at room temperature for replacing medium, subculturing, etc., but it is important to grow cells in a well-controlled incubator. Although cells will tolerate temperatures down to about 10°C reasonably well, they are killed at very low temperatures, e.g. freezing is lethal. It is possible to freeze cells and keep them alive but this requires the use of an antifreeze to protect them.

Sterility

The usual cell culture media are not only ideal for growing human cells but are also ideal for growing bacteria, fungi and other micro-organisms. Bacteria and fungi will usually grow more rapidly and aggressively than human cells. To prevent micro-organisms adversely affecting the growing cells, it is important to keep the culture medium free from contaminants. Simple sterile procedures are the best defence but are usually backed up by including penicillin and streptomycin in the medium to inhibit bacterial growth.

Because of the complexity of the formula and the difficulties of maintaining sterility during preparation, most laboratories buy their medium ready made up and sterilized, rather than preparing it themselves. This is the easiest and most reliable way to get well-balanced and reliable growth media.

Preparation of stained smears

Cells can be stopped in metaphase to obtain more mitotic cells in the smear

The purpose of growing cells in culture is to obtain cells in mitosis. Most cells, even in culture, will not be in mitosis itself but in interphase when the chromosomes are not visible. Mitosis normally only lasts between 1 and 2 h, and even in culture many cells only divide once every 24–48 h, so as few as one in a hundred cells may be in mitosis at any one time. Some laboratories like to enhance the number of cells in division by adding a mitotic spindle inhibitor to the medium some hours before the smears are prepared. This stops the cells in metaphase, when the chromosomes are aligned along the cell equator. Thus, if colchicine is added for the final 24 h of culture, all of the cells that enter mitosis will be held in metaphase. This increases the number of mitoses seen but the chromosomes are at their shortest and thickest in metaphase, which limits the resolution of banding patterns. Thus, other workers prefer to leave the cells alone so that all stages of mitosis will be present. Metaphase is the best stage to prepare chromosome spreads for simple counting, but prophase, when the chromosomes are longer, allows better banding resolution.

Cells are made to swell to separate the chromosomes

Just before smears are made, the cells are stripped from the bottom of the flask and treated with a hypotonic solution. Cells in hypotonic solution will absorb water and swell. This causes the chromosomes to separate and makes counting and identifying the chromosomes easier. The hypotonic treatment needs careful timing and control to prevent the cells from bursting since once the cell membrane bursts individual chromosomes may be lost, making accurate counting impossible. The ideal situation is maximum swelling without rupturing of the cells.

Chromosome spreads are fixed in methanol/acetic acid

The swollen cells are fixed in suspension using methanol/acetic acid. This fixative is a good nuclear fixative but is a poorer cytoplasmic fixative so the chromosomes are well preserved but some of the cytoplasmic protein is lost. This loss of protein is an advantage for this application since it makes the final preparation less obscured by protein. The smears can then be made by placing a drop of the suspension of fixed cells on to a slide and air-drying. Drying is accelerated if the slide is warmed on a hotplate before dropping on the suspension.

Banding patterns are stained using Giemsa

Staining to produce the bands can be done by a variety of techniques but the commonest is using Giemsa staining, often with extra treatments such as enzyme digestion or salt treatment to enhance the banding pattern. The banding pattern produced with Giemsa is referred to as G-banding. Fluorescent banding techniques, e.g. using quinacrine dyes, produce a slightly different pattern of banding and are referred to as Q-banding. These fluorescent probes attach to the adenine/thymine-rich regions of DNA (see Chapter 8). Specific techniques are also available to stain the centromere.

Chromosomes are counted and arranged in order

After staining, the slides are observed under very high magnification and the chromosomes are counted and measured. By taking photographs, it is

---

Box 13.6 Brief history of chromosome counting

Chromosomes were recognized in the 19th century but the correct number of human chromosomes was not determined until 1956 (by Tjio and Levan). Until the discovery of banding in the late 1960s, chromosomes could only be grouped into seven groups and could not be recognized individually.

Q-banding was the first to be introduced in 1968. Giemsa banding was first used in 1971 with warm saline treatment to enhance the bands. Trypsin was introduced in the same year and is now the most popular method.

possible to cut out each chromosome from the photograph and pair it with its partner chromosome. The pairs can then be lined up in order (see *Colour plate 36*). This is known as the **karyotype**. The chromosomes are numbered to identify them. The larger chromosomes are numbered first so chromosome number 1 is the largest human chromosome. Cutting out the photographs is slow and tedious so computer-aided techniques are becoming more common. These not only make it easier to assemble the chromosomes but also help in identifying the chromosomes by using image analysis techniques (see Chapter 15). The appearances are vague and need an experienced eye to ensure that all abnormalities are detected. This is especially true of structural abnormalities.

13.2 THE EFFECTS OF ABNORMAL CHROMOSOME NUMBER

The normal human chromosome number is 46, which consists of 23 pairs of chromosomes. One set of chromosomes comes from each parent and this double set is referred to as the **diploid** number. Abnormalities of chromosomes occur quite frequently in human reproduction with about 7.5% of conceptions being chromosomally abnormal. This high level of abnormality falls to about 0.6% of pregnancies at birth since many of the abnormal embryos cannot survive and spontaneously abort. Chromosomal abnormalities are the commonest cause of spontaneous abortions, with about 60% of spontaneous abortions showing abnormal numbers of chromosomes. Abnormalities can occur in a number of ways, each of which has its characteristic set of syndromes. These changes vary in their severity; the most severe is dealt with first here.

Euploid variation

Euploid variation involves a change in a complete set of chromosomes with the total number of chromosomes following the pattern: total number of chromosomes = $n \times 23$. Thus:

- $n = 1$ is **haploid** and the total number is 23;
- $n = 2$ is **diploid** (normal) and the total number is 46;
- $n = 3$ is **triploid** and the total number is 69;
- $n = 4$ is **tetraploid** and the total number is 92.

Haploid and polyploid foetuses do not survive

All euploid abnormalities are inviable in human beings although they occur frequently in plants. Although humans as a whole cannot survive abnormal numbers of chromosomes, some human cells are often polyploid (e.g. liver). More than 99% of triploid conceptions abort during early pregnancy and the few live births that have occurred did not survive long after delivery. No tetraploid conceptions have survived to birth.

Euploid variations may be due to abnormal divisions or abnormal fertilization

There are probably several different causes of euploid variation. Haploid states could occur due to development of an unfertilized egg but seem totally inviable even as embryos and do not occur even in aborted embryos. Polyploid states may be due to non-separation of the chromosomes in gamete formation resulting in diploid gametes. Normally the meiotic division reduces the number of chromosomes in the gametes to a haploid state. About 10% of polyploid conceptions occur due to the extra set of chromosomes coming from diploid ova and about 24% of the extra chromosomes come from diploid sperm.

An alternative way of getting polyploid conceptions is by double fertilization. There is normally a mechanism in the ovum to prevent more than one sperm head penetrating into the ovum but if this fails then several different sperm may each supply a complete set of chromosomes resulting in polyploidy. Double fertilization seems to occur in about two-thirds of all triploid conceptions. Triploid abortions may be recurrent in some women and seem to run in some families, suggesting a genetic susceptibility to this type of abnormality. Euploid variation is easily diagnosed from chromosome spreads since it is obvious that there are large numbers of extra chromosomes. Euploid variations will normally only be seen in aborted foetuses.

Autosomal aneuploid variation

Variation of less than a complete set of chromosomes is termed **aneuploid variation** or **aneuploidy**. Autosomes are those chromosomes that are identical in both sexes and are numbered from 1 to 22. Aneuploidy is usually a variation of only one or two chromosomes at most and multiple chromosome variations are uncommon. The change of only one chromosome results in the chromosome number being 46 ± 1. Thus, 46 − 1 is termed **monosomy** (e.g. 45, −7) and 46 + 1 is called **trisomy** (e.g. 47, +21), with the missing or additional chromosome indicated after the chromosome number.

The presence of an extra set of genes seems to alter the cell's metabolic balance and control. An aneuploid foetus is affected by multiple abnormalities due to the imbalance, affecting a large number of genes on each chromosome. The larger the chromosome, the greater the burden of defects and each chromosome has a characteristic set of metabolic abnormalities related to the genes contained on that chromosome (i.e. a characteristic syndrome; see *Box 13.7*).

Box 13.7 Syndromes

The occurrence of a set of symptoms or conditions together is called a syndrome. A syndrome may not always be a single disease but the symptoms commonly occur together. Syndromes are often recognized before the underlying cause is determined that would allow them to be described as a disease.

Autosomal monosomy is inviable and most affected embryos abort spontaneously, often very early in pregnancy, and are rarely seen even in abortions. This lack of the abnormality ever being seen suggests that the embryo is unable to implant or even that the zygote is totally inviable. Occasionally, foetuses that are 45, −21 have survived through to birth but they did not survive long after being born.

Autosomal trisomy is the commonest abnormality of chromosome number. Most of the affected foetuses do still abort and probably over 95% do not reach the end of pregnancy and instead miscarry. Trisomy is also the commonest form of abnormality in spontaneous abortions with nearly one-third of all abortions being trisomic.

The commonest form of trisomy at birth is **Down's syndrome** where there is an extra chromosome 21 (see *Box 13.8*). Down's syndrome occurs with a frequency of about 1 in 700 live births. Although it is the commonest abnormality at birth, over 60% of Down's syndrome foetuses still spontaneously abort during pregnancy.

Box 13.8 Dr Down and his syndrome

Dr John Langdon Haydon Down was the superintendent at the Earlswood Asylum for Idiots in Surrey. He published a short paper on the 'Ethnic Classification of Idiots'. He held a view that would nowadays be held to be 'politically incorrect'. Down thought that male Europeans were the highest level of evolution and he looked at his 'idiots' (a term that was then a technical term rather than the more general meaning it has assumed today) as lower forms of humans. Down classified them into different, and in his view lesser, racial types. He identified Ethiopian, Malay and other idiocies. One type, however, has proved to outlast his simplistic and unfounded philosophy of the hierarchy of races and that is his classification of 'Mongolian idiocy'. This real syndrome is still often referred to as 'Mongolism' although it has no real link to oriental races except perhaps the epicanthal fold over the eyes. Ironically, his name has been used to try to replace this 'non-PC' name, yet he was the originator of the ill-thought epithet.

Down's syndrome has many genetic abnormalities

Chromosome 21 is a very small chromosome so it carries fewer genes than most chromosomes. The smaller number of genes is probably the reason that so many Down's syndrome children survive. Yet even with this tiny chromosome the number of defects is large. Down's syndrome patients have characteristic facial features including a generally flattened facial profile, a small low-bridged nose and an extra fold of skin over the eye (epicanthal fold). They also have an enlarged protruding tongue and their mouths are not held closed. They have redundant skin folds around the neck and misshapen low-set ears.

They have a shorter than normal stature and their limb bones are short. The middle phalanx of their little finger is abnormal making it incurving. The palm of their hand shows only a single crease instead of the more usual double crease. They also have an extra-wide gap between the first and second toes ('sandal gap'). Their joints are more flexible than normal. The tone of their muscle fibres is less than in normal muscles and they have pelvic abnormalities.

Mental retardation is probably the single most important feature of the syndrome and Down's syndrome patients are one of the largest groups of mentally retarded people in institutional care. Their intelligence may in some cases be within the normal range but most have an IQ of less than 70.

Female Down's syndrome patients have reduced fertility but any children are usually normal and not affected by Down's syndrome. Males are usually infertile.

They suffer from an increased incidence of certain diseases: endocardial defects 40%; cataracts 2%; epilepsy 10%; hypothyroidism 3%; and leukaemia 1%. Alzheimer's disease is common in Down's syndrome patients who survive beyond 40 years old.

This is a large list of symptoms so the syndrome is quite complex and involves the imbalance of many genes.

Trisomic foetuses other than Down's syndrome rarely survive

Other trisomic foetuses that sometimes survive to birth are Patau syndrome, which is a trisomy of chromosome 13 and occurs with frequency of around 1 in 5000 births, and Edwards' syndrome, a trisomy of chromosome 18 with a frequency of 1 in 3000 live births. Most other trisomics abort and do not reach birth. The incidence of most trisomies shows a link with maternal age (see *Box 13.9*). Other factors pre-disposing to the incidence of trisomy include exposure to radiation, hypothyroidism, viral infections and familial tendency.

Sex chromosome aneuploidy

The sex chromosomes X and Y have unique features that make them more likely to produce viable aneuploidy syndromes than most of the autosomes.

Box 13.9 Effect of maternal age

A number of chromosomal abnormalities including Down's syndrome have a strong link with maternal age. The incidence rises with the age at conception. Mothers over the age of 40 have a 20- to 40-fold increased risk of having a Down's-affected child compared with a 20-year-old mother. This indicates a non-disjunction in ovum formation possibly due to the long meiotic prophase.

Girls are born with all of the ova in their ovary already partially in the first meiotic prophase. The meiotic division only goes to completion during ovulation. This means that some eggs may remain in the middle of cell division for 40 or more years. It is hardly surprising that occasionally this results in chromosomes sticking together and not separating. Because of the non-disjunction, one of the daughter nuclei is effectively trisomic and the other monosomic.

In Britain, the number of women delaying the birth of children until later in life is increasing. This results in an increase in chromosomally abnormal conceptions. However, the availability of pre-natal diagnosis and elective abortion of affected embryos means that the number of affected live births is falling. This means that published figures for the frequency of chromosomal abnormalities often differ depending on whether they consider only live births and the years that are included in the survey.

The Y chromosome is a very small and insignificant chromosome that has no function except for determining sex. The Y chromosome converts the embryonic gonad into a testis and does very little else. The testis then produces testosterone that controls the main body structure and produces either a male or a female type of body. The Y chromosome is, however, dominant and if present will turn the foetus into a 'male', regardless of how many X chromosomes are present.

The X chromosome is large and important and contains many genes totally unrelated to gender. However, in adults only one X chromosome is ever active in any cell. Any extra X chromosomes above the single one that is needed for normal cell activity are 'switched off' during early embryonic life between day 12 and day 16. This inactivation of any supernumerary X chromosomes is called Lyonization. This results in a visible heterochromatic (dark-staining) structure close to the nuclear border in epithelial cells (see *Colour plate 37*). This structure is called the **Barr body** and provides a convenient way of determining the number of X chromosomes within a cell (see *Box 13.10*).

If only one X chromosome is present (e.g. normal male), then no Barr bodies are seen. If two X chromosomes are present (normal female), then one Barr body is seen as the unwanted X is switched off. The number of X chromosomes is thus the number of Barr bodies plus one. Abnormal numbers of Barr bodies are found when the phenotypic (body) sex is different from the chromosomal sex, e.g. Klinefelter's, Turner's and 47XXX syndromes.

Barr bodies can be visualized by taking a buccal (cheek) smear and staining with a basic dye such as cresyl fast violet. The Barr bodies are then seen as small dark-staining structures inside the nucleus close to the nuclear border. Not all cells allow the Barr body to be identified but about one-third of cells should show distinct Barr bodies, so examination of about 30–40 cells should give a good indication of their presence.

Barr body

Klinefelter's syndrome

This syndrome is associated with an extra X chromosome giving a complement of 47XXY or less commonly 48XXXY. It can also occur as a mosaic in which only some of the cells of the body have an abnormal chromosome number. Klinefelter's syndrome has a frequency of around 1 in 1000 live births so it is slightly less frequent than Down's syndrome.

Klinefelter's syndrome patients appear to be male, since they have the dominant Y chromosome, but they are usually infertile. Investigation of

---

Box 13.10 Sex determination in sport

The use of Barr bodies to determine chromosomal sex was introduced into athletics to prevent cheating by men masquerading as women. It was first used in Mexico in 1968. This is at first glance a good test for sex since buccal smears are a better and less intrusive test than physical examination of the external genitals of female athletes, which was the previous method for determining the sex of athletes.

What has happened in practice, however, is that the test has not detected any cheating where men (XY) have tried to compete as women (XX), but it has, perhaps unfairly, disqualified athletes who have genuine medical conditions such as XX/XY mosaics and androgen insensitivity. Androgen insensitivity is a condition in which the receptors for the male hormone are abnormal resulting in the inability of cells to respond to testosterone. Although they are Barr body-negative (they have only one X chromosome), they are, if anything, at a disadvantage since they have no response to testosterone (an anabolic steroid) whereas 'normal' women have a low level of testosterone, which would enhance athletic performance.

---

infertility may be the first time they are diagnosed and about 10% of all infertile males turn out to have Klinefelter's syndrome. Klinefelter's syndrome patients usually have a lower than normal testosterone level and have small testes and poorly developed secondary sexual characteristics. They tend to have long limbs and may develop slight breast enlargement, which is called gynaecomastia. They are more likely to develop diabetes mellitus and as group they have a lowered average IQ although individuals may be more intelligent than average. There is one (or more) Barr body present, despite the person being apparently male.

There is no major link between the incidence of Klinefelter's syndrome and maternal age; about 60% of the extra chromosomes are of paternal origin and 40% of maternal origin.

Turner's syndrome

In this syndrome there is only one sex chromosome. Thus, they are usually designated as X0 (X nought). Turner's syndrome often occurs as an incomplete form of the disease with about 57% of affected individuals being 45X0, 16% being mosaic with only some cells affected, 10% having deletion of part of the X chromosome and 17% having their X chromosomes fused to form an isochromosome X. Cases of Turner's syndrome are less common than Klinefelter's syndrome with around 1 in 5000 live births being affected.

Turner's syndrome patients appear female but have primary amenorrhoea and never menstruate. They have redundant skin around the neck with a short stature and this gives them a very stocky appearance. Their intelligence is normal and they have a normal life span. Congenital heart disease is more common in Turner's syndrome patients, with up to 20% of patients being affected, and they also suffer more commonly from hypertension (27%). Over 75% have only the maternal X and 25% only the paternal X, suggesting that a defect in sperm formation is more common in this syndrome than ovarian defects. The effects on the patient vary in severity. Mosaic and deletional variants of the syndrome often show relatively mild effects. There is no Barr body present in the buccal smears, despite the person being apparently female, although Barr bodies may be present in some cells of mosaics since the defect only affects some cells in these individuals.

47XXX, superfemale or supernumerary X syndrome

In these patients, there are more than two X chromosomes present and although 47XXX is the most common form, it is also possible to get 48XXXX and 49XXXXX. They occur in about 1 in 1000 births. This syndrome often goes totally unrecorded since the affected female is apparently quite normal but there may be some slight reduction in IQ, especially with XXXX and XXXXX variants, although this would usually be within the normal range for an individual. Affected females are usually fertile and, despite being chromosomally abnormal themselves, their children are quite normal. There does seem to be a maternal age effect. Buccal smears show multiple Barr bodies present depending on the number of X chromosomes present.

47XYY double Y syndrome

The majority of these patients are asymptomatic and are never diagnosed. XYY occurs with a frequency of around 1 in 1000. Although there are no distinctive signs, their IQ may be reduced and they may be more aggressive and have behavioural problems. This is borne out by the reported finding of XYY at a rate of 20 per 1000 of the prison population compared with 1 in 1000 in the general population. Thus, XYY patients were 20 times more likely to end up in prison than a normal male in this study. This link with behaviour is controversial. Patients with XYY are usually fertile and have normal offspring.

Box 13.11 Syndrome symptoms may be corrected by therapy

Early diagnosis of affected children is becoming more common and treatment can be given to correct abnormalities. Thus, growth hormone treatment of a Turner's syndrome child would mean that the characteristic short stature would be prevented. Similarly, plastic surgery can correct some abnormalities such as webbing of the neck. Thus, the symptoms described are often missing and the descriptions may apply only to untreated patients.

Structural abnormalities of chromosomes

Structural abnormalities involve changes of less than one complete chromosome (see *Fig. 13.1*). Different types of abnormality occur but the overall incidence is about 1 in 200 live births. The number of different possible changes means that a shorthand description is often used (see *Box 13.12*).

(a) [A B C D E F G H I J K L M N O P]

(b) [A B C D K L M N O P]

(c) [A B C D E F G H I J K L]

(d) [A B C D E F G H I J F G H I K L M N O P]

(e) [A B C D E F G H I v w x y z J K L M N O P]

(f) [A B C D E F G M L K J I H N O P]

Figure 13.1
Structural abnormalities of chromosomes: (a) normal chromosome; (b) internal deletion; (c) terminal deletion; (d) duplication; (e) translocation; (f) inversion

---

Box 13.12 Nomenclature of chromosomal abnormalities

The position and form of chromosome abnormalities are described in a shorthand form such as 46, XX, t(9:22)(q34;q11), which shows the Philadelphia chromosome in a woman. The first figure is the total chromosome count (in this case 46, normal diploid number). The next gives the sex chromosomes (in this case XX, female). The letter 't' indicates a translocation (del = deletion, dup = duplication, inv = inversion, fra = fragile site). The next pair of numbers in brackets indicates the chromosomes involved and the last set indicates where on the chromosomes the changes occur. In this case, chromosomes 9 and 22 are involved with the short arms (q = short arm, p = long arm) being affected at positions 34 and 11 in the banding patterns.

The complications of nomenclature have increased since the technology has improved the resolution of chromosome bands. Whole books on nothing but nomenclature have been written. Details can be found in *ISCN 2005. An International System for Human Cytogenetics Nomenclature.*

Deletions

Deletions involve the loss of part of the chromosome and act like incomplete monosomy. The symptoms are usually similar to the full monosomic syndrome but with a reduced range and intensity of effect. The severity is dependent on the extent of the deletion, e.g. deletion of part of chromosome 5 allows survival to birth as Cri du Chat syndrome, whilst monosomy of chromosome 5 is lethal. Smaller **microdeletions** show less widespread defects and are linked to single diseases (e.g. malignancy) rather than a syndrome of symptoms.

Duplications

Duplications are small increases in the amount of chromosomal material and act as incomplete trisomy. Again the range of symptoms and severity vary with the size of the duplication.

Translocations

Translocations involve transfer of genetic material from one chromosome to another. If the translocation goes in both directions, it is described as a

reciprocal translocation. If there is no loss or duplication of material, then the effects are minimal as they constitute a **balanced translocation**. Although balanced reciprocal translocations are not deleterious, they can result in problems during meiosis when the balance can be upset and the offspring may be affected by **unbalanced translocations**.

Robertsonian translocations involve the fusion of the long arms of two chromosomes, often with the total loss of the short arms. Translocation Down's syndrome is typical of such translocations. **Isochromosomes** are formed by the fusion of the long arms of both isologous chromosomes.

Translocation Down's syndrome. This involves the translocation of part of chromosome 21 on to another chromosome. The commonest form (about 4% of Down's cases) involves a Robertsonian transfer of the long arm of chromosome 21 on to the long arm of chromosome 14 giving a large abnormal translocation chromosome.

The loss of the short arms does not seem to cause any major problems and people with the chromosome can appear quite normal, i.e. they have a carrier status. The carriers are, however, easily detected cytogenetically as they have only 45 chromosomes and the abnormal chromosome is much larger than normal. Carriers can transmit the disease to their children

Figure 13.2
Inheritance of translocation Down's syndrome. This shows the chromosomes of a carrier at the top with a translocation 14, 21 chromosome and a normal 14 and a normal 21 chromosome. The two lower sections show the gametes produced depending on the pairing of chromosome 21. If the normal chromosome 21 ends up in the same nucleus as the normal chromosome 14, then after the addition of a normal set of chromosomes from the other gamete, the embryo will be diploid. The other nucleus formed from this pairing will contain only the translocation chromosome and after fertilization with a normal gamete will produce a translocation carrier. If the normal chromosome 21 ends up in the same nucleus as the translocation chromosome, then one nucleus would produce a Down's syndrome-affected child and the other would produce a monosomy of chromosome 21 that is inviable

depending on how the chromosomes transfer into the gametes. The chromosomes pair, with chromosome 14 dominating the pairing. There are four gametes that are likely to be produced and these are shown in *Fig. 13.2.*

The translocation Down's syndrome-affected patients have 46 chromosomes (unlike the 47 of trisomic Down's syndrome) and have the large abnormal chromosome. Translocation Down's syndrome shows a familial pattern of inheritance and is not connected to maternal age.

The risk of a carrier having an affected child is not a simple 1:4 Mendelian ratio as the Down's syndrome foetus is less viable than a normal foetus and abnormal gametes are likely to be less fertile (especially abnormal sperm). If the male is carrying the 14:21 translocation chromosome, then the risk of having an affected child is about 1%, whilst if the female is the carrier the risk rises to 15%.

Inversions

Inversions occur when a chromosomal segment becomes reversed. Provided there is no loss or gain of chromosomal material in the inversion, then the person will be normal. Problems only arise during gamete formation and only then if a crossover occurs at meiosis.

If a crossover occurs within the inverted segment, then abnormal gametes will be formed. The severity depends on whether the inversion includes the centromere (called a pericentric inversion) or is entirely within one arm of the chromosome and does not include the centromere (paracentric inversion). Paracentric inversions will give recombinant chromosomes, one of which is acentric (no centromere), whilst the other is dicentric (two centromeres) and both nuclei would produce inviable cells. Crossovers affecting pericentric inversions produce abnormal offspring due to the chromosomes having both a deletion and a duplication.

In female carriers of an inversion, about 8% of the offspring will be affected and in male carriers 4% of the children will be abnormal.

Chromosome 9 is unusual and shows a relatively high incidence (about 1% of the population) of a small pericentric inversion but no abnormal offspring have been reported as being associated with this inversion.

Fragile sites on chromosomes

These are sites on chromosomes that are particularly vulnerable to damage. These fragile sites occur in some inherited diseases.

The commonest disease associated with a fragile site is **Fragile X syndrome** (see *Box 13.13*). This occurs in about 1 in 2000 males and 1 in 4000 females. The cause is an abnormality of the distal end of the X chromosome where there is a multiple repeat of the CGG sequence of bases. In a normal X chromosome, there are less than 50 such repeats but in affected individuals there are more than 200 such sequences. These sequences render the chromosome more fragile than normal and can cause loss of part of the chromosome. The affected individuals show mental and physical handicaps. The abnormality can be detected cytogenetically or by Southern blotting using the restriction enzymes *Eco*RI and *Eag*I.

Box 13.13 Fragile X Syndrome

Fragile X syndrome is the commonest form of inherited mental retardation with an estimated incidence of 1 in 1000 males. It is sex-linked with the incidence figures being lower for females. The true incidence is not known as there have not been any large-scale population studies. It is possible that around 60–90 % of people with Fragile X syndrome are not yet correctly diagnosed.

Fragile X syndrome patients may show some physical features associated with the disease including a long narrow face and prominent ears, jaws and forehead but these are not seen in all patients. Up to 80% of boys who inherit Fragile X syndrome have some mental impairment. The majority are only mildly to moderately retarded. Girls are less affected with only about 30% having some degree of mental retardation; this is because the faulty gene is supplemented by the other X chromosome.

Up to 20% of those with Fragile X syndrome may show some autistic behaviour, e.g. poor eye contact, hand-flapping, hand-biting and poor personal skills. Behaviour problems and speech or language difficulties are also frequently associated with Fragile X syndrome.

Other fragile sites also occur in Huntingdon's chorea and myotonic dystrophy. All show the phenomenon of **anticipation** where the disease gets worse from generation to generation, presumably as the number of trinucleotide repeats increases making the site more fragile.

Mosaicism

Most chromosomal abnormalities in foetuses occur due to defective meiosis or fertilization and result in all cells of the embryo being affected. However, it is possible that, in the early embryo, mitosis may be defective resulting in only some cells being chromosomally abnormal. Such individuals are termed **mosaic**. The effects of mosaicism are similar to the full chromosomal abnormality but in a milder form. The severity of the symptoms is related to the proportion of cells affected.

The extent of the cells affected depends on how early in embryogenesis the abnormal mitosis occurs. If it is an early division, then many organs can be affected, whilst a later abnormal division may affect only a few tissues. If the abnormal mitosis was the very first division of the fertilized ovum then about half of the cells in the final foetus would be affected. This would give a more severe syndrome than if the abnormality occurred in the second division when only one quarter of cells would be affected.

About 1% of Down's syndrome cases, 16% of Turner's syndrome and 5% of Patau syndrome cases are mosaic rather than the full syndrome. In mosaics, several tissues may need to be karyotyped to detect the abnormality since only a few tissues may have developed entirely from the defective cell in the embryo.

13.3 MOLECULAR GENETICS

The sequence of bases in DNA specifies the protein structures and is the basis of the transfer of genetic information from one generation to the next.

The role of the double helix and the specific pairings of bases (adenine pairing with thymine and guanine pairing with cytosine) are well known and the details can be found in any modern biochemistry or genetics textbook. The manipulation and control of this base-pairing mechanism is the basis of most molecular biology techniques. The accuracy of the pairing allows specific sequences of bases in DNA to be identified and localized. This can be used to identify the position of mutations and therefore genetic disease in cells.

Pairing with RNA is also possible and allows the detection of mRNA with specific base sequences to be localized. The detection of specific mRNA sequences enables the molecular biologist to identify which cells are using a particular gene and changes in the activity of particular genes with time. Hybridization of DNA sequences requires that the DNA is denatured before annealing, whereas mRNA is not double-stranded and does not need this step. In this chapter, DNA techniques will be used as an example, but similar methods are applicable to detecting RNA sequences.

DNA hybridization

DNA hybridization involves 'melting' and 'annealing' of two DNA strands

DNA consists of two complementary strands that can unite to form a double helix and this is the usual form of DNA in human cells and in fixed tissue samples. The helix is held together by hydrogen bonds that are sufficiently weak to be broken by raising the temperature ('melting' or denaturation of DNA) or by using mild chemical treatment. Different DNA samples will melt at different temperatures. The more G–C base pairs there are, the higher the melting temperature required, since G–C pairing involves three hydrogen bonds whereas A–T pairs have only two hydrogen bonds. A temperature of 90–95°C will usually melt mammalian DNA. If the temperature is then lowered to 60–70°C, any complementary sequences will realign and reform the double helix ('anneal') using specific hydrogen bonding. Annealing is most stringent (i.e. requires the best match) if the annealing temperature is 20–30°C below the melting temperature of the DNA. If the sequences are not complementary, they will not anneal in this way since the specific hydrogen bonding will not be correctly aligned. Thus, if annealing occurs then the two sequences must be identical or at least extremely similar. This very specific bonding is made use of in hybridization techniques to identify specific DNA base sequences.

In situ *hybridization is more applicable to sections than blotting and PCR*

Nucleic acids in sections can be identified using blotting techniques or the very powerful **polymerase chain reaction** or **PCR** (see *Box 13.14*), which are very important techniques in molecular biology. These techniques use the

Box 13.14 Polymerase chain reaction

The polymerase chain reaction (PCR) is a method of cloning DNA very rapidly. It uses short primers that are known to bind either side of the DNA to be cloned. The sample is incubated in a solution containing the primers, DNA polymerase enzyme and the four deoxyribonucleotide triphosphates. The DNA is heated to separate the two strands of the DNA helix and then cooled to allow hybridization with the primer oligonucleotides. The DNA polymerase then forms a new strand on each of the old strands so there will now be two DNA helices. By repeating the sequence, each of the two will split and now form four DNA helices. Every time the cycle (heating to separate the strands, cooling to allow hybridization and finally producing a new strand) is repeated, there will be a doubling of the amount of DNA. Twenty to 30 cycles generates a huge number of copies of the original DNA. In histology, PCR will give copies of DNA in the cells but the new DNA molecules will be in solution rather than localized in the tissues. The reaction can be useful to detect very small amounts of DNA that might be missed using *in situ* hybridization. This might occur in viral infections where perhaps only one or two cells in the tissue might have the viral genome. PCR will allow the virus to be detected although it will not indicate which cells are infected.

tissue section simply as a source of DNA and extract the DNA from its position. This ignores the ability of histological sections to identify exactly where specific sequences are located. PCR is also so sensitive that extremely high levels of care and careful controls are required to ensure that there is no contamination. The benefit of a histological approach is that it will not only detect whether a sequence is present but will also locate which cells have the sequence. This is achieved by a range of methods that leave the nucleic acid in position (*in situ*) and are referred to as *in situ* hybridization methods.

In situ *hybridization uses a labelled probe DNA*

In situ hybridization techniques use labelled strands of DNA of a known sequence to identify whether the complementary sequence is present within the tissue. The known DNA sequence is labelled in some way that allows it to be identified and localized. The labelling problems and solutions are in many ways similar to the labelling techniques used with proteins, as outlined in Chapter 8. The original methods used radioactive labelling (see Chapter 11) and were often difficult to apply, but more recently the DNA has been labelled with biotin or fluorescent materials (known as fluorescent *in situ* hybridization, or FISH) or colloidal gold. The choice of method is determined by the speed and sensitivity required and if electron microscopic detection is needed. Fluorescent labels are quicker but less sensitive, gold is needed for electron microscopy and biotin is more sensitive but can give a higher background staining. Radiolabelling is rarely performed now because it has few advantages and several drawbacks (it is slow and expensive and radioactivity is a problem for handling and disposal). Commercially available probes are available for many important genes and these are often available with a range of different labels.

Figure 13.3
Denaturation and reannealing of DNA

The two DNA strands are separated by heating

Having obtained the labelled nucleic acid probe, it is first necessary to separate the two strands of DNA in the tissues (see *Fig. 13.3*). Separation can be achieved by heating the DNA to 95°C for 15 min. The labelled probe DNA is added and then annealed to the tissue DNA at 60–70°C. The labelled probe DNA is at a much higher concentration than the natural DNA, so the added probe is more likely to bind than the natural DNA strand.

This is a powerful technique and can localize defective genes or detect the absence of genes in cells. The length of the DNA probe is critical for the correct result. If the probe is much shorter than about 18 bases, then the sequence of bases that the probe DNA will anneal with will not be unusual or unique and may be repeated at many places in the DNA. Short sequences of bases will occur in almost all genomes and all chromosomes. If the probe is very long, then hybridization will be much slower and some hybridization may occur even when there are mismatches between the probe and the tissue DNA. Thus, longer probes will not detect genes that are altered by a single base-pair mutation, e.g. in sickle cell anaemia.

The amounts of DNA used are quite small

Labelled DNA probes are expensive and difficult to produce in large quantities so the technique needs to be done with very small amounts of reagent. The reactions are often performed under a coverslip to prevent evaporation and using as little as 50 µl of labelled probe. The whole slide is also kept in a humidity chamber of some sort to minimize evaporation at the raised temperatures used in hybridization.

Nuclease enzymes need to be inactivated

The amounts of DNA being used are very small and can be destroyed by even slight nuclease enzyme activity. The reagents and the sections must be kept free of all nucleases. Ribonuclease is resistant to heat so it needs inactivating chemically. This can be done with the inhibitor diethylpyrocarbonate (DEPC). The safest way is to add DEPC to all solutions, including distilled water, and to treat all glassware before use. Nucleases also need calcium ions for their activation so the addition of EDTA to solutions also helps to prevent nuclease activity.

DNA may need unmasking after fixation

In the same way that antibody techniques use enzyme treatment to remove any blocking proteins, *in situ* hybridization methods use proteinase K to unmask the DNA. The proteinase K also helps to destroy nuclease enzyme activity so it helps protect the nucleic acid. It is, of course, essential that the enzyme used is pure and is not contaminated with nucleases. Proteinase enzymes will not destroy DNA but it is still necessary to restrict the digestion or the tissue structures will be affected and some DNA may be lost because its tissue links are removed.

The stringency of hybridization can be controlled using additives

Formamide is a reagent that destabilizes the hybridization complex. Formamide can be used to supplement the effects of heat. The higher the concentration of formamide, the lower the annealing temperature that is needed (about 0.6°C for every 1% formamide). The balance between temperature and formamide concentration is often the critical factor in controlling the formation of precise hybridization complexes.

Sodium chloride can also alter the stringency of hybridization. High salt concentrations will mask the electrostatic repulsion between probe and tissue DNA allowing less stringent annealing, whilst low salt levels will favour very stringent matching. (This masking of repulsion is reminiscent of the salting-on seen with dyes.)

Fragmented non-specific DNA, usually salmon sperm DNA, can be applied to stop non-specific binding of DNA to tissues in the same way that normal serum is used to block non-specific protein binding in immunotechniques. Dextran sulphate can also be used to block non-specific binding.

DNA hybridization is likely to become more important in the future as DNA probes become available commercially. At present, much of the work being done with *in situ* hybridization uses DNA probes prepared 'in house' since suitable commercial probes are not available. There are some probes available but they do not cover the full range of probes needed. The number of available probes is, however, increasing rapidly. Once reliable probes and simple reliable *in situ* hybridization methods are available, it seems highly likely that they will be used for many diagnostic situations.

SUGGESTED FURTHER READING

Kiernan, J.A. (2001) *Histological and Histochemical Methods*, 3rd edn. Oxford: Hodder Arnold.

Lamar Jones, M. (2002) Molecular pathology in-situ hybridization. In *Theory and Practice of Histological Techniques*, 5th edn (eds J.D Bancroft. and M. Gamble). Edinburgh: Churchill Livingstone.

Shaffer, L.G. and Tommerup, N. (eds) (2005) *ISCN 2005. An International System for Human Cytogenetics Nomenclature*. Basel: Karger.

SELF-ASSESSMENT QUESTIONS

1. Explain what the term cytogenetics means.
2. How can cytogenetics be useful in clinical practice?
3. Outline the preparation of chromosome spreads from human lymphocytes. How are the chromosomes made to separate?
4. How can the banding patterns on human chromosomes be demonstrated?
5. Give the karyotype of a normal human female. What would a karyotype of 47 XY, +21 mean?
6. Approximately how common are chromosome abnormalities at conception and how common are they at birth?
7. Why do alterations in the sex chromosome numbers occur more frequently than abnormalities in the number of most other chromosomes?
8. What are the differences between the usual Down's syndrome and the translocation form of Down's syndrome?
9. What is a pericentric inversion and how will it affect the individual?
10. Outline the principles of the *in situ* hybridization method. What is its application in histology?

Infective agents and amyloid

Infection of tissue is a common finding in cellular pathology and the ability to recognize the causative agent can be invaluable in diagnosis. Identification from tissue sections is not the best method available and whenever possible identification should be done by microbiological techniques, which allow greater sensitivity and accuracy. Most microbiological identification relies on growing the organism and detecting its growth requirements, sensitivity to inhibitors and biochemical tests. Identification from histological sections suffers in comparison with these culturing methods since the organisms are killed by fixation. Formaldehyde fixation in particular is a very effective method of killing infective organisms. All of the useful microbiological growth methods are lost once the tissue is fixed. Identification of the organism may still be possible but is less certain or more difficult, or both.

In infected tissues the causative organism may be relatively uncommon and unevenly spread. This will mean that in an individual section there may be only a few organisms. Unless the staining technique makes these pathogens stand out strongly, it is easy to miss them altogether. The use of fluorescent techniques (see Chapter 15) where the organism is the only material staining against a dark background can help to identify their position in these cases.

Organisms can also be altered by processing and care may be needed. The simple staining techniques of microbiologists often need adapting to cope with formalin-fixed sections, e.g. Gram-positive bacteria may lose their positive reaction in sections and appear Gram-negative.

Finally there may be the possibility of harmless bacteria proliferating in the tissues unconnected with the disease (see *Box 14.1*).

Box 14.1 Commensals

Accurate identification is often crucial since bacteria are common in many sites. Non-disease-causing organisms are called **commensals** and these are common and may even be beneficial. Innocuous commensals need to be eliminated as only the pathogenic organisms are of concern in disease. Rapid fixation of the tissues is needed since many organisms will continue to grow after death and in a few hours or days they can completely destroy the tissue making diagnosis impossible.

Commensal organisms can also mask pathogens by their sheer numbers. One slightly different pathogenic organism in a group of commensals may easily be missed. This can be a problem in post-mortem material where the growth of a harmless commensal may overwhelm the pathogenic organism.

14.1 IDENTIFICATION OF CAUSATIVE ORGANISMS

Although simple histological staining may be limited, there is often other information available or other tests that can be tried if a diagnosis is needed. The attempt to diagnose an agent in fixed tissue can use the following strategies:

- **Clinical diagnosis and symptoms** may be helpful. Often a clinical diagnosis may already have been made and all that is needed to identify the organism is to confirm the clinical assessment. The patient's history may also be helpful with regard to recent travel abroad, ethnic origin, medication and immune status.

■ **Appearance of the section.** The body may respond in a characteristic way to certain organisms. Langhans' giant cells (see *Fig. 14.1* and *Colour plate 38*) are very strongly linked to tuberculosis, even if the organism itself is not easily seen in the standard haematoxylin and eosin stain. The appearance of the tissue may not be specific but may limit the possibilities and thus simplify identification.

Figure 14.1
Giant cells. These are large cells, often more than 200 μm in diameter, with a large number of peripheral nuclei

■ **Special stains or histochemical tests.** The stains may be fairly general (e.g. Gram stain) and may simply identify whether the organism belongs to one particular group or they may be more specific indicating a limited range of organisms.
■ **Immunofluorescent or immunochemical detection.** This method will identify any organism very selectively and can be absolutely specific. The only difficulty is that this can only be used as a confirmatory method since you need to know which antisera to try. Once you have narrowed the options down to a very limited range of possible organisms, this is probably the best way to identify and confirm an individual organism. The use of immunotechniques is also a good way to spot organisms that are too small to be visualized with the light microscope (e.g. viruses).
■ **Nucleic acid hybridization techniques.** In many ways, these resemble the antibody techniques in their applicability. They are excellent confirmatory methods provided you know what you are looking for. They do have the advantage over immunotechniques for virus detection in that they will detect the nucleic acid incorporated into the cell even when no virus particles are present. Some viruses can insert their own nucleic acid into the genome of the host cell resulting in a latent infection. Herpes simplex virus does this and can regularly reactivate, causing repeated bouts of cold sores. These latent infections can be quite important and the use of DNA hybridization allows the detection of the virus even when the infection is latent and not active.

14.2 TYPES OF MICRO-ORGANISM

Infective agents can be of a variety of types and these vary in their size and life history. Only the major types of organism are dealt with in this chapter although others exist and can be important. Mycoplasmas, for example, are considered to be sufficiently different from the classical bacteria to have their own classification and are important in causing up to 10% of community-acquired atypical pneumonia (caused by *Mycoplasma pneumoniae*).

The main groups of organisms are:

■ **Viruses.** These are very small, obligate intracellular parasites. Individual virus particles can usually only be seen with the electron microscope.

■ **Bacteria.** These are larger organisms with most being between 1 and 10 μm in size. Bacteria are visible with the light microscope and a few types can be stained selectively, although not usually identified positively, using simple staining methods. They are probably the most important group in histological identification although not necessarily the most important in terms of disease.

■ **Fungi.** These are found in two forms: **yeasts**, which are single-celled forms, and **hyphae**, which are groups of cells forming threads. They are often larger than bacteria and vary from about 2 to 200 μm. They have a distinctively different cell wall to bacteria.

■ **Protozoa.** Tropical diseases such as malaria and sleeping sickness are caused by protozoa. Although once uncommon in Britain, these diseases are becoming increasingly important as a result of immigration and international travel. Some previously minor diseases have also become important in immunosuppressed patients.

■ **Helminthic infections.** These are caused by parasitic worms and are more common in countries where hygiene is poor. They are usually quite large and can be recognized by their morphology alone.

Box 14.2 Smallpox

Viral diseases are often more difficult to treat than many other forms of infection, so identification may only be of academic interest rather than clinically useful. Viruses can be prevented from causing disease by immunization. This was extremely effective in the case of smallpox, which has been completely eradicated by a World Health Organization programme that started in 1967 and ended in 1969 after 2 years with no reported cases. The disease was once prevalent in many countries with 15 million cases and up to 2 million deaths. The organism caused a distinctive inclusion body called a Guarnieri body in infected cells.

By contrast, there has been a rise in the incidence of human immunodeficiency virus infections but this virus is best seen in cultured cells and cannot be identified easily in tissue sections.

Viral infections

There are many viruses that cause disease (see *Box 14.3*) and so can occur in tissues. Recognition of viral infections is often possible on haematoxylin and eosin sections since they can have distinctive effects on the cells. Although individual viruses are very small, they may occur as aggregates

---

Box 14.3 Pathological effects of viruses

Viruses can cause damage to the host in three ways. Firstly, the virus may directly damage or kill the cell in which it replicates. This **cytopathic effect** is found with hepatitis A virus, which kills liver cells.

Secondly, the virus may trigger an immune response in the host. The infection results in viral antigens appearing on the surface of the cell and these initiate an immune response. The result is that the cell is killed but it is the host's response that causes the damage. Since without a host response the virus causes very little damage, it allows the development of carriers who have a weak or non-existent immune response to infection. The host remains healthy but infective, i.e. is a carrier of the disease. This can occur with hepatitis B virus.

Finally, the virus may transform the cell into a tumour cell. This can occur if the virus carries an **oncogene** or if it interferes with gene regulation. The Epstein-Barr virus and some human papilloma viruses can affect cells in this way.

---

where the viruses clump together within the tissue forming **viral inclusion bodies**. The inclusion bodies are rich in both proteins and nucleic acids so they stain very strongly. These inclusion bodies can often be better seen with trichrome stains (e.g. Lendrum's phloxine tartrazine) where the differences in acidophilia and basophilia of the inclusion body can be exaggerated. Inclusion bodies often have individual names after the person who first described them. Inclusion bodies can be in the cytoplasm (e.g. Negri bodies in rabies) or in the nucleus (e.g. herpes virus) or in both (e.g. cytomegalovirus). In some cases, such as with the surface antigen of the hepatitis B virus (HBsAg, previously also called Australia antigen), there are more selective methods available. HBsAg can be demonstrated by using an orcein stain after permanganate oxidation, which converts sulphur-containing protein into sulphonate residues that then react with the orcein.

Electron microscopy is one of the most useful methods for detection of viruses as many viruses have distinctive shapes, although this will often only indicate the type of virus involved rather than the individual species. The use of antisera against viral proteins is probably currently the best method in widespread use but the use of *in situ* hybridization techniques may become more important as they can be even more specific and have the advantage of detecting viral DNA hidden inside the nuclei of cells.

The **rickettsiae** are intermediate between the viruses and bacteria in that they are more bacteria-like in structure but are obligatory intracellular parasites. Like viruses, they produce inclusion bodies in the cell rather than extracellular colonies and so their demonstration in tissues is more related to viruses than bacteria.

Important virus types causing human diseases

Herpes viruses. These are DNA viruses that are often acquired during childhood and then become latent when they integrate their DNA into the host's DNA. They may re-erupt into active disease in later life. All are similar in structure with a roughly spherical shape of about 120 nm and are covered with a lipid membrane. Individual diseases include varicella-zoster virus, which initially causes chickenpox but can re-emerge from latency in dorsal root ganglia as shingles; herpes simplex virus 1, which causes cold sores; herpes simplex virus 2, which causes genital herpes; Epstein–Barr virus, which causes glandular fever; and cytomegalovirus, which often occurs as an opportunistic infection in AIDS.

Retroviruses. These viruses contain RNA rather than DNA and include human immunodeficiency virus, which causes AIDS, and human T-cell leukaemia virus.

Paramyxoviruses. These are RNA viruses and include the viruses that cause measles and mumps.

Rhinoviruses. These are RNA viruses and include the common cold virus.

Togaviruses. These are RNA viruses and include rubella virus, which causes German measles.

Rhabdoviruses. These are RNA viruses and include rabies virus.

Enteroviruses. These are RNA viruses and include poliovirus. Although best known for its paralysing effects from infecting the anterior horn cells of the spinal cord, poliovirus is an enteric virus that first infects the gut; only in some cases does it get into the blood stream and affect the nerve cells.

Papillomaviruses. These are DNA viruses and include human papilloma viruses, which cause warts. Some types have also been linked to cervical cancer.

Box 14.4 Prions

The causative agent of spongiform encephalopathy can survive fixation and processing and needs special precautions. The spongiform encephalopathies include Creutzfeldt–Jakob disease and bovine spongiform encephalopathy (BSE). The causative agent, however, is not believed to be an organism in the conventional sense but an infective protein (**prion**). The agent can be inactivated by formic acid. There is currently no way of recognizing the agent in tissues and the only identification method is from the characteristic spongy degeneration of the brain.

Bacterial infections

The principal method used for bacteria is the Gram stain or one of its modifications. The Gram stain detects a difference in the cells of the two types of bacteria although there are several possible explanations for the differential staining. The permeability of the cell wall differs (Gram-positive cells have thicker walls) and this is the simplest reason and explains the staining well. The dye (usually methyl violet or crystal violet) penetrates the cell wall and is then aggregated by adding iodine. The large dye aggregates are still easily removed from the more permeable Gram-negative bacteria by a decolorizing agent such as alcohol or acetone but are retained by the more impermeable Gram-positive bacteria. The difference is only in the rate of removal and prolonged washing in acetone will decolorize all bacteria. The Gram-positive nature also alters with fixation and processing. Usually a modified Gram stain is used rather than the simple technique but the method is similar.

Some bacteria can be stained more selectively

Mycobacteria can be stained using the Ziehl–Neelsen (ZN) stain for acid-fast bacilli. The original method used hot carbol fuchsin to stain the mycobacteria followed by differentiation in acid/alcohol. The presence of a hydrophobic material (mycolic acid) in the wall of these organisms is the usual explanation for their retention of the dye. The ability of mycobacteria to resist decolorization is called acid fastness and the organisms can be referred to as AFBs (acid-fast bacilli) or AAFBs (alcohol- and acid-fast bacilli). The acid fastness varies with the species. *Mycobacterium tuberculosis* (which causes tuberculosis) is more robust than *Mycobacterium leprae* (which causes leprosy) and will show stronger acid fastness. The ZN technique is often modified to retain the acid fastness by avoiding strong hydrophobic solvents that would extract the mycolic acid. It has also become popular to use variations of the staining technique that do not involve the use of hot carbol fuchsin and are often referred to as a 'cold ZN'.

The technique can also be performed using the fluorescent dyes auramine O and rhodamine. This makes it easier to spot isolated bacteria, which fluoresce bright yellow against a dark background (see *Colour plate 39*).

Selective methods have been published for *Helicobacter pylori* (which can occur in the stomach and is linked to ulceration, gastritis and stomach cancer) and the use of silver staining for spirochetes. Details of these methods are available in many books on staining techniques.

Box 14.5 Bacterial morphology

The shape of bacteria and their method of associating together can also be useful indicators of the type of organism present. **Cocci** are rounded, whilst **bacilli** are rod-shaped. These two forms of bacteria are the commonest. Other shapes such as comma-shaped (**vibrio**) and spiral forms are less common, so if seen they can be more informative. If the organisms form chains they can be called streptococci (or streptobacilli), whilst clustering indicates staphylococci.

The shape needs to be examined carefully since sections will often slice through the organism so that rods can appear as cocci. If there are many organisms present, then some will lie entirely within the section and the shape and grouping will be identifiable, but if there are only a few bacteria in a section, it becomes more difficult.

Important organisms seen in tissue sections

Gram-positive organisms. *Staphylococcus aureus* is a common pathogen and can cause boils, infections in wounds, abscesses and septicaemia. It is a great problem in hospitals where some strains are becoming resistant to several antibiotics including methicillin (methicillin-resistant *Staphylococcus aureus* or MRSA). The clumps of Gram-positive cocci are fairly distinctive. *Streptococcus* species are also Gram-positive but form chains rather than clumps and include *Streptococcus pneumoniae*.

Lactobacillus acidophilus is a commensal found in the vagina ('Doderlein's bacillus'). *Corynebacterium vaginale* may cause cervicitis and is fairly common in cervical tissues (5–7% of women). *Corynebacterium diphtheriae* was once a common disease causing a severe form of laryngitis but effective vaccination has made it a rare disease in modern Britain.

Clostridia species are associated with a variety of diseases including gas gangrene (*Clostridium perfringens*), botulism (*Clostridium botulinum*), tetanus (*Clostridium tetani*) and pseudomembranous colitis (*Clostridium difficile*).

Mycobacteria are also Gram-positive but only weakly so. Although leprosy and tuberculosis are the main mycobacterial diseases in humans, other mycobacterial species may become opportunistic infections in AIDS patients.

Gram-negative organisms. The Gram-negative 'gonococcus' *Neisseria gonorrhoeae* is the causative organism in gonorrhoea. The organisms are difficult to find in sections of infected tissues although easier to find in smears. *Legionella pneumophila* is a small coccobacillus that causes the pneumonia associated with droplets of water from air-conditioning units. It has a high mortality and is also known as Legionnaire's disease. This is again difficult to see in sections. It is easier to stain with silver techniques than with dyes.

The spirochetes are an unusual group of long, slender, spiral, rod-shaped organisms. They cause the diseases syphilis (*Treponema pallidum*) and Weil's disease (*Leptospira interrogans*). The slender rods are difficult to see in sections and need to be stained with a silver technique to see them easily. Suitable silver techniques include the Dieterle's, Warthin–Starry, and Steiner and Steiner methods.

Fungal infections

Fungi are extremely common organisms in the environment but only a few are pathogenic in humans (see *Box 14.6*). The commonest site of infection is on a surface such as skin or in the mouth. The general term for fungal diseases is **mycoses**. Superficial mycoses such as athlete's foot and ringworm are usually fairly mild diseases but systemic mycoses, where the disease is more widespread inside the body, can be dangerous.

Fungi can occur as a yeast or hyphal form. The hyphae are often distinctive, with features such as the presence or absence of cross-walls (septae) and the degree of branching being useful indicators. Yeast forms are less easy to differentiate on morphological criteria.

Fungi can be stained and demonstrated by the periodic acid–Schiff (PAS) technique, which detects their polysaccharide cell walls. The use of chromic acid as an oxidizing agent (Gridley's technique) or methanamine silver (Grocott's technique) are essentially similar to the PAS method but are still used instead of a simple PAS.

Important fungi seen in tissue sections

Aspergillus fumigatus is a very common organism in soil and can be a commensal in the upper respiratory tract. If it invades the lung, as happens in some AIDS patients (see *Box 14.6*), it may cause pneumonia.

Candida albicans is found in small numbers as a common commensal on wet mucous membranes but can become pathogenic following antibiotic therapy that kills the normal suppressive bacterial flora. It then causes the condition known as **thrush**. In immunosuppressed patients, it can also become systemic.

Cryptococcus neoformans and *Histoplasma capsulatum* can both be acquired from bird droppings and cause systemic disease but are only significant in immunosuppressed patients.

Pneumocystis carinii again is an organism that has only become important in immunosuppressed patients and is a major killer of AIDS patients where it can cause pneumonia.

Parasitic infections

Parasites are large enough and distinctive enough for most diagnoses to be made on the shape and structure of the organism and the nature of the host's response. A haematoxylin and esoin stain may be supplemented with the Romanowsky method (such as Giemsa) or stronger haematoxylins (iron or phosphotungstic acid haematoxylin) or even using PAS to show glycogen, but there are no staining techniques specific for the organisms.

Entamoeba histolytica causes amoebic dysentery. The organism is up to 50 μm in diameter and may contain the remains of ingested blood cells.

Toxoplasma gondii is common in cat faeces and can cause an acute inflammatory condition in lymph nodes (lymphadenopathy) but the infection is often unnoticed (a subclinical infection). In immunosuppressed patients, it can be more dangerous causing brain infections and inflammation of the meninges.

Plasmodium species cause the various forms of malaria. Malaria is common in tropical countries and is regularly seen in immigrants and travellers from these countries. The parasites are usually diagnosed from blood films but they can also be seen in tissues. The associated malarial pigment is similar to formalin pigment and can be removed by alcoholic picric acid. Removal of the pigment allows the malarial parasites to be seen more easily.

Leishmania donovani causes the systemic disease kala-azar, whilst *Leishmania tropica* causes the skin disease 'oriental sore'. The infection is spread by the bite of the sandfly and the organisms can be seen in infected areas in the cytoplasm of enlarged macrophages.

Trichomonas vaginalis is found in the urinogenital tract of both sexes. It is commonly seen in smears but less often in sections.

14.3 AMYLOID

Amyloid is an abnormal protein that accumulates between cells in many organs and can be associated with different pathological conditions. Fresh amyloid has a waxy appearance and absorbs acid dyes although only very weakly. This name is inaccurate as there is no chemical resemblance to starch and it is mainly protein (see *Box 14.7*).

Box 14.7 Origin of the term amyloid

The name amyloid is misleading since it suggests a starch-like material. The eminent pathologist Rudolph Virchow found that amyloid reacted with iodine/sulphuric acid and produced a blue colour and since this is reminiscent of the blue colour given by starch when treated with iodine he introduced the name **amyloid** (*amylo* = starch).

The later finding that it is in fact protein has led to people suggesting other names but in an attempt to be more descriptive these names have often been clumsy. One suggestion was **idiopathic fibrillar glycoprotein**. This name is certainly more accurate than amyloid but such names are unlikely to replace the succinct, if inaccurate, amyloid, which is much easier to say and remember.

Composition and structure of amyloid

Component	Percentage by weight
Water and salts	75
Protein (including plasma protein)	25
Polysaccharides (mainly mucins)	1–2
Lipid	0–3

Amyloid protein is a β-pleated sheet

Despite always having a very similar appearance and sharing staining properties, amyloid protein is very variable in its amino acid composition. All of the different forms of the protein have a β-pleated sheet structure and this seems to be the common link between these different materials. Although amyloid has little structure when viewed with the light microscope (i.e. it is **amorphous**), it does form fibrils that are visible with the electron microscope. These fibrils are 7.5–10 nm in diameter but are variable in length and are striated at 10 nm intervals. The β-pleated sheet structure is unusual in human proteins (although it is found in silk). This structure is very resistant to enzyme degradation and this probably accounts for its accumulation and deposition in tissues since the enzymes cannot remove the deposits quickly enough.

The different amyloid proteins are related to normal proteins

There are several types of amyloid that have been identified but not all of them are considered to be pathological. ASc-type amyloid is common in old people but does not seem to be linked directly to any disease. Only two of the pathological types are common (AA and AL) and the others are included

Table 14.1

Amyloid type	Normal protein the amyloid resembles	Diseases with which the amyloid is associated
AL Amyloid light chain immune-associated amyloid	Immunoglobulin light chain	Multiple myeloma, Waldenström's disease
AA Reactive amyloid	Serum amyloid A (acute phase reactant, apolipoprotein of high-density lipoprotein)	Rheumatoid arthritis, tuberculosis, Hodgkin's disease, familial Mediterranean fever
AE Endocrine-related amyloid	Peptide hormones (calcitonin, insulin)	Insulinomas, medullary carcinoma of the thyroid
β-Amyloid	Membrane glycoprotein	Alzheimer's disease
AS Senile amyloid		Old age (80+)
ASc	Transthyretin (pre-albumin)	
ASc1	Atrial naturetic peptide	
AF Familial amyloid	Transthyretin (pre-albumin)	Familial amyloidosis
AD Dermal amyloid	Keratin	Lichen amyloidosis
Haemodialysis-associated amyloid	β2 microglobulin	Renal failure with haemodialysis

for completeness. The two common pathological amyloid types occur mainly as a secondary effect to other diseases and amyloidosis may be the first clinical finding that indicates an underlying disease. The different types of amyloid have amino acid sequences that are similar or identical to normal body proteins and each amyloid type has a set of diseases or conditions with which it is often associated. *Table 14.1* lists the different types of amyloid.

Amyloid P is associated with all amyloids

In addition to the main fibrillar amyloid, there is a minor protein component that is found in all amyloid deposits except for those in the brain. This component is called amyloid P. It is derived from blood proteins (serum amyloid P, SAP) and is an acute-phase reactive protein. The normal blood form of the protein (SAP) appears to bind to amyloid deposits, hence its accumulation, but instead of forming fibrils it forms a 9 nm ring structure made up of five subunits of SAP with a central hole of about 4 nm.

Distribution of amyloid

Amyloid distribution varies with the disease

Amyloid can occur in many organs and the exact distribution varies with the associated disease. Three types of distribution have been identified:

1. **Systemic primary.** Amyloid is mainly found in the heart, gastrointestinal tract, tongue, skin and nerves. This is seen in cases of primary amyloidosis and neoplasms of B lymphocytes. The amyloid type is usually AL but this primary distribution pattern can occur with AA amyloid in rheumatoid arthritis.
2. **Systemic secondary.** In this case the amyloid is found in the liver, spleen, kidney, adrenals, gastrointestinal tract and skin. This distribution is associated with cases of chronic inflammatory diseases. The amyloid type that is found is usually the AA variety.
3. **Localized.** Localized tumour-like nodules occur in tongue, bladder, skin or lung and are associated with localized endocrine neoplasms. The β-amyloid in Alzheimer's disease is also localized but occurs as plaques rather than nodules.

Amyloid can be found in many organs but the frequency with which a particular organ is involved varies and there is no single site that is always affected. Taking a single biopsy sample is therefore never fully reliable as the organ may not be affected in that patient. Common sites include the liver (48%), kidney (87.5%), gingiva (19%) and rectum (75%). Rectal biopsies have become a popular method of investigating possible cases of amyloidosis because of their less-invasive nature (often an endoscopic biopsy) and frequent involvement.

Amyloid accumulates between cells and causes their death

The first accumulation of amyloid occurs between the cells and often close to the basement membranes of a blood vessel. As the deposit increases, it

---

Box 14.8 Treatment of patients with amyloid

Amyloid deposition has no direct cure but effective treatment of any underlying disease will often slow down or even stop the deposition. Amyloid diagnosis before death has become much more common than in the past due to better biopsy techniques and a greater awareness of the deposition of amyloid. Most patients are now detected in the early stages rather than late in the disease. Whilst this is often beneficial to the patient, it has made life more difficult for the laboratories. The large deposits in organs that are easy to find and easy to stain are being replaced with small biopsies containing less amyloid, which is more difficult to detect.

---

gradually infiltrates into tissues and can trap and destroy the cells. There is still doubt about the mechanism cell death. It may be due to simple mechanical 'strangling' by cutting off the cells from their blood supply or it may involve a toxic effect of the amyloid. Amyloid has been found to be toxic to nerve cells in cultures but whether it is also toxic *in vivo* is not known.

Effects on organs

Kidney. Amyloid is first deposited in the glomerular mesangium and the basement membrane of blood vessels. As the accumulation continues, it eventually obliterates the capillary lumens and destroys the glomerular cells. The amyloid deposit can eventually completely replace the glomerulus. Renal arterioles can also be affected leading to ischaemia and tubular atrophy. The destruction of the renal tissue produces proteinuria and eventually the **nephrotic syndrome**. Renal involvement is usually fatal (see *Box 14.8*).

Spleen. The spleen becomes enlarged (splenomegaly) and the deposits may be of two types: (i) generalized deposits in both the red and white pulp ('lardaceous spleen'), and (ii) deposits only in the white pulp ('sago spleen'). If only the spleen is infiltrated and other organs are not affected, it is not usually fatal.

Heart. Usually deposits in the heart are smaller than in other organs. The deposits occur in the subendocardium, with more generalized deposits in

---

Box 14.9 Origin of deposits

The deposition of amyloid in the tissues probably reflects a generalized problem with the destruction and removal of large amounts of unusual proteins. The wide range of proteins involved and the relationship with excess protein secretion suggests that during the degradation of the extracellular protein, the protein alters its conformation and forms the β-pleated sheet form. The β-pleated sheet form is then more difficult for enzymes to destroy. If other proteins can similarly change their form during degradation, then it is likely that other forms of amyloid will continue to be discovered. There is already a suggestion that in Creutzfeldt–Jakob disease the prion protein (see *Box 14.4*) may undergo a similar change and produce a specific amyloid type.

---

the myocardium. The deposits may cause pressure atrophy of the heart cells and cardiac amyloid often leads to cardiac arrhythmia.

Liver. The amyloid deposits cause massive enlargement (hepatomegaly) and the liver becomes pale and waxy. Amyloid appears first in the space of Disse and progressively squeezes the adjacent hepatocytes to death. If only the liver is involved, then it is rarely the cause of death.

Staining

Since amyloid deposits vary in their composition, they will not all stain in the same way. A technique that works well with one sample of amyloid may stain a different case of amyloidosis only very weakly or not at all. A negative staining reaction should be considered inconclusive rather than definitely negative. If an amyloid deposit fails to stain with one technique, then it may be worthwhile trying a different one, which may give a much better result.

There are a variety of methods that have been used to demonstrate amyloid and some of these are outlined below.

Iodine/sulphuric acid

This method is mainly of historical interest although some pathologists still use it as a macroscopic method on whole organs whilst performing a post mortem. The mechanism is still unclear, with the original idea of a carbohydrate in the amyloid acting in a similar way to starch being largely replaced by the concept that it is the β-pleated sheet arrangement that traps the iodine.

Methyl violet metachromasia

Methyl violet has been used for a long time but how it produces metachromasia is not apparent. Amyloid deposits often contain mucinous materials that might explain the metachromasia but methyl violet does not produce metachromasia with any carbohydrates or mucins. Amyloid is not metachromatic with other dyes such as toluidine blue that give strong metachromasia with mucins. The results with methyl violet are inconsistent and often difficult to observe. This has led to the suggestion that the methyl violet contains an impurity that is simply more selective for amyloid. This would be analogous to the trichrome methods where differences in staining are relative rather than absolutely selective. It is no longer as popular a method as it once was.

Congo red

This is the preferred method in most laboratories. Most amyloids react and give some staining. The red colour (see *Colour plate 40*) may be weak and some other materials may occasionally stain slightly, but it is still probably the best of the current methods. It is even more specific if the section is examined using crossed polarizers in a polarizing microscope (see Chapter 15). The amyloid fibrils will show up as a dichroic green/yellow colour (see

Colour plate 41). Only chitin and cellulose show a similar reaction and these look quite different to amyloid in sections so there should be no confusion. The section thickness and orientation can be crucial to this colour – too thin and the colour is red, too thick and it becomes yellowish. The fibres need to be oriented correctly relative to the plane of polarization of the light to see the full effect so only a proportion of the amyloid will be seen at any one time (see *Colour plate 41*). The remaining amyloid deposits can be seen by rotating the section. Congo red is also fluorescent so the extent of the amyloid can be seen using this property. (Sirius red is an alternative to Congo red for staining amyloid but is not fluorescent.)

Pre-treatment of the section with potassium permanganate destroys the congophilia of AA amyloid but AL amyloid is resistant so this property can be used to distinguish the two types.

Thioflavine

This is possibly more sensitive than Congo red because of its intense fluorescence but it can be non-specific. It still remains popular as an alternative or complementary method to Congo red and is excellent for detecting very small deposits that are easily missed with Congo red staining.

Other methods

Other methods include immunotechniques, staining for tryptophan and X-ray crystallography but these tend to be limited to research into amyloid rather than reliable and easy identification techniques.

SUGGESTED FURTHER READING

Bancroft, J.D. and Cook, H.C. (1994) *Manual of Histological Techniques and their Diagnostic Application*. Edinburgh: Churchill Livingstone.

Kiernan, J.A. (2001) *Histological and Histochemical Methods*, 3rd edn. Oxford: Hodder Arnold.

Sheehan, D.C. and Hrapchak, B. (1980) *Theory and Practice of Histotechnology*. St Louis: Mosby.

Swisher, B.L. (2002) Microorganisms. In *Theory and Practice of Histological Techniques*, 5th edn (eds J.D. Bancroft and M. Gamble). Edinburgh: Churchill Livingstone.

Vowles, G.H. and Francis, R.J. (2002) Amyloid. In *Theory and Practice of Histological Techniques*, 5th edn (eds J.D. Bancroft and M. Gamble). Edinburgh: Churchill Livingstone.

SELF-ASSESSMENT QUESTIONS

1. Explain why it is better to identify bacterial infections from microbiological specimens rather than using paraffin wax sections.

2. Outline the types of method that can be used to help identify micro-organisms in tissue sections.
3. What are the major types of infective organism that can occur in sections? Name one example in each group.
4. What is amyloid? Why is amyloid not destroyed in the body?
5. List the different types of amyloid that are usually recognized and give an example of an associated disease or condition for each.

Light microscopy

Learning objectives
After studying this chapter you should confidently be able to:

■ **Describe the principles of simple and compound microscopes.**
Simple microscopes consist of a single lens, which bends the light from a specimen and thus produces a magnified image. A compound microscope uses two or more lenses held a calibrated distance apart. The combination produces a greater magnification than is possible with a single lens, as the first lens (the objective lens) produces an image (virtual image) inside the tube, which is then further magnified by the eyepiece lens.

■ **Describe the importance of numerical aperture and correction of aberrations.**
Numerical aperture (NA) is a measure of the light-gathering power of the lens. The greater the NA, the greater the resolution of the lens. The NA also affects the depth of field of the lens. The NA thus indicates the usefulness of a lens for a particular application.

■ **Outline the principles of darkground and polarizing microscopy.**
The darkground microscope uses oblique illumination. This oblique light does not directly enter the objective, resulting in a dark background. Objects that diffract light into the objective show brightly against the dark background. Polarizing microscopes use two polarizing filters. One filter is below the specimen and the other is between the specimen and the eye. The two filters are rotated so that no light passes through and only objects capable of rotating the polarized light appear bright in a dark field. This allows the eye to detect rotation of the plane of polarized light, which is not detected by the unaided human eye.

■ **Outline the principle of the fluorescent microscope.**
The fluorescent microscope uses two filters. A filter below the specimen absorbs all of the long-wavelength light so the specimen is illuminated only with short wavelengths. The second filter blocks this short-wavelength light leaving a dark background. Only specimens that fluoresce (i.e. shift the wavelength of the light to a longer wavelength) are visible.

■ **Outline the role of digitization in microscopy.**
Digitization is used for photographic recording where the speed and low cost of digital technology are useful. Digitization also allows the direct importation of images into computer programs for measurement and analysis.

Box 15.1 A brief history of microscopes

The term lens comes from the Latin for lentil. The lenses that were first used looked like lentils in shape and the name has stuck. Glass lenses were first used sometime before 1300 but were used mainly as a method for aiding failing vision rather than extending human vision to see minute structures. The idea of a compound microscope was first proposed around 1600 and compound microscopes were used by Robert Hooke (first person to use the word 'cell' in microscopy) in the mid-1600s.

Early lenses were badly ground so for a long time the use of single lenses was often better as they produced fewer aberrations. Antoni van Leeuwenhoek used single lenses with magnifications greater than 200×. The lenses had such short focal lengths that they were used virtually touching the eye and almost touching the object on the opposite side. Lenses were used mainly at lower powers for examining insects and were known as 'flea-glasses'.

In the 19th century, development continued with better correction of lens aberrations and better resolution. Thus, by the beginning of the 20th century routine light microscopes were almost as good as those used today (see *Box 15.4*).

Most human cells are so small that even a very large cell, e.g. 100 μm in diameter, is only just about visible as a tiny speck to the unaided human eye and no internal detail can be seen. Smaller cells, such as erythrocytes or bacteria, are far too small to be seen at all. This means that to observe cells in histology and cytology we must use a microscope to make the image larger (see *Box 15.1*).

15.1   HOW A MICROSCOPE WORKS

The size that an image appears to the human eye is controlled by the angle the light makes as it enters the eye. Objects that produce a large angle appear bigger, so we can make an object appear larger by altering the angle of light entering the eye. This happens when we get closer to an object and its apparent size increases. Glass, water and transparent plastics can bend light passing through them (see *Fig. 15.1*) by **refraction** and this bending can be used to magnify the image. A piece of glass with one or two convex curved surfaces can refract the light to a single focal point and this acts as a magnifying lens or **simple microscope**.

The nature of light

Although in most optical diagrams light is shown drawn as a straight line this is just a convenient way to represent it. Light is an electromagnetic wave and as it travels through any medium it vibrates at right angles to the direction in which it is travelling. Light has properties associated with this wave nature that are crucial in the theory of optics including microscopy. The important properties for understanding resolution are the wavelength, frequency and amplitude. In *Fig. 15.2*, the amplitude and wavelength are shown.

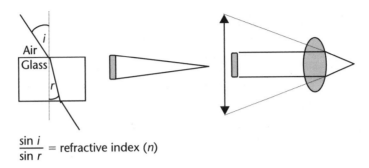

$$\frac{\sin i}{\sin r} = \text{refractive index } (n)$$

Figure 15.1
On the left, the light ray bends on entering and leaving the glass block. This bending is refraction. In the centre, the object is seen as a small structure with only a small angle subtended at the eye, whilst on the right, the lens bends the light and makes it appear larger

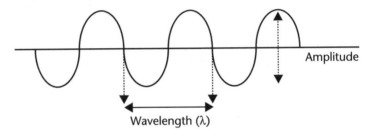

Wavelength (λ)

Figure 15.2
The wavelength (λ) and amplitude of a light wave

The amplitude is detected by the human eye as the intensity or brightness of the light, whilst the wavelength is detected as the colour of the light. The frequency of the light is the number of vibrations of the beam in 1 s. Since the speed or velocity of light in a vacuum is constant, the frequency and the wavelength of light are linked:

$$\text{Velocity } (V) = \text{frequency } (f) \times \text{wavelength } (\lambda)$$

In the case of light in a vacuum, the velocity is approximately 3×10^8 ms^{-1}. Although electromagnetic waves can have any wavelength, only certain ones are visible to the human eye. These wavelengths are the visible spectrum of colours and are shown in *Fig. 15.3*.

The wavelength of light varies depending on the medium

When light enters a medium that is denser than a vacuum, it is slowed down but the frequency remains the same. Likewise, light travels more slowly in glass than it does in air. The frequency of vibration remains the same, so in glass the wavelength must become shorter because of the relationship between velocity, wavelength and frequency. For this reason, physical

Figure 15.3
The electromagnetic spectrum. The longer wavelengths are on the left and shorter on the right with the visible spectrum in the middle. The diagram is not drawn to scale and the visible spectrum in reality occupies a much smaller part than shown

scientists prefer to use the frequency of light rather than the wavelength since frequency is constant, regardless of whether the light is travelling in air, glass, water or any other medium. Most microscopists prefer to use the wavelength of light since the length of the wave relates to characteristics such as resolution, which are also measured as lengths.

The slowing of light causes the light to bend as it passes from one medium to another depending on their densities. The amount of bending is measured by the **refractive index** (RI). Air has an RI only a little higher than 1, water is 1.33 and glass is about 1.5.

Microscope lenses

Simple microscopes are limited to low magnifications
Simple single-lens microscopes are very useful and are widely used for low magnifications such as reading lenses and watchmakers' eye loupes. Single lenses suffer from the problem that they need to have a highly curved surface (which makes the lens very small) in order to get high magnifications and they need to be used close to the specimen and close to the eye. It is inconvenient and impractical to use a simple lens of more than about 20× magnification.

Compound microscopes use more than one lens to increase magnification
To get larger magnifications than is convenient with a single lens, it is possible to magnify the image produced by one lens by using a second lens to produce a higher magnification. This type of system is called a compound microscope. The lens that does the initial magnification and which is close to the object being viewed is the **objective lens**, whilst the lens at the other end through which the eye looks is the **eyepiece**. The lenses are held in a tube that keeps out stray light and holds the two lenses the correct distance apart for optimal performance and allows us to see the image clearly. This is the basis of all compound microscopes.

Other parts are usually added to make life simpler when using the microscope or to improve the stability and brightness of the image (see *Fig. 15.4*):

Figure 15.4
Parts of a microscope

- A **mechanical stage** that holds the specimen and allows it to be moved slowly and smoothly across the field of view.
- A rigid stand **to eliminate vibrations.**
- A **lighting system** to illuminate the specimen and a condenser **to focus the light on the specimen.**
- A **focusing system** to allow the specimen to be focused smoothly and easily.
- Adaptations to allow binocular viewing, or **tilted (inclined) eyepieces.**
- A **turret** to hold more than one **objective.** By rotating the turret, the overall magnification of the microscope can be easily changed.

There is no reason why more lenses could not be added to magnify the image further to give any magnification required (1,000,000× would be possible in theory). However, there is no point in magnifying much beyond 2000× as there are other limits on the microscope image that make high magnifications useless. In particular, the **resolution** of the lens limits the usefulness of the image. Resolution is the ability to see two structures that are very close together as separate structures (see *Fig. 15.5*). The resolving

Original objects | Objects at limit of resolution | Unresolved image

Figure 15.5
The original objects on the left are quite separate. In the middle, they can just about be resolved as two overlapping images and on the right they are unresolved and appear as a single image

---

Box 15.2 Increasing the angle of light captured by a lens

The resolution relates to the aperture as the amount of light, or more particularly the angle of light, that enters the lens. The greater the angle of light trapped, the better the resolution. This is usually more obvious when dealing with telescopes. Most people readily accept that to see the detail of stars more clearly you need a bigger telescope. A telescope with a 10 cm diameter lens will see more detail than one with a 5 cm lens. The same applies to microscopes but instead of making the lenses larger, the microscope manufacturers usually move the lens closer. This increases the angle of light captured from the specimen without making the lenses too large and cumbersome. This reduces the distance between the lens and the specimen making manipulation difficult. Therefore, specialized microscopes are made with larger 'working distances' for purposes such as fine surgery where microscopes are needed that allow fine manipulation.

---

power is measured as length (e.g. 1 µm), with smaller distances representing better resolution since objects that are very close together can then be resolved as two separate structures. Thus, a resolution of 0.2 µm is better than a resolution of 1 µm.

The numerical aperture is a measure of the resolving power of a lens

The resolution of a microscope lens is measured by the **numerical aperture** (NA) of the lens. This measures the light-gathering power of the lens (see *Box 15.2*). The greater the angle of the light, the better the resolution. For microscopists, the NA is more important than the magnification and is always engraved on the barrel of the lens.

In mathematical terms:

$$NA = n \times \sin \alpha$$

where n is the refractive index (RI) of the medium below the lens (air is 1, water is 1.33 and microscope oil is 1.4) and α is the half-angle of the cone of light that can just enter the lens. The sine of an angle is always less than 1. Therefore, since the RI is 1 for an ordinary dry lens (one that has air between the objective and the specimen), it follows that the NA of a dry lens is always less than 1. In practice, it is usually less than 0.9. For an oil-immersion lens where the RI is higher (RI of oil is 1.4–1.5), the NA is always less than 1.4, usually 1.25–1.3 for a high-power lens.

The resolution of a lens is given by the mathematical relationship:

$$Resolution = (0.61 \times wavelength)/NA.$$

With a NA of around 1.2–1.3, this means that the resolution of an oil-immersion lens is about half the wavelength of light ($0.61/1.2 \approx 0.5$).

The light microscope cannot resolve objects closer than 200 nm

Thus, the ultimate resolution of a light microscope is limited by the nature of light and is roughly half the wavelength of the light used. The shortest wavelength that the human eye can see is about 400 nm (0.4 µm) so the best resolution that a light microscope can achieve is about 200 nm (0.2 µm). No matter how good the microscope, this limit is imposed by nature and cannot be overcome when using visible light. Better resolution can only be achieved by using different types of microscope that use shorter-wavelength radiations such as the electron microscope.

Optimum resolution with 1000× NA

The best resolution for the human eye is achieved when the total magnification of the microscope is about 1000× the NA of the objective. If a much higher magnification is used, the image gets larger but no more detail is seen by the human eye. This phenomenon is termed **empty magnification**. Instead of improving the image, any extra magnification makes the quality gets worse (rather like the way that getting too close to a television or cinema screen makes the image larger but less clear, although the physical reasons for the degradation are slightly different).

Immersion oil improves resolution by increasing NA

Oil is used in microscopy to improve the resolution by acting as a waveguide for light. Without oil, light travelling from the specimen goes through extra refractions and some of the light is lost. Immersion oil has a similar RI to glass and so minimizes the refractions (see *Fig. 15.6*). This allows a greater angle of light to be trapped and so increases the NA. Oil is only needed between the front of the lens and the top of the specimen and should be cleaned off after use to prevent it hardening. Oil should only be used with lenses designed to use oil (it is always marked on the lens, although it may be in a foreign language, e.g. oel if the microscope is German). Using oil with a dry lens results in degradation of the image rather than an increase in resolution, as does *not* using oil with an oil-immersion lens (see *Fig. 15.7*).

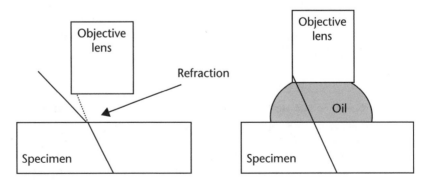

Figure 15.6
On the left in the absence of oil, the refraction as the light leaves the specimen causes it to bend and not enter the objective. On the right, the oil prevents the refraction and the light enters the lens

Figure 15.7
Effect of omitting oil with an oil-immersion lens. The lenses are designed to focus light that has not been refracted. If oil is omitted, then refraction occurs and the lens focuses the light as if it was not diffracted. This results in extra images at different focal planes. This smears the image and gives a blurred overall effect. With a dry lens, the opposite would be true as the lens is designed to correct for refraction and again extra images are produced that blur the specimen

Lens aberrations

The objective lenses used in microscopes do suffer from optical problems and these are called aberrations. Aberrations are distortions of the image caused by refraction in the objective lenses. There are seven types of aberration that can occur and that need to be considered when the microscope manufacturer designs the lenses in a microscope.

Chromatic aberration. When light passes through glass at an angle, the different wavelengths of light are not all bent (refracted) to the same extent. This can be seen using a glass prism where a spectrum of light emerges from the prism when a beam of white light is shone on to it (see *Fig. 15.8*). This property of producing a spectrum is referred to as **dispersion**. Although dispersion and refraction are related phenomena, they are not identical so the simple RI is not a measure of dispersion. In a lens, dispersion results in different colours of light being brought to different focuses. Thus, if the red light is focused there are green and blue images that are out of focus. This aberration is usually corrected in good-quality microscopes. The correction is achieved by using two lenses of different materials that differ in their ability to disperse the light into a spectrum. Two levels of correction can be

---

Box 15.3 Better lenses are needed for photography than for visual microscopy

For high-quality photomicroscopy, the lenses need to be of the best quality and as fully corrected as possible but for simple viewing by the human eye this is less essential. This is partly because the human eye and brain are good at ignoring slight defects in the image. This is useful since the lens in the human eye suffers from the same aberrations. The brain, for some reason, does not ignore things in the same way when they are present in a photograph. This phenomenon results in photographs that show people with telegraph poles apparently growing out of their head. They looked all right in real life but look dreadful in a photograph. Thus, photographic corrections need to be of a higher quality than for simple visual microscopy.

(a) With a prism white light is split to give a spectrum

(b) With two prisms there is no spectrum and the light remains a beam of white light

(c) The cross-section of a lens resembles two curved prisms

(d) A concave and convex lens doublet can reduce chromatic aberration

Figure 15.8
Chromatic aberration. White light can be split into a spectrum by a prism or by a lens, which, in cross-section, resembles two prisms on top of each other. Two inverted prisms prevent dispersion and a lens doublet can have the same effect

achieved called **achromatic** and **apochromatic**. Apochromatic correction is a better but more expensive option.

Lateral chromatic aberration. Here the effect is that, although all the different colours of light are brought into focus at the same place, the blue image is a different magnification. This results in colour fringes around objects. This is difficult to correct in the objective lens and is usually corrected in good-quality microscopes by using **compensating eyepieces**. The compensating eyepieces have a lateral chromatic aberration built in as part of their design. This aberration is exactly opposite to the aberration in the objective so the two aberrations cancel out. Compensating eyepieces are matched exactly to the objectives and should not be swapped from one system to another or they will introduce chromatic aberrations.

Spherical aberration. This is a consequence of the lenses having a curved (spherical) surface. This aberration is always fully corrected in any decent microscope.

Distortion. Distortion results from lenses having slightly different magnifications at the centre and at the edge of the lens. The effect can cause barrel or pincushion shapes from a square object (see *Fig. 15.9*). Usually there is

Pincushion distortion   Original square object   Barrel distortion

Figure 15.9
The effect of distortion on a square object

some residual barrel or pincushion distortion in high-power lenses but it is minimized by the manufacturer and is not usually a problem, especially since biological specimens are never exact square shapes so the distortion is not noticed.

Astigmatism. This is where objects at different orientations are at different focal planes so that radial objects will be in a different focal plane to tangential objects. Astigmatism is always fully corrected in a good microscope.

Coma. This produces a 'tail' coming away from bright objects. Coma is often only minimized in most laboratory microscopes rather than being fully corrected. Coma only affects the periphery of the field of view and is not observable in the centre of a lens.

Curvature of field. Here the edges of the field of view are out of focus when the centre is in focus and vice versa. Curvature of field is usually fully corrected in lenses that are intended for photography but otherwise it is only minimized.

Although it is possible to fully correct each aberration, it results in a more complex lens. Each aberration requires the lens designers to have at least

---

Box 15.4 Modern lens improvements

The best available resolution of the light microscope has not greatly altered since the last century and has possibly even diminished, since electron microscopy can now resolve so well that it is unnecessary to push the light microscope to the very limits of resolution. Instead, lens designers have concentrated on improving other characteristics of the light microscope. The use of special glass and modern plastics has improved the clarity and brightness of the image. There has also been an increase in the field of view seen down the microscope. Older lenses suffered greatly from aberrations at the edge of the field of view so lens manufacturers only made use of the central part of the image. Now better corrections allow more of the image to be acceptable.

One advance has been in the **blooming** or coating of optical components, which reduces flare. Flare is light that passes through the lens but plays no part in the image. The light is scattered over the whole image making it appear as a **'soft focus'**. The same effect is seen with a dirty lens or even a dirty window or windscreen in strong sunlight where there is a lot of light coming in through the glass but it interferes with the clarity as it spreads the light. The coating of lenses means that flare can be reduced to very low levels. The result is a brighter, clearer image but coating of lenses does not increase the resolution.

one lens face for each correction. Thus, fully corrected lenses have many optical elements all fitted into one barrel. The more lenses, the higher the cost, so full correction of every aberration is expensive and most microscopes are not fully corrected (but see *Box 15.3*).

The distance light travels between the lenses is the optical length

Lenses are usually made to fit a standard type of microscope with a standard optical tube length. The standard is now often 160 mm although other lengths have been used in the recent past. The optical path length is usually inscribed on the barrel of an objective and altering the tube length of a conventional microscope will increase the magnification.

More recently, most high-quality microscopes have been made with optics that have no fixed tube length. Instead, the light travels along the microscope tube as a parallel beam. The tube length can therefore be extended without altering the magnification. Such optics are called **infinity optics**.

The optical path length is often different to the physical tube length since prisms are often used in modern microscopes to make inclined eyepieces and binocular heads. These fold the light path, making the distance the light travels longer than the simple physical distance between the objective and the eyepiece.

Most microscopes allow all of the objective lenses fitted on the turret to be **parfocal**. Changing one lens for another by rotating the turret will leave the lenses approximately in focus and only fine adjustments need to be made. This is very convenient and is the best reason for not mixing lenses from different microscopes. Mixing lenses may mean that **correction collars** are needed to match the lenses and retain the parfocal ability.

Illumination

The illumination system of a microscope is part of the optical system and needs to be correctly set up to allow the best resolution. Below the stage is a condenser that concentrates and focuses the light on the specimen. Condensers, like objectives, have their light-concentrating power rated in NAs. The condenser NA should be matched to the lens NA to allow maximum resolution of the image. The condenser is usually fitted with an iris diaphragm to prevent unwanted light entering the lens. This substage iris should be adjusted to the point where it gives maximum illumination but closing the iris any further would result in a reduction of the light intensity. This is the **threshold of darkening** and gives optimum resolution. Although altering the iris diaphragm can be used to change the brightness of the image, this is not a good idea since it also reduces the resolution by reducing the NA of the condenser. Most microscopes have a knob to control the light source intensity and this is the recommended method to make the image comfortably bright for your eyes. Closing the iris can occasionally be useful with low-contrast objects where the increase in contrast outweighs the loss of resolution.

Most modern laboratory microscopes use a variation of Köhler illumination. The exact method of adjusting it varies with the make and model, but learning how to set up the microscope properly is an essential skill needed to getting the best from the instrument.

15.2 SPECIAL FORMS OF MICROSCOPY

The human eye can only detect two changes in light. One is a change in intensity (how bright something appears) and the other is a change in wavelength (the colour that something appears). There are other aspects of light that can be seen by some animals but not humans; however, these can be made visible to the human eye by manipulating the conditions. The microscope with its defined illumination can be used in this way so that, as well as being an instrument to magnify, the microscope can show things that are normally not seen by the human eye. These include very slight differences in RI, phase changes in the light waves and polarization of light. These specialized forms of light microscopy make it possible to see living cells without the need to fix or stain them.

In normal microscopy, the image is seen against a bright background and is referred to as **brightfield microscopy**. In brightfield microscopy, only objects that absorb light can be seen. Usually specimens are coloured (absorb some wavelengths of light) and so can be seen by the change of colour.

Many of the special forms of microscopy involve a dark background with the objects showing up brightly against the darkness. This contrast makes best use of the human eye's sensitivity. It is easy for the human eye to pick out very small amounts of light against a dark background, whilst the same intensity would be invisible if the background was light. The human eye is extremely adaptable and adjusts to the current illumination. Thus, the human eye can detect stars against a dark background, yet the same stars are invisible if the sky is bright. The stars are still there, it is just that the difference in intensity is so slight compared with the overall intensity that the human eye cannot detect the difference; in technical terms the signal-to-noise ratio is too small.

Darkground microscopy

This uses oblique illumination. The light, instead of coming from directly below the specimen and then entering the front lens of the objective, is arranged to come from an angle such that the light will not enter the objective (see *Fig. 15.10*). The oblique angle is achieved by using an annulus in the substage condenser or a special darkground illuminator, both of which produce a hollow cone of light.

Since no direct illumination enters the objective the background remains dark (see *Colour plate 42*). Only if something in the specimen bends the light will any light enter the objective and be seen. For darkground

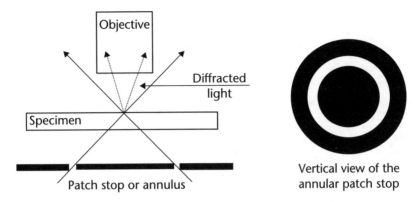

Figure 15.10
Darkground illumination. Only a small circle of light can pass through the clear area of the patch stop and this light is angled to ensure that undeviated light will not enter the objective. If diffraction occurs, then the diffracted light will enter the objective forming a bright image on a dark background

microscopy diffraction gives the greatest effect, so diffracting objects appear bright against the dark background. This allows the eye to see them clearly and enables the microscope to produce an image of objects that are smaller than the usual resolution limit (see *Box 15.5* for an alternative illumination technique). The same effect as darkground microscopy can be seen with a bright beam of light such as the projector in a cinema when very small specks of dust can be seen dancing in the projector beam but in even illumination the specks of dust are invisible.

Polarizing microscopy

Polarization is a description applied to the wave motion of light. In polarized light, the vibrations (wave pattern) occur in only one plane (see *Fig. 15.11*). This is unusual. In light produced by most light sources there is a mixture of light with many different directions of vibration. Such unpolarized light can be polarized by passing it through a filter that selectively

---

Box 15.5 Rheinberg illumination

Rheinberg discs are an alternative to simple darkground illumination. Instead of the annulus being a combination of totally opaque and totally transparent, the two parts are made of different-coloured filters. The annulus can be red, giving oblique red light, and the rest green. Diffracted light will be red and the background green. This gives a 'prettier' image than simple darkground illumination and is popular with illustrators and natural history filmmakers. The colours of the discs can be any pair of contrasting colours so the image can be quite varied. It does not give any extra information about the specimen compared with plain darkground microscopy – it just looks nicer. There are some even more complex variants with different parts of the filter in different colours.

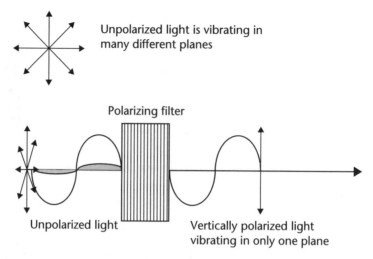

Unpolarized light is vibrating in many different planes

Polarizing filter

Unpolarized light

Vertically polarized light vibrating in only one plane

Figure 15.11
Polarization of light. Unpolarized light has its waveform vibrating in all planes. The top view shows a few of the vibrations seen looking along the direction of the light ray. The light would be coming straight out of the page and the wave vibrations would be at right angles to the line of travel. When unpolarized light is passed through a polarizing filter, all the vibrations except one are removed leaving, in this case, vertically polarized light

absorbs light vibrating in every direction but one plane. Such a filter is termed a polarizing filter. Longer wavelengths of radiation (microwaves and infrared) can be filtered using parallel fine wires that are aligned accurately. For visible light, it is usual to use either crystals of calcite (Nicol prisms), which were the original method of polarizing light, or more commonly nowadays polarizing filters that have precisely aligned crystals (see *Box 15.6*).

Human eyes cannot see the polarization of light so objects that alter the polarization without altering the colour or intensity of the light appear transparent and lack contrast. The polarization changes can, however, be converted into intensity or colour changes to which the human eye is sensitive by using two polarizing filters. In the microscope, one filter is placed

---

Box 15.6 Polarizing filters

Polarizing sunglasses use the same principle as polarizing microscopy. The polarizing lens absorbs all the light except that which is vibrating in one particular plane. This absorption of a large fraction of the light has a darkening effect that is useful for sunglasses and has the advantage of not altering the colours. It is essentially a **neutral density filter**.

It also alters the way we see reflected light. Light reflected from a surface is polarized by being reflected. Thus, polarizing sunglasses can apparently remove reflections such as those from the surface of water and allow the viewer to see into the water. Polarizing filters are used in photography for reducing reflections and enhancing colours by reducing the reflections.

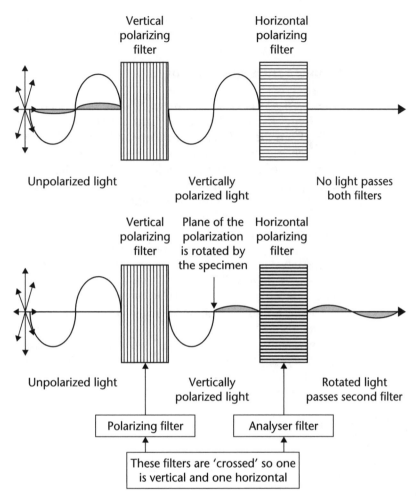

Figure 15.12
Arrangement of filters for polarization

between the light source and the specimen (polarizer) and one between the specimen and the eye (see *Fig. 15.12*). Thus, the object is illuminated by polarized light. If the analyser is then rotated to a direction at 90° to the polarizer (crossed polars), it will absorb the already polarized light giving a dark background.

Anything rotating the plane of the polarized light will appear bright and coloured against the dark background. This type of microscopy is excellent for crystals (see *Colour plate 43*) and regularly spaced materials such as the myofibrils in muscle fibres. Materials that cannot rotate the light are said to be **isotropic** (e.g. muscle I bands = isotropic bands) and those that can rotate the plane of polarization are **anisotropic** (e.g. muscle A bands = anisotropic bands). They are also referred to as birefringent or sometimes called doubly refractile since they have two different RIs depending on the plane of polarization. These terms are not absolutely synonymous to physical scientists but tend to be used interchangeably in biological microscopy.

Fluorescence microscopy

Fluorescence occurs when a material absorbs light and then quickly re-emits it. If some of the energy of the light is lost then the emitted light differs in energy from the absorbed light. The wavelength of light is related to its energy. Lower energy light has a longer wavelength than higher energy light. Thus, when some of the light energy is lost, the emitted light has a longer wavelength than the absorbed light. This change from short-wavelength excitation light to longer-wavelength fluorescent light is called the Stokes shift.

By using two filters it is possible to observe only the longer-wavelength fluorescent light against a dark background (see *Fig. 15.13*). The first filter, the excitation filter, is placed between the light source and the specimen. This allows only short-wavelength light to be transmitted. This short-wavelength light will excite the emission of the fluorescence. The second filter, the barrier filter, is placed between the specimen and the eye (or camera). This absorbs all of the short-wavelength light and transmits longer wavelengths. Thus, it transmits the emitted fluorescence.

It is worth noting that the position of the filters is the same in both polarizing microscopy and fluorescent microscopy. One filter is between the light

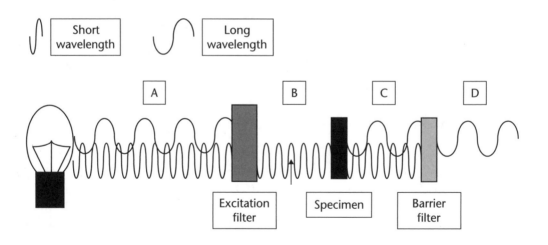

Figure 15.13
Arrangement of filters for fluorescent microscopy. The light from the lamp at A is a mixture of long and short wavelengths. After passing through the excitation filter, there are only short wavelengths of light (B). The fluorescent specimen converts some of the short wavelength light to longer wavelength fluorescent light (C). The barrier filter removes the short-wavelength light leaving only fluorescent light (D)

Box 15.7 Fluorescence in everyday life

Fluorescence is widely used in areas other than microscopy. **Brighteners** are materials added to washing powders and detergents to make the washed clothes brighter. These compounds absorb short-wavelength light invisible to the human eye and convert it into visible light. The effect is that in sunlight the clothes glow and seem 'cleaner'. The effect is best seen in short-wavelength 'disco' lights, which have a violet colour that shows the white clothes literally glowing.

Fluorescent pens are used to identify valuables such as computers and video recorders by marking them invisible to the human eye but visible under UV light.

---

source and the specimen to control the illuminating light and the other between the specimen and the eye to control the transmitter light.

The filters are complementary and in the absence of a specimen they should stop *all* of the light. Only if fluorescence occurs will anything be seen with the microscope. This technique is widely used in immunofluorescence (see Chapter 10), for the detection of neurotransmitters (see Chapter 9) and when using ion-selective dyes (see Chapter 9).

Filters can be manufactured in two ways:

1. **Absorption filters.** These are simply dyes in a suitable matrix (gelatine or glass). They are cheaper but give broad transmission peaks since the dyes have limited absorbing ability.
2. **Interference filters.** These produce their colour by the thickness of a special coating. The thickness and material used in the coating control the wavelengths of light that are transmitted and reflected. This type of colour is seen when there is a thin layer of oil on the surface of water. Neither the oil nor the water need be coloured, yet when the angle of light is right the surface of the oil film appears in rainbow colours.

Interference filters are more expensive than absorption filters but can have very sharp cut-off points in the light that they transmit. Absorption filters are suitable for many simple applications but interference filters are needed for precision fluorescence. Interference filters can also be made into **dichroic mirrors**, which transmit long wavelengths and reflect short wavelengths. This allows **epifluorescence**.

Epifluorescence microscopy

Epifluorescence illuminates from above using a dichroic mirror and uses the objective as a condenser. As can be seen in *Fig. 15.14*, the light source is situated above and to one side of the specimen and the objective. A dichroic mirror is placed in the optical path and angled at 45°. The light from the lamp impinges on the dichroic filter. Short-wavelength light is reflected down the objective to illuminate the specimen. Any long-wavelength light is transmitted through the filter and absorbed by the black wall of the microscope. The short-wavelength light hits the object and elicits the fluorescence. The fluorescent light is emitted in all directions so some of the

Unwanted long wavelengths absorbed by the wall of the microscope

Objective lens

Dichroic mirror

Specimen illuminated by short wavelength light

Figure 15.14
Epifluorescence microscopy

light will enter the objective and be magnified. This light reaches the dichroic filter but since the fluorescent light is a long-wavelength light, it will be transmitted by the angled filter and will reach the eyepiece. Most of the incident short-wavelength light will pass through the specimen and not be reflected back into the objective. Even if some short-wavelength light is reflected, it will not be able to pass through the dichroic filter and will instead be reflected back into the lamp house.

Epifluorescence has several advantages over transmission fluorescence

The epifluorescent microscope gives a clearer and brighter image and is the main form of fluorescence microscopy used in laboratories as it has significant advantages compared with transmitted light fluorescence:

- The image is brighter, especially at high magnifications, since all of the incident light is concentrated on the area being viewed and not spread over the whole specimen as it would be in normal fluorescent microscopy. The intensity of the excitation is greater and this gives a brighter image.
- There is less fading since only the area being viewed is illuminated so only a small area fades at any one time.
- There is better resolution of detail since the light only has to pass through the coverslip and not through the slide. The brightest part of the image will be the part nearest to the objective and this reduces flare.
- There is less risk of eye damage. With a conventional brightfield microscope it is possible to omit the barrier filter so that short-wavelength light reaches the eye. UV light is dangerous to the eye and such a mistake could cause eye damage. The dichroic filter is both an excitation and a barrier filter. If it is left out, then no light will enter the microscope; if it is in place, then it acts as a barrier filter. The epifluorescent arrangement is much safer.
- Since there is only one filter, it is easier and quicker to change filter combinations.

- Filters are more accurately matched.
- It is possible to have conventional brightfield microscopy illumination set up to illuminate from below the specimen and have the incident light microscopy coming from above. It is quite simple to see the same field with both forms of illumination. Simply switching the brightfield lamp off will allow the dimmer fluorescence to be examined and if the fluorescence is bright and the brightfield illumination is kept low, it can even be possible to view both forms of illumination at the same time.

Confocal microscopy

The latest addition to the range of fluorescent microscopes is the confocal microscope, which uses lasers as a coherent light source. The lasers are used to illuminate a single very small point on the specimen and the fluorescence from this point is measured accurately. Since both the illumination and the observation are focused concurrently on one small spot, the method has become known as **confocal microscopy**. To cut down the extraneous fluorescence and scattered light, the confocal microscope uses a very small aperture at the secondary focus of the objective. This aperture has the effect of restricting or eliminating any out-of-focus light. The confocal microscope produces a very clean signal from the spot examined with virtually no noise from out-of-focus materials. Since only one spot can be examined at any one instant, it is necessary to scan the laser beam across the specimen and reconstruct the full image using a video display.

By taking several exposures at different settings, the confocal system can be used to produce a composite image. This can be combining different labels to co-localize different materials, or to reconstruct a three-dimensional image from individual optical slices through the specimen, or to combine images in time to form a movie of the cellular changes.

Confocal microscopes are considerably more expensive than conventional fluorescent microscopes but the quality of their results means that they are becoming increasingly common for research and are likely to become used more commonly in diagnostic applications.

Interference microscopy

Interference is a phenomenon of the electromagnetic nature of light. As it travels along, the electromagnetic wave has an electric and a magnetic field that vibrate; hence it is called electromagnetic radiation. Since the vibration is a waveform, the peaks and troughs of the waves can be displaced. This gives waves that are said to be either in phase or out of phase (see *Fig. 15.15*).

Light from a single source is coherent when the propagating waves have the same wavelength and are in phase with each other. If two such coherent waves are combined, they will interact and produce a new wave with the same wavelength and phase but increased amplitude or brightness. This is **constructive interference**.

Figure 15.15
Light waves that are in and out of phase. The three waveforms shown above show the alteration of phase. All three waves have identical wavelength and amplitude and will appear identical to the human eye. They differ in phase but the human eye cannot directly see the phase of the light. Waves a and b are exactly in phase, with peaks and troughs coinciding exactly. Waves b and c are exactly out of phase (180° out of phase) with peaks coinciding with troughs

If two beams of the same wavelength but different phases are combined, then **destructive interference** occurs. The two beams interact but the combined wave has a lower amplitude and is dimmer than either of the two original beams. This is not as obvious as constructive interference. The beams effectively cancel each other out. If two beams have the same wavelength and amplitude but are completely out of phase, then the effects of their electric and magnetic fields will be equal but opposed and hence

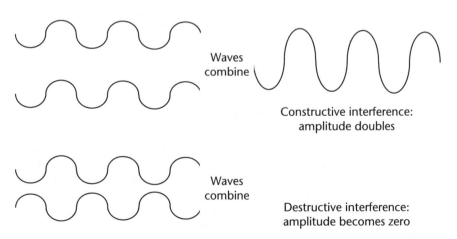

Figure 15.16
Interference. The two waves at the top combine with increased amplitude because they are in phase, whilst the two equal but out-of-phase waves in the lower half cancel each other out when they are combined

there will be no net magnetic or electric field; the light waves have cancelled each other out (see *Fig. 15.16*).

Interference can be used as a method of converting changes in the phase of light, which are invisible to the human eye, into intensity changes that are visible. **Interference microscopy, differential interference contrast** and **phase-contrast microscopy** (see below) make use of this phenomenon but are quite different in the final image produced.

Phase changes are not visible to the human eye

The human eye cannot detect phase changes in light so if we wish to observe whether a specimen changes the phase of light, we need a method of converting the phase change into an amplitude change. This is what interference microscopy achieves. By splitting a coherent beam of light into two beams and passing one beam through the specimen, we can detect whether the phase has changed by combining it with the other beam again. If the phase is altered, then it will result in interference. The interference alters the amplitude that the human eye can see.

The interference microscope (see *Fig. 15.17*) or interferometer microscope is a very precise measuring instrument that can effectively measure the dry weight (mass) of very small objects. It is an unusual type of microscope and requires very careful setting up and calibration. It uses two beams of light that are separated by a beam splitter; one passes through the specimen, whilst

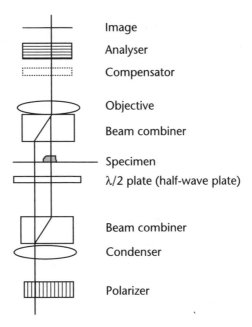

Figure 15.17
Path of the light beams through an interference microscope. A single coherent light beam is split into two beams, which travel through different parts of the specimen before being recombined

the other passes through a blank area of the slide. When the two beams are recombined, they interfere depending on the degree of phase difference. The amount of phase difference is itself dependent on the dry mass of the specimen. The two beams must have identical path lengths so when they are combined again they would still be in phase. Only if the specimen alters the phase of the light does the image appear.

Polarizers and analysers (as used in polarizing microscopy), a half-wave plate (which effectively reverses the polarization of light) and a compensator are also needed. The adjustment of all of these components changes the image and it is this complexity that limits the use of the interference microscope.

The differential interference contrast microscope (e.g. Nomarski) uses a smaller separation of the light beams (comparable in size to the resolution of the microscope). These give a false three-dimensional image and have a much smaller halo than the phase-contrast microscope. This small offset halo gives the impression of a three-dimensional image, which is a characteristic of Nomarski microscopy. These microscopes are generally used in a similar way to phase-contrast microscopes but are more expensive.

Phase-contrast microscopy

The phase-contrast microscope is in many ways related to the darkground microscope but the hollow cone of light produced by the annulus in the substage condenser is arranged to enter the objective, whereas in darkground microscopy it completely misses the front lens of the objective. The ring of light is arranged so that it is focused on a phase plate at the back focal plane of the objective. The phase plate is a simple circle of glass with a groove cut into it that alters the phase of light relative to the ungrooved region (see *Box 15.8*). Light passing through the thicker region of glass will have its phase retarded relative to the light that passes through the grooved region (see *Fig. 15.18*).

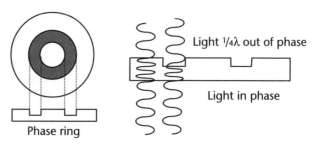

Figure 15.18
A phase ring as used in phase-contrast microscopy. The phase ring is situated in the back focal plane of the objective and consists of a grooved piece of glass. The groove is darker than the rest of the glass. As light passes through the glass, the wavelength alters. The light passing through the groove has its phase altered relative to the light passing through the full thickness of glass

> **Box 15.8 Negative phase-contrast**
>
> The phase ring can be made in the opposite way with a raised platform of glass instead of a groove. This means that undiffracted light is retarded rather than the diffracted light being retarded. This is sometimes referred to as **negative phase-contrast**.
>
> The amount of retardation can also be varied from $1/4\lambda$ through $1/2\lambda$ to $3/4\lambda$. The most common application is for $1/4\lambda$ difference with positive phase-contrast.
>
> The phase-contrast microscope was developed by Fritz Zernicke in 1932 at around the same time as the interference microscope was developed. In more recent years, the **modulation contrast microscope** has been developed. This uses a slit rather than an annulus and a different level of absorption rather than a phase delay. Phase objects are still visualized but the modulation contrast microscope is better for thick objects and the phase-contrast for thin flat objects.

Light that passes straight through the specimen is focused on the groove, whilst any diffracted or refracted light will pass though the thicker areas. The two beams are recombined in the eyepiece and interfere. This produces interference and hence an image, even in unstained specimens (see *Fig. 15.19* and *Colour plates 42* and *44*).

There is much less refracted light than direct light so the grooved area also has some light-absorbing material deposited so that the refracted light and undeviated light have similar intensities and the interference is then more apparent.

Phase-contrast microscopy is relatively cheap as phase plates can be built into objectives fairly simply and will not seriously impair the lens for normal microscopy when normal illumination is used. It then only requires an annulus to be placed in the substage condenser and phase-contrast illumination is achieved. Substage condensers with rotating filters and annuli are

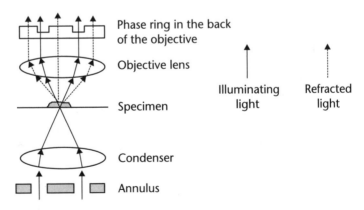

Figure 15.19
Phase-contrast microscopy. Light passing through the annulus forms a ring of light that will pass through the groove of the phase plate. If any light is diffracted or refracted, it will pass through the full thickness of the glass and have its phase retarded compared with the undeviated light

common so that switching from brightfield to phase-contrast or darkground microscopy is as simple as rotating a ring on the condenser. Phase-contrast does introduce a distinctive halo that reduces the resolution slightly, but the increased contrast it produces in living cells makes it a popular method in tissue culture work.

The differential interference microscope detects phase shifts introduced by the specimen, whilst phase-contrast really introduces the phase changes to detect slight changes in RI. In practice, they tend to be used in similar ways to look at living cells without the need to fix and stain them.

15.3 PHOTOMICROGRAPHY

The ability to record what you see is just as important in histology as in any other walk of life, but to record a microscopic image the usual camera lens is replaced by the microscope and the camera body must be attached to the microscope.

Photomicrography has its own advantages and disadvantages compared with normal photography. The advantages are that for most histological specimens the specimen does not move so exposures can be quite long and this allows slow films to be used. Slow films often have better contrast, better colour rendition and finer grains so the quality of photographs taken with the microscope can be excellent. The disadvantages are that the microscope is not as versatile as most camera lenses (see *Box 15.9*). There is no equivalent of the aperture control, which is available on most cameras. This means that there is no control over the depth of field (the amount that is in focus) and exposure is entirely controlled by time. The microscope is also a fixed focus lens so the image cannot be framed differently by moving closer or farther away as it can with a normal camera.

There are two types of system used to produce photomicrographs: one is a dedicated system built by the manufacture to match their microscopes,

---

Box 15.10 Microphotography

Photomicrography is the taking of photographs of small objects and making them bigger. Microphotography is taking photographs of large things and making them smaller. This is done using very fine grain film and has its main use in taking photographs of documents. Many documents need to be stored in detail but are difficult and expensive to keep in their full format. These can be photographed on film and the film takes up much less space. This is done for newspaper archives in libraries where the information is held on microfilm rather than as the full newspaper.

Microphotography is therefore quite different to photomicrography although the two words often get confused.

---

whilst the alternative is to attach a standard single-lens reflex camera to a microscope using a simple adapter.

Use of digital photography

Photomicrography is increasingly using digital technology instead of conventional photographic film. The advantages of using digital imaging are:

1. Speed. Since there is no development needed, the image can be transferred to a computer and printed within a few minutes. Single images can be downloaded and printed and there is no need to use a whole film as with conventional films.
2. Images can be transferred quickly. The transfer can be to another site using the Internet or into a computer application such as a word processor (e.g. Word) or an audiovisual system (e.g. PowerPoint).
3. The images are easily corrected or modified. This partially overcomes one limitation mentioned earlier as editing the image can mimic zooming and differential focusing. This type of modification needs to done responsibly. Overuse of modification of the image can come close to fabrication of data rather than just recording what is actually there.
4. Ease of measurement using image analysis as the image can be imported directly into image analysis programs.

File types and digital images

Since digital images can generate very large computer files, it is often necessary to reduce the size for storage or sending over the Internet. Files can be compressed in a variety of ways, some of which degrade the image and some of which do not. For routine photographs or snapshots, a slight degradation is often not visible but for scientific purposes the files must not be degraded. Formats that degrade the image are referred to as **lossy compression** as some information is lost in the process. Formats that retain all of the information are referred to as **lossless compression**. Sometimes some formats are not recognized by individual computer programs so the choice of image format is often crucial. The different file formats can be recognized as they use a file suffix to aid recognition, e.g. image.jpg is a jpeg file.

File formats for digital photographs include:

- **Bitmap** (suffix .bmp). This is an uncompressed image and so contains all of the information (lossless) but can result in a very large file. It is used only if no better file format is available.
- **GIF** (suffix .gif). This is produced by CompuServe as a method of transferring pictures. It gives a good compression but it is a lossy compression. It is limited to 256 colours and so will not give a good record of a colour photograph. It is excellent for graphics.
- **JPEG** (suffix .jpg). This is a lossy compression but gives a good saving in file size. It produces good results from routine photographs but is not suitable for scientific images that are to be analysed. It is very widely recognized.
- **TIFF** (suffix .tif). This is a lossless compression but does not compress files as much as JPEG. This is the preferred format for most scientific images.

In addition, there are many less-common formats such as RAW, PNG, PSD, PCT and TARGA, which have specialist or restricted applications.

15.4 OPTICAL ILLUSIONS AND MICROSCOPY

The microscope is a magnifying system but it is not complete without something or someone to use its image. In most cases it is used by a human being for visual examination of specimens. The human visual system is therefore part of the optical system. The human eye can introduce its own aberrations into the system, but provided any major aberrations are corrected by spectacles or contact lenses they will not interfere with the optical quality of the final image. Most microscope manufacturers offer high eyepoint eyepieces that allow spectacle wearers to wear their spectacles whilst using the microscope so that the optics of the human visual system do not degrade the image.

One very neglected part of microscopy is the role of the human visual system in interpreting the image once it has been received by the retina. The retinal image is interpreted by the visual system and the visual system can be fooled. The human visual system is not a passive viewer but interprets what it sees and attempts to identify structures and patterns in any image projected on to the retina. The human visual system is extremely good at interpreting normal visual images and making assumptions about the nature of the real object that is producing that image. It is not, however, perfect and psychologists have catalogued a wide variety of different **illusions** that fool or confuse the human eye. These illusions can sometimes occur in the microscopic image and be misinterpreted. The confusion is perhaps easier in microscopy than in everyday life because the microscopic image is unusual. The appearance of a section is only two-dimensional rather than having the usual three dimensions. The human eye unconsciously tries to interpret the flat, even plane of a section using the same techniques that it uses to interpret the three-dimensional world of normal life.

The eye–brain system can be fooled in a number of different ways, each of which causes significant illusions or mistakes.

Geometric illusions

These are illusions that occur when the size, shape or orientation of objects is wrongly perceived. Size distortions are the simplest and most extensively investigated illusions. The Müller–Lyer illusion is one of the best known of the geometric illusions (see *Fig. 15.20*).

Figure 15.20
The Müller–Lyer illusion. Both horizontal lines are equal in length but the upper line appears longer than the lower line due to the presence of angled fins

In the Delboef illusion, the size of circles is misinterpreted when they are part of concentric pairs. This illusion does not rely on the circles being symmetrically arranged and the figures do resemble cells with nuclei so the appearance could affect interpretation of important parameters such as nucleocytoplasmic ratio (see *Fig. 15.21*).

Figure 15.21
The Delboef illusion. The inner circle on the left appears to be larger than the outer circle on the right due to the effect of the other circles present. An outer circle apparently enlarges the inner enclosed circle and an inner circle shrinks the outer circle

In the Titchener illusion, the presence of non-overlapping circles alters the apparent size of an inner circle (see *Fig. 15.22*).

Figure 15.22
The Titchener illusion. The inner circles are equal but the one on the right surrounded with smaller circles seems larger than the one surrounded by larger circles

The Poggendorff illusion may lead to the wrong tracing of nerve or connective tissue fibres (see *Fig. 15.23*).

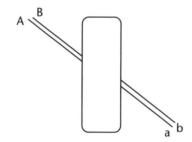

Figure 15.23
The Poggendorff illusion. Line A appears to connects with line a and line B with line b. However, the only straight connection is the line B–a

---

Box 15.11 Optical illusions can kill

Optical illusions are not just trivial party games but have very real applications in life. The use of elongated letters that appear to stand upright is used as advertising at sporting events and as warning signs on roads. In at least one case, an optical illusion (the Poggendorff illusion) was given as a major factor in a fatal air crash. In other areas of science such as astronomy and radiography, the study of illusions is taken more seriously. In microscopy, there have been very few papers or articles directly related to the subject.

Illusions are still used in microscopy, e.g. in the shadowing of objects where a false impression of depth is achieved by deliberately printing the negative of the photograph rather than the positive (see *Fig. 16.5* in Chapter 16).

Contrast illusions

Contrast illusions occur when there is a false impression of the brightness of an area due to its surrounding areas. An example of this is the White illusion (see *Fig. 15.24*).

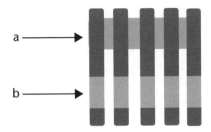

Figure 15.24
The White illusion. The extra bars (a) and (b) are the same brightness (20% grey) but (a) seem less bright than (b) because of their position between the darker lines, whilst (b) seem brighter as they are in the dark lines

Organizational illusions

The human brain always tries to organize images even when there is no real pattern. This gives rise to the children's game of seeing pictures in the fire or in cloud patterns. The use of ink blots by psychiatrists (the Rorschach inkblot test) to probe the human psyche is well known and the images seen are taken as an indicator of the person's mental state and not the physiology of the visual system. Different patients will see different images in the same pattern. Early microscopists often saw objects differently to how we would see them today (see *Box 15.12*).

The Kanitsza figure (see *Fig. 15.25*) consists of three dark circles with segments removed but there is a strong impression of a triangle that seems

---

Box 15.12 Errors in early microscopy

Organizational illusions are one of the most insidious forms of illusion because they involve a definite interaction between the brain and visual system. We not only have the problem of seeing things in error but also of imposing our own structure on things that are unconnected.

An early microscopist named Hartsoeker examined human sperm and interpreted what he saw in the light of current theories. He drew a perfect image of a small embryo in the head of the sperm.

This fitted in with the **animist** idea of human conception. The theory proposed that the father's sperm provided the embryo, whilst the mother simply provided a suitable place for the sperm-borne embryo to grow. The microscope Hartsoeker was using was not up to the standards of a modern microscope so he 'organized' the vague pattern of light and dark into the shape he expected. I do not think he was being deliberately misleading; it was an honest mistake. But it was a mistake and he believed what he thought he saw.

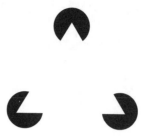

Figure 15.25
The Kanitsza figure. The three dark circles with missing segments give a strong impression of a triangle

brighter than the surrounding paper. There is no triangle, yet the human visual system forces it on our consciousness. The non-existent triangle even seems brighter than the surrounding paper. The Kanitsza figure can be a very strong illusion and using stereo images the imaginary figure can appear as a three-dimensional tilted triangle.

Colour illusions

Colour-blindness is a well-known example of individual variation in colour perception and affects a substantial proportion (over 8%) of the male population. The affected person sees objects quite differently to the rest of the population. This can mean that a colour-blind person may miss a critical feature. For example, observing the standard Ziehl–Neelsen technique (red mycobacteria) is enhanced for a normal sighted person if the background is a contrasting green colour, but the red–green contrast is the worst possible option for a person with red–green colour blindness. It is usual to consider that a person who cannot see a particular colour contrast is seeing things 'wrongly' but it is as well to remember that all colour vision is an illusion since humans only have receptors for three regions of the spectrum. It is quite possible to produce any colour with only three monochromatic lights, yet we consider colour to indicate the wavelength of light. Anyone with a known defect should take care to use the appropriate colour contrasts to avoid missing significant features. The use of special variants of staining techniques is often useful, e.g. replacement of fuchsin in the Ziehl–Neelsen technique with victoria blue makes it easier for a red–green colour-blind person to see the tuberculosis mycobacteria.

Although artefacts and technical mistakes are more common sources of error than the human visual system, it is as well to be aware of visual illusions. This is particularly true when trying to measure the size of objects. If we need to be sure that one object is larger than another, we should measure it objectively rather than relying on our subjective judgement.

15.5 MEASUREMENT AND MICROSCOPY

Measurement in microscopy is not as easy as in normal life because the magnification alters the size and the specimens are too small to be measured directly using a ruler. It can, however, be even more important to measure objects since there is no obvious scale for humans to relate to the cell size.

Not only is the microscope itself a problem in measurement but also the preparation of tissue for microscopy alters the size of objects. The techniques for measuring in microscopy always suffer from the difficulties associated with preparation of sections, so that any measurement always has a degree of error and the size of this error is often unknown.

Tissue limitations

The preparation of the section introduces problems in measurement and these include:

■ **Shrinkage/swelling.** These are commonly associated with processing. Shrinkage is the most likely result and tissues may lose 20% or more of their original volume in the preparation of paraffin wax sections. Most of the shrinkage is due to a combination of the fixative, dehydration and the heat from the wax bath. Although it is possible to measure the tissues before and after processing to gain some idea of the extent of the shrinkage, it still does not guarantee an accurate correction factor since different parts of the tissue may have shrunk to differing degrees.

■ **Section thickness.** This is a problem since it is rarely known with any accuracy. It is also difficult to measure thickness once the section has been cut. Microtomes are not reliable enough to use the thickness settings on the microtome feed mechanisms. Firstly, there is no guarantee that the settings were ever anything more than a rough guide and secondly, any wear on the microtome or any slight slackness in any part can lead to alternate thick and thin sections. This is commonly found during cutting and it is likely that sections may vary by 20–30% between one section and the next, even when the ribbon seems quite even.

Measurements that can be made include size (length, area and volume), the number of objects in a given volume and optical density.

Direct measurement of structures

Size: length or linear measurement

The length or breadth of an object is probably the simplest microscopical measurement and can be done in a number of ways.

Estimating size by comparison with a known object. Biologically, exact size is often not critical and an approximate size is all that is needed. For example, the size of a superficial cell in exfoliative cytology is considered to be between 40 and 60 μm. It is not critical to know the size of a cell to

---

Box 15.13 Estimating the size of a microscopic object

It is possible to measure using an ordinary ruler and the magnification. It is easiest to do with a monocular microscope. Look down the microscope with one eye and keep the other eye open. You will now see an image of the specimen with one eye and an image of the bench with the other. A ruler held 250 mm away from the eye will appear in focus at the same time as the specimen. Measure the specimen in millimetres by mentally merging the two images and then simply divide by the total magnification and you get a reasonable approximation of the size. This also means that if you have a good sense of scale, then a very approximate size can be guessed. Thus, if a cell looks to be 10 mm at a magnification of 1000, then the real size is 10 μm.

---

fractions of a micrometre as long as the size is somewhere in that range. By comparing to a cell of known size, it is possible to get a sufficiently accurate idea of the size for many purposes. In most sections, the best cell for comparison is the red blood cell, which is 7–8 μm. Thus, if a cell is about three times the diameter of a red cell, then its diameter is about 20–25 μm. This technique is widely used and is very easy with a little practice. It essentially gives an idea of the relative size of objects. A similar approximation can be done using an ordinary ruler (see *Box 15.13*).

Using a graticule. Graticules are transparent discs of glass etched with a pattern. The pattern can be a graduated linear scale that can be used as a ruler, circles of different sizes, square grids or a multiplicity of other types. Linear-ruled graticules can be placed in the eyepiece so that the ruled patterns are visible at the same time as the magnified image of the slide. The eyepiece scale can be calibrated against a known size using a stage micrometer, which has an accurate 1 mm rule divided into 100×10 μm graduations. Once the eyepiece graticule has been calibrated, it is possible to measure lengths very accurately and yet quite simply. Graticules are comparatively cheap (only a few pounds) and, provided only a few measurements are needed, they are reasonably quick. The variety of styles of graticules make it possible to measure circles, distances, separation of lines, etc.

Taking a photograph and measuring the photograph. Provided you can calculate the magnification accurately (e.g. by photographing a stage micrometer at the same magnification), it is possible to measure the photograph using an ordinary ruler and then calculate the size of the original object. The measurement of photographs is widely used in electron microscopy, but can also be useful in light microscopy for moving objects since the photograph freezes the action and allows measurements to be performed.

Size: area

Area can be calculated if the object is a reasonably simple shape by measuring length and breadth and using geometry, but if the shape is complicated this can be difficult or impossible. The area can be calculated by using a photograph and then cutting out the shape and weighing the cut-out part.

Provided it is calibrated and heavy paper is used, this is surprisingly accurate. (If the photograph itself is cut out then the paper should be bleached of silver since the silver deposit makes the weight irregular.) Generally, however, it is very tedious to measure areas by these direct methods.

Size: volume

Volume is even more difficult to measure by direct methods since volume needs to be measured in three dimensions so multiple sections are needed and the exact thickness of the sections needs to be known. By using thick board or plastic, an image can be built up from photographs. This is extremely tedious.

Number

This is at first sight apparently easy. For example, to count how many cells are dividing all we need to do is take a measured area and count how many cells are in that area. The normal field of view of a microscope is a standard area so it is not unusual to estimate the numbers of objects relative to one standard field. For example, you can count the number of mitotic figures in a high-power field to get an estimate of the numbers of dividing cells in a tissue. This is often done but it is only a relative count, not an absolute figure. Provided it is only used to see whether there are more or fewer mitoses than usual, then simple counting can be useful. If the exact number of mitoses is needed, then counting becomes more difficult. The actual number is not only related to the numbers seen in the measured area but also related to the size of the objects being measured, the thickness of the section and the distribution of the objects. These are related by the equation:

$$N = n\,\frac{t}{(D + t)}$$

where N = true count, n = observed count (cells are only counted if the centre of the cell is in the section), D = diameter of the cells and t = section thickness. However, exact calculation requires careful corrections.

Density

Density measurements are again apparently easy but in reality are more difficult. Simply shining a light through a section and reading the result in a colorimeter or spectrophotometer is inaccurate since the distribution of coloured objects is not uniform or even regular. It is the equivalent in a biochemical measurement of not mixing a tube of solution before trying to measure the concentration. The results are not consistent and can be very misleading.

The Beer–Lambert law relates the incident and transmitted light:

$$log\!\left(\frac{I}{I_0}\right) = -\varepsilon dc$$

where I = intensity, d = thickness, ε = absorption coefficient and c = concentration. If the thickness is constant and the material is the same then:

$$log\left(\frac{I}{I_0}\right) \propto c$$

Since the change in transmission is logarithmic, it follows that doubling the concentration does not double the absorption. Thus, if a material has an absorption A such that only one tenth (0.1) of the light gets through when it is evenly distributed, then when it is unevenly distributed the results can be quite different.

If a section has four separate areas:

A	A
A	A

there will be a quarter (0.25) of the incident light falling on each block. Of this light one tenth will be transmitted (0.025), so the total transmittance is $0.025 + 0.025 + 0.025 + 0.025 = 0.1$:

0.025	0.025
0.025	0.025

and the overall transmission is **0.1**.

If the same quantity of material is concentrated in one sector then the total transmittance will be more (the absorbance will be less) than with an even distribution.

0	0
0	$4 \times A$

The transmittance will be 100% in the three empty sectors but 0.0001 in the sector with all of the material.

0.25	0.25
0.25	0.000025

Only the one area absorbs at all and since it is now four times the concentration virtually no light is transmitted through this area but the overall transmittance is **greater than 0.75**, much greater than that in the case where the same amount of material is evenly distributed. Thus, in this example the same amount of material ($4 \times A$) can give a transmittance of 0.1 or 0.75. The same amount of material can give transmittances as high as 99% depending on how small an area it occupies.

The only remedy is to measure large numbers of small areas and then integrate the result. This is more difficult and if the areas are small and highly concentrated, it may still be inaccurate.

Box 15.14 Statistical sampling

The idea of point counting is similar to that in opinion surveys. Rather than having to ask the whole population what they think about a topic, the pollsters ask a thousand people and then extrapolate to get an approximate answer, with about a 3% error. This is quicker, easier and cheaper than asking everybody and is reasonably accurate.

Pollsters do, however, sometimes get it wrong but they do have extra problems in that some people refuse to co-operate and distort the result.

Statistical micrometry

Statistical micrometry does not attempt to measure the actual size directly but attempts to get an estimate of the size and to **calculate how accurate that estimate is**. Absolute accuracy may not be possible but fortunately a high degree of accuracy is often not needed. As there is wide variation in the normal sizes of cells and structures, not only between normal individuals but also within the same specimen, and provided an estimate is within a few per cent of the true size, then it is usually good enough for even the most critical applications in biology. Statistical estimates are not only easier to apply but can give any required degree of accuracy. One example is point counting to measure cross-sectional area (see *Box 15.14*).

Point counting

Imagine a carpet with a complex pattern of red and green. If you throw a coin randomly on to the carpet, the chances of it falling on a green part rather than a red part are directly related to the areas of both colours. If the red and green have equal areas, then the probability of the coin landing in a green area is the same as it landing in a red area, i.e. a half (0.5). If the red area covers three-quarters of the carpet, then it is more likely that the coin will fall on the red area than the green. The probability of landing on a red area is 0.75 and on a green area is 0.25, the same as their relative areas. If you throw the coin often enough, then the areas can be guessed by counting how many times the coin falls on a red area and how many on a green area. This is the principle of point counting.

If a graticule with a large number of dots on is superimposed on a section containing two components, A and B, then the chances of the point falling on A is A/(A + B) (i.e. A/total area). If the number of dots counted is large enough, then it is possible to estimate A and B as a ratio and this is the **area fraction** or **area proportion**.

A typical graticule will have 25 or 100 such points. Crosses are often used instead of simple dots as they are easier to locate when seen against a section. Only the centre of the cross is counted the arms just help to identify the centre point. Using a 100-point eyepiece graticule and a section of kidney, the calculation might be something like the example shown in *Fig. 15.26*.

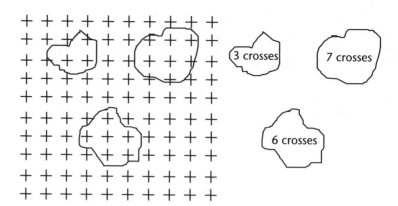

Figure 15.26

The graticule is used with a section of kidney and in the cortex 16 of the crosses of the graticule are superimposed on top of glomeruli. The area of glomeruli is therefore 16/100 of the area of the graticule. Thus, in a cross-section of kidney, the cross-sectional area of the glomeruli is 0.16 or 16%

Whether the dots fall on an object or not is a random statistical event so it is also possible to get an estimate of the accuracy of the measurement. The accuracy is measured by calculating the relative standard error (RSE). Thus, if an RSE of 1% is achieved, we can be reasonably sure that the true measurement is within 1% of our estimate. The RSE can be calculated from the following formula:

$$\text{RSE} = \sqrt{\frac{1 - \text{area proportion}}{\text{hits}}}$$

In the example used in *Fig. 15.26*, the RSE would be:

$$\text{RSE} = \sqrt{\frac{1 - 0.16}{16}} = 0.23$$

This means the estimate is only 23% accurate. If we wanted 5% accuracy, we would need to count more grids. A single count is not accurate enough. By assuming that the proportion will not change greatly, we can tell how many grids are needed. Thus, taking an RSE of 5% (0.05), we can use the equation:

$$0.05 = \sqrt{\frac{1 - 0.16}{\text{hits}}}$$

Solving this suggests that we need to count about 20 grids to get an estimate accurate to 5%. If we need to know the actual areas rather than just the area proportion, we need to know the area the graticule covers on the section and then by proportion we can calculate the actual area in square metres. This area of the graticule can be measured using a stage micrometer.

Volume measurement

Unlike the direct methods, measuring volume using point counting is no more difficult than measuring area, provided the following conditions are met:

1. The objects are homogeneous (evenly arranged) in the tissues.
2. The sections are thin compared with the objects.
3. More than one level (i.e. section) is measured.

Then the following applies:

Area proportion = volume proportion   (theorem of Delesse)

Thus, in the example of the kidney above, we could estimate that the volume proportion of glomeruli is 16% of the total volume of the cortex. To get the total volume of glomeruli, we only need to know the volume of the renal cortex and it can be calculated by simple ratios. In this case we could *not* use the volume of the kidney as a whole, since glomeruli are not evenly distributed within the kidney; there are no glomeruli in the renal medulla, although they may be reasonable regular within the cortex.

15.6   IMAGE DIGITIZATION

Digital cameras have become much cheaper and better in recent years and it is now quite simple to produce a computer file of the image in digital form. This has advantages not only for photomicrography as mentioned earlier but also in image analysis. Each number represents one dot on the screen and is called a pixel ('picture cell' or 'picture element') and the image is called a 'bit-mapped image'. Bit mapping needs three pieces of data for each pixel:

1. A number representing how far across the screen the pixel is (x position).
2. A number representing how far down the screen the pixel is (y position).
3. The intensity of the pixel.

The more pixels a picture has, the greater the resolution and detail in the image but the more data that needs to be stored. The intensity data for each pixel may be a single byte or several bytes. Monochrome images typically use only 1 byte (equivalent to 256 shades of grey from black to pure white), whilst colour images typically use more than 1 byte. For colour, 3 bytes is common, 1 byte for each of the three primary colours of the display, and this gives 16,777,216 possible colours ($256 \times 256 \times 256$).

The x and y positions are not usually stored as separate numbers. Since the pixel values are stored in order as a list, the x and y position of each pixel can be calculated from its position in the list. Thus, the position of the pixel is implied rather than stored in memory.

A 1024 $\times$ 1024 monochrome image will therefore need 1 Mbyte of memory and a colour image will need 3 Mbytes. Many applications do not need colour and monochrome image processing is still common.

Box 15.15 Image digitization

Digital imaging is widely used in the film industry to merge computer-generated material with live action shooting, to add or remove objects and to quickly change aspects of a scene without needing to completely reshoot it. It is also becoming increasingly used in business to read documents automatically (using character-recognition programs), for speed cameras and other types of law enforcement (reading number plates) and for quality control.

The leaders in the field of videodigitization are NASA who use digitization to send pictures back from space. The Hubble space telescope is a great example of the data collection that can now be achieved with high-resolution cameras.

The image can easily be modified in the following ways to allow the detail in the image to be more easily seen by the human eye:

1. **Intensity shifting.** If the image is too dark or too light overall, the intensity can be shifted by adding or subtracting a constant from the intensity value for each pixel.

2. **Contrast stretching.** The difference between grey shades can be exaggerated by using a mathematical operation (e.g. multiplying by a factor or taking the logarithm of the number).

3. **False colouring.** Grey shades are converted into colour differences rather than shades of grey. This uses a **look-up table** to convert each pixel. Each possible shade of grey is simply assigned a particular colour and this is stored as a table of colours in the computer. As each pixel is being displayed, the computer 'looks up' the colour corresponding to the value of the pixel in the table and displays that colour instead of a grey shade. There does not need to be any regularity in a look-up table and colours are often chosen simply to look attractive or to enhance contrast. False colouring is quite effective if a particular set of objects can be shown to stand out from the background. If a histochemical test has been done and the colour is fairly difficult for the human eye to see, computer enhancement will allow the colour to be boosted by using a look-up table.

4. **Inverting**. This alters the image from a positive to a negative form.

The computer can also be used for measurement. This is often complex but commercial programs are available and are becoming more common. Image analysis is now one of the most rapidly expanding areas of computer

---

Box 15.16 Image analysis expertise

It is difficult to find out exactly how good current technology has become as the most advanced systems are those used by military forces. These are used for automatic recognition of enemy aircraft, tanks and soldiers. The details are classified as secret, but it seems likely that they are better than the current commercial recognition systems. However, some transfer is occurring. In 2001, QinetiQ was formed as a private company from parts of the British Ministry of Defence research sections. QinetiQ is using its expertise to develop medical image interpretation software. As this technology filters out of the secret military area, it is revolutionizing microscopy.

technology. The analysis is not restricted to histology and is also used in industry, commerce and everyday life (see *Box 15.15*).

In computer recognition, objects are often classified differently to the way a human would normally describe them. Several different measurements can be used that are relatively easy for a computer system to measure but would be less easy for the unaided human eye. With complex shapes, there are a variety of parameters that can be measured by simple formulae including:

- area;
- Feret diameters (or 'calliper diameters'), where the largest Feret diameter is the length and the smallest is the breadth (see *Fig. 15.27*);
- length/breadth (maximum Feret/minimum Feret);
- convex perimeter (like pulling a string around the shape);
- roundness [= $\text{perimeter}^2(4\pi \times \text{area})$];
- radius of an equivalent circle;
- convex perimeter [= $2\tan(\pi/2n) \times \Sigma n\text{Feret}$];
- roughness (= perimeter ÷ convex perimeter).

Feret

Figure 15.27
Diagram illustrating a Feret diameter and convex perimeter

The application of this type of technology may well revolutionize the whole of cellular pathology with automatic analysis of sections and computer diagnosis. The question is not so much whether this will happen as when. The systems are currently too unreliable for accurate diagnosis, but with the advances currently occurring it is possible that for some specialist purposes computer technology could be diagnosing sections within a decade or two. They are already used in some laboratories for recognizing chromosomal disorders or screening cytology smears.

SUGGESTED FURTHER READING

Aherne, W. (1970) Quantitative methods in histology. *Journal of Medical Laboratory Technology* **27**, 160–170.

Bancroft, J.D. (2002) Light microscopy. In *Theory and Practice of Histological Techniques*, 5th edn (eds J.D. Bancroft and M. Gamble). Edinburgh: Churchill Livingstone.

Cook, D.J. (1983) Optical illusions in microscopy. *Microscopy* **34**, 533–552.

Floyd, A.D. (2002) Quantitative data from microscopic specimens. In *Theory and*

Practice of Histological Techniques, 5th edn (eds J.D. Bancroft and M. Gamble). Edinburgh: Churchill Livingstone.

Slayter, E.M. and Slayter, H.S. (1992) *Light and Electron Microscopy*. Cambridge: Cambridge University Press.

Spencer, M. (1982) *Fundamentals of Light Microscopy*. Cambridge: Cambridge University Press.

SELF-ASSESSMENT QUESTIONS

1. Why is the numerical aperture of a microscope important?
2. What is meant by empty magnification?
3. What is an achromatic lens?
4. Outline the principle of a darkground microscope.
5. Why do crystals of urea appear bright in the polarizing microscope?
6. How are the filters in a fluorescent microscope arranged so that the fluorescence can be observed?
7. Why is it unreliable to estimate the size of an object 'by eye'?
8. In a section across the bronchus of a person who had chronic bronchitis there are some mucous glands. A point count is made of 200 points: 110 points fall on the glandular tissue and 90 fall on other tissues in the wall. What is the proportion of mucous glands in the tissue?
9. What are the problems associated with measuring density in a section of stained tissue?

Electron microscopy

Learning objectives
After studying this chapter you should confidently be able to:

■ **Describe the principle of the transmission electron microscope.**
The electron microscope uses a beam of electrons rather than visible light to examine and magnify the specimen. The electron beam has a much shorter wavelength resulting in a much greater resolution than the light microscope. The electron beam can be focused to form a highly magnified image by using magnetic fields instead of solid glass lenses. Specimens for electron microscopy need to be very thin and dry and the electron microscope needs a very high vacuum to work. This means that the cells are always dead.

■ **Describe how specimens can be prepared and stained for the conventional transmission electron microscope.**
Specimens need to be fixed very promptly (typically with osmium tetroxide or glutaraldehyde) to preserve the cell structure. The specimens are then dehydrated and impregnated with a plastic monomer, which is then hardened by polymerization. The plastic allows much thinner sections as it gives firmer support to the tissues. The sections can be cut on an ultramicrotome using glass or diamond knives. The sections are finally stained using heavy metal salts to increase the contrast.

■ **Describe the principles of the scanning electron microscope.**
The scanning electron microscope uses a thin beam of electrons, which scans across the specimen in a raster. The beam illuminates one spot on the specimen and all of the electrons that bounce back from the specimen are collected and counted. The number of electrons is used to alter the intensity of the beam in a cathode ray tube, which is scanning in synchrony with the illuminating beam. This produces a three-dimensional image of the surface of the specimen.

■ **Outline the methods of preparing specimens for the scanning electron microscope.**
The specimens do not need to be embedded and sectioned as they are for the transmission electron microscope. They do need to be dried and coated to make them electrically conductive. Drying must not distort the specimen so critical point drying is preferred to simple desiccation.

■ **Describe the principles of X-ray analysis in electron microscopy.**
When an atom is struck by a high-energy electron, it will dislodge an electron from the outer electron orbit of the atom. The dislodged electron may then fall back into the outer orbit and loses energy as X-rays in the process. The amount of energy is related to the orbit and is characteristic of each element. By measuring the energy of the X-ray it is possible to identify the nature of the element undergoing the transition. By scanning the beam across the specimen, it is possible to map the occurrence of elements in the specimen.

There are two quite different forms of electron microscopy. The first is transmission electron microscopy (TEM), which was the first type to be produced, with the first commercial models appearing in the 1930s, so when people refer to the electron microscope they are usually referring to this type of microscope.

Since the 1960s, another form of electron microscopy has become commercially available; this is scanning electron microscopy (SEM), and subsequently scanning transmission electron microscopy (STEM) has become available. Since TEM is in many ways similar to conventional light microscopy it is also sometimes called conventional transmission electron microscopy (CTEM) to distinguish it from STEM. In biology and medicine, CTEM is still probably the most common and most useful form of microscope, but SEM is becoming ever more useful and certainly gives very striking images for illustrations.

16.1 CONVENTIONAL TRANSMISSION ELECTRON MICROSCOPY

Light microscopy has always been limited since it cannot resolve features of less than about 200 nm apart. Attempts to overcome this resolution limit continued for many years with people trying UV light (see *Box 16.1*), X-rays and similar short wavelengths related to light. These were generally either very little improvement on the ordinary light microscope or difficult to use, and often both. The electron microscope was developed using electrons rather than electromagnetic radiation and has proved to be much more successful. It can be used with only a little more difficulty than the light microscope.

Electron microscopes are much more expensive than light microscopes and need a special electrical supply because of the high voltages and currents used. They need a large water supply to remove the excess heat and a very strong and rigid floor to enable them to be used since even slight vibrations can seem huge when highly magnified. They are generally much larger and require a room of their own and basically are not able to be moved. Throughput of specimens is much slower and running costs are much

---

Box 16.1 Ultraviolet microscopy

The UV microscope is different to the fluorescent microscope, which also uses UV light. In the fluorescent microscope, UV light is used to make the specimen glow visibly (fluoresce). The microscopist looks at the visible light and the UV light is removed by a barrier filter and never forms part of the final image. A true UV microscope uses UV light as the illuminating light and it is the UV light that forms the image. Using UV light is difficult since UV light is absorbed by glass so all of the lenses need to be made of quartz instead of glass and all of the slides need to be quartz. This is expensive. The image cannot be viewed directly since UV light is not visible and is also dangerous to the human eye, so all examinations must be done on photographs. This is expensive. The increase in resolution afforded by UV light is simply not worth the trouble.

higher and because of this electron microscopes are much less common than light microscopes.

Electron microscopy is made possible since electrons, although often considered as particles, can also have wave-like properties. The wavelength of an electron beam is related to the energy used in the production of the electron beam. Very short-wavelength electron beams can be produced using very high voltages. The same underlying laws govern the light and electron microscopes. Thus, as with the light microscope, good resolution is achieved by using short wavelengths. The extremely short wavelengths of the electron beams used in the electron microscope make it possible to achieve very high resolution. The modern electron microscope has a resolution of around 2 nm for biological specimens and is almost to the point of resolving individual atoms with crystalline materials. In practice, the resolving power of the modern electron microscope is so great that in biology the limiting factor is not the wavelength or the resolution of the microscope but the tissue preparation. Biological preparations cannot be prepared of sufficiently high quality to make use of the available resolution and, in any case, the resolving power is greater than any biologist would reasonably need.

Components of the electron microscope

The electron microscope is quite similar in principle to the light microscope, but instead of a lamp to produce a beam of light there is an **electron gun** producing a beam of electrons. The electron gun consists of a tungsten filament, which is heated to emit electrons and surrounded by a negatively charged shield. The shield has an aperture so as the electrons are repelled from the shield they can only escape through the aperture. The electrons are then accelerated using an anode, which produces a strong electric field between the electron source and the anode itself. This accelerating voltage is what determines the wavelength of the electrons and is usually between 20 and 120 kV. The electrons are then focused using magnetic lenses.

The general layout is similar to the light microscope (see *Fig. 16.1*) with a **condenser** focusing the electron beam on to a specimen and an **objective lens** focusing the electrons that have passed through the specimen and magnifying the image. The image is then further magnified by a **projection lens** (equivalent to an eyepiece in light microscopy) and finally viewed on a fluorescent screen or photographed using standard photographic techniques. Although the principle is similar, there are often modifications in commercial instruments. In most electron microscopes, there are extra lenses in the system, such as a second condenser focusing the electron beam on to the specimen and extra diffraction and intermediate lenses magnifying and focusing the light after it has passed through the specimen.

Several significant differences exist between electron and light microscopy

Although there are similarities to the light microscope, there are also several differences. Some are advantages but some make electron microscopy more difficult and more expensive:

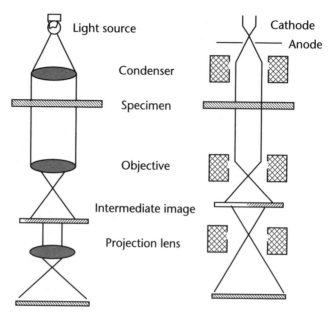

Figure 16.1
Comparison of the light microscope (left) and electron microscope (right). The light microscope is shown inverted for easier comparison. This schematic diagram shows that the two forms of microscopy share many similarities

- Electrons have a much shorter wavelength so resolution is improved. This allows high magnification without it becoming empty magnification. Factors other than simple resolving power limit the magnifications used. For biological specimens, it is not normally possible to achieve resolutions better than about 10 nm.
- The lenses are magnetic and not glass. Each lens is a coil of wire that generates a strong magnetic field. Electrons are charged particles so are deflected by passing through a magnetic field. This is similar in some ways to the refraction of light when passing from air to glass. The field can be shaped using **pole pieces** to produce the same magnifying effect on electron beams that a convex glass lens produces with a light beam.
- The shaping of the magnetic field cannot be as complex as the shaping of a glass lens and this limits the ability of magnetic lens designers to totally control lens aberrations. To overcome this limitation, the electron microscope usually works at much narrower apertures (see *Box 16.2*) than the light microscope since most aberrations are worse when a large aperture is used. Since the wavelength of the beam is so small, the reduced apertures do not seriously diminish the resolution and aperture size is less critical than in the light microscope where aperture size (numerical aperture) is the limiting factor in resolution.

Box 16.2 Apertures in electron microscopy

The apertures in the electron microscope are pieces of molybdenum or platinum with a small hole (200–300 μm) in the centre. This limits the size of the electron beam. The small apertures can be easily contaminated and so become asymmetric. This results in **astigmatism**. This must be compensated for, especially at high magnifications. The compensation is carried out with a **stigmator**, which is a special multipole magnetic lens that can produce a correcting magnetic field. The control of this a correction is one of the key skills for an electron microscopist. Regular cleaning and polishing of these apertures is an important part of regular maintenance.

The small apertures do increase the depth of field so the electron microscope is actually able to focus more of the thickness in a specimen than an equivalent light microscope lens. The greater depth of field and the very thin specimens used in electron microscopy mean that the whole of the specimen can be in focus at once so there is not the constant readjustment of focus that is needed in light microscopy.

- The magnification is altered by changing the electrical current through one or more of the lenses rather than changing lenses, which is the usual way of increasing the magnification in light microscopy. Electrons spiral in an electric field so altering the magnification results in the image rotating as well as getting larger.

- Electrons are easily absorbed or deflected by many substances including air and water. To avoid this absorption, the whole microscope tube must be kept in a very high vacuum. The electron microscope requires complex pumps to remove all of the air and it must be kept under vacuum since if it is returned to atmospheric pressure the microscope will need to be 'outgassed' for several hours to remove all traces of air.

- Special air locks are needed to put specimens into the microscope without losing the vacuum in the main microscope tube. This slows down specimen changes.

- The specimens must be very thin and dry. This invariably means that electron microscopy specimens are dead. There is no electron microscope equivalent to techniques that allow living cells to be examined by light microscopy.

- The intense energy of the electron beam in the high vacuum of the electron microscope can be quite destructive to specimens. Even dead cells need to be well protected by embedding in plastic to survive being examined in the electron microscope and unlike light microscopy the plastic is left in place and is not removed for staining or viewing.

- Electrons are deflected by any material with a static electrical charge. The specimen is constantly being irradiated with a beam of electrons during viewing and without special precautions this would very rapidly charge the specimen and make viewing impossible. For this reason, the specimen must be put on to an electrically conducting copper grid (see *Box 16.3*) to disperse electric charge, which may be coated with carbon to help conduct the charge. The spaces in the grid allow electrons to pass through while the copper bars act as a mechanical support and electrical earth to disperse any static electricity.

Box 16.3 Copper grids for electron microscopy

The copper grids used in electron microscopy are more intrusive than the glass slides used in light microscopy. It is impossible to arrange the specimens on the grid so it is pure chance where the individual cells lie. The grids all too often interfere with visualization of the area of the tissue that is most interesting. The grids are quite small but have an apparently large area when highly magnified and searching across a grid can seem very tedious. There are no real shortcuts since the position is controlled solely by a very fine mechanical *x*–*y* movement. The bars on some grids are made slightly different to allow the operator to know roughly which part of the grid they are observing by providing some 'landmarks' to navigate by.

- Electrons are not visible to the human eye and must be viewed using a phosphorescent screen. This phosphorescent screen uses a similar material to the phosphor used in television screens, which also use electrons to produce an image. The alternative is to produce a permanent record using photography. Electrons will directly affect photographic emulsion so placing a sheet of film in the plane of the image will produce a negative. More recently, digital photography technology has been adapted to allow it to be used in the electron microscope. The electron microscope screen is visible immediately but is mainly used for identifying which area of the specimen is to be photographed. Photographs are used as the main image in electron microscopy as they can be further enlarged and are more convenient to view and handle (e.g. to measure sizes).
- The image is always a monochrome image. Coloured electron microscope images are artificially coloured, often using computer techniques.
- The contrast between the nucleus, cytoplasm and other structures is enhanced using heavy metals rather than dyes. Most dyes will not deflect or absorb electrons sufficiently to act as 'stains'. There are only a few heavy metal salts that are suitable for electron microscopy so the range of reagents is more restricted. The fact that only shades of grey are possible also limits the amount of contrast that can be achieved.

Preparation of tissues for the electron microscope

The general principles of histological preparation are similar to light microscopy, but the need for very thin sections and the greater detail required in the final preparation mean that there are significant differences in the actual procedures.

Fixation

The general principles of fixation that apply to light microscopy are still valid for electron microscopy but fixation is even more critical since subcellular changes can occur within seconds in some conditions. Usually the tissue must be fixed within minutes and becomes almost useless for critical work if left for a few hours. By contrast, post-mortem specimens for light microscopy are often left intact within the body for more than 24 h before the specimen is placed in fixative.

To speed up fixation for the electron microscopy, the specimen is either perfused *in vivo* or if this is not possible it is cut into very small pieces by chopping with a razor blade. Each fragment may be less than 0.5 mm in size. This allows rapid penetration of fixative. Fixation is often carried out at low temperature to slow down degeneration. Fixatives that are used in electron microscopy include:

- **Osmium tetroxide.** This preserves lipids very well and is the main fixative for membranes and membranous organelles.
- **Glutaraldehyde.** This preserves proteins well and is the main method of preserving the cytoskeletal materials.
- **Formaldehyde.** Formaldehyde for electron microscopy use needs to be much purer than for simple light microscopy. It is usually prepared by depolymerizing pure paraformaldehyde rather than using the impure formalin solutions that are usual in light microscopy. Since formaldehyde results in fewer cross-links than glutaraldehyde, it is often useful in histochemical and immunological techniques. Stronger cross-linking would chemically alter the tissues making these techniques useless.

Fixatives can also be mixed to give a compound fixative (e.g. Karnovsky's fixative uses formaldehyde and glutaraldehyde) or the fixatives can be used in sequence to give a secondary fixation (e.g. glutaraldehyde followed by osmium tetroxide). The fixative must be buffered, usually to pH 7.2–7.4, but occasionally a higher or lower pH is used. The buffers used include phosphate buffers, cacodylate buffers and collidine buffers. Some fixatives such as glutaraldehyde may react with some buffers. The fixative solutions must be carefully controlled to give optimum results.

Osmolality is also important. Often a slightly hypotonic solvent is used (290–320 mOsm).

The fixation time for electron microscopy is usually much shorter than for light microscopy, often just 1–4 h. This is partly a reflection of the much smaller block size, which means that diffusion is not a major limiting factor.

Although fixation is important, most laboratories have slightly different techniques that work well in that laboratory so there is no single recognized technique used by everyone.

Processing

The waxes used in light microscopy are useless for electron microscopy as they would rapidly vaporize in the electron microscope due to the vacuum and electron beam. Instead, plastics are used to embed and support the tissues. These plastics can be acrylics or epoxy resins. Acrylics were used in early electron microscopy techniques but have largely been replaced by epoxy resins. The use of these materials has already been covered in Chapter 4.

Box 16.4 Microtome knives for electron microscopy

Originally glass knives were made by hand and this required great skill to obtain a good edge. Nowadays, knife-making machines are available. These machines take pre-cut strips of glass, lightly score them and apply even pressure to fracture the glass. This produces rectangles of glass, which are then cut diagonally to produce triangular knives with the fine cutting edge across the thickness of the glass. The angle of the cutting edge can be varied: 45° is suitable for most materials, 35° is better for soft blocks and 55° is better for hard blocks.

Glass knives are the commonest and cheapest way to cut sections but diamond and sapphire knives can also be bought. These are harder and sharper than glass knives but considerably more expensive. They come with special holders that act as the floating-out bath.

Diamond knives are made from industrial diamonds and polished to give a fine cutting edge. The edge is fragile so care is needed to avoid damage but if used carefully they are very long lasting and can give months of use. As they are used repeatedly the edge will build up a layer of debris if not cleaned regularly. This can be done with the pith from an elder plant, which is rigid but soft and will gently scrape away the dirt without damaging the edge. Diamond knives can be resharpened when they become blunt but this is expensive.

Sectioning

Sectioning of the plastic-embedded tissue is done using a glass knife (see *Box 16.4*) and an **ultramicrotome**. The glass knives are made by breaking a sheet of glass to give a fresh and extremely sharp edge (see *Fig. 16.2*). The knives are disposable and have a very short but useful life. Two or more knives may be needed to cut a single block depending on the material being cut.

The basic components of the ultramicrotome are the same as for a normal microtome but the feed mechanism is much finer. The feed may be mechanical or by thermal expansion of a metal rod attached to the microtome chuck. An electric heating coil surrounds a metal rod holding the chuck and as the rod expands it pushes the chuck forward. The thermal expansion is easily altered by varying the current through a heating coil and can give very fine advancement of the chuck. The degree of advancement is, however, less predictable than a mechanical feed so that section thickness cannot accurately be set in advance. Instead of relying on the settings on the microtome, the section thickness is measured by the interference colours seen when the section is viewed at an angle. Sections may appear pale gold

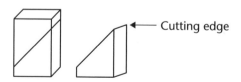

Cutting edge

Figure 16.2
Glass knives for electron microscopy. A small rectangle of glass is scored and then fractured to give a triangular knife

← Water bath made by
wrapping adhesive
tape around the
knife

Figure 16.3
Water bath attached to a glass knife

(approx. 90–120 nm), silver (approx. 60–90nm) or grey (less than 60 nm). Other sections are too thick to be useful.

As sections come off the edge of the knife they are floated on to a small waterbath attached directly on to the knife (see *Fig. 16.3*). The sections can be flattened on the waterbath by allowing some chloroform or xylene vapour to soften the plastic and then gently teasing the section with a hair probe.

Sections are picked up on a fine copper grid (2.3 or 3 mm diameter), which supports them in the electron microscope. The grids have one side shiny and one side dull. Although it probably makes little difference to the result, it is probably best to standardize on one orientation (e.g. shiny side up) so that you always know on which side of the grid the section has been placed. Grids come in a variety of different grid patterns and hole sizes that are a matter of personal preference rather than being critical in use. Grids may need to be coated for some applications. The coating is a thin film of plastic or carbon or even both. This gives extra support but the coating film can sometimes interfere with the clarity of the final preparation. After being picked up on the grid, the section is then dried by placing in a closed container on top of filter paper. Plastic petri dishes are a cheap and convenient container for grids but commercially produced holders are available.

Staining

Unstained plastic sections are usually low in contrast, so no detail can be seen with the electron microscope. Contrast can be introduced into the specimen by staining with heavy metal salts that can absorb or deflect the electrons.

Staining can be done at any stage in the preparation. Osmium tetroxide is a stain as well as a fixative so staining often starts during fixation. Other stains can be added during the processing of the block, e.g. during dehydration. Both of these techniques stain all of the tissue in the block and are referred to as block staining. The difficulty with block staining is that penetration of the reagents may be a problem since the large ionic heavy metal stains used in electron microscopy do not penetrate easily through intact cell membranes. In addition, the reagent may interact with one or more reagents in the processing (e.g. phosphotungstic acid reacts with epoxy resin).

The finished section on the grid can be stained by immersion in reagent and this is probably the commonest method for staining. Penetration is very

Table 16.1 Selectivity of various metal salts used in electron microscopy

Metal salt	Selectivity
Lead salts	General contrast enhancement
Uranyl salts	General contrast enhancement but more selective for DNA
Phosphotungstic acid	Polysaccharides
Osmium tetroxide	Lipids including membranes

poor since the section is embedded in plastic. Only the surface really absorbs the stain but this is usually sufficient to give a good contrast. Stains must be filtered just before use since heavy metals tend to precipitate easily and even tiny precipitates appear as the size of boulders when magnified by a factor of 100,000×.

Different metals have slightly different affinities for tissue components so that the final image can be altered to some extent (see *Table 16.1*). Their specificities, however, are probably even less reliable than with dyeing so interpretation is not straightforward. It is probably better to think of electron microscope stains as making materials more readily visible rather than identifying materials by their staining reaction. The metals can also be used in combination to increase contrast but, unlike dyes in light microscopy, which have different colours, they all just alter the tone of grey so they cannot be easily distinguished.

Specialized electron microscopy techniques

Shadowing

Shadowing can give an impression of three dimensions and is used in measuring height. TEM is only capable of giving a two-dimensional image, much like an X-ray or photograph, but by choice of preparative technique it is possible to give an impression of three dimensions (see *Box 16.5*) and to measure the height as well as the length and breadth of an object. This is usually used with discrete objects deposited on the grid by drying from a suspension (e.g. bacteria, viruses or crystals) rather than being used on sections. The object is coated with a heavy metal but instead of it being

---

Box 16.5 Shadowing makes use of illusions

Shadowing is the technique of deliberately using an optical illusion to show the structure in three dimensions. The only problem is that some structures are ambiguous. The human brain always assumes that light comes from above and interprets shadows in that way. If a picture is viewed upside down, then the result is that grooves become ridges to correlate with the shadows and ridges become grooves. Thus, the whole relief becomes inverted and can be misinterpreted.

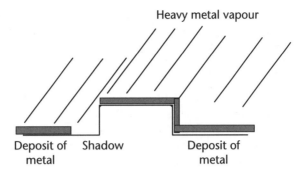

Figure 16.4
Shadowing with heavy metal vapour. The metal is deposited at an angle so that a shadow occurs

evenly coated from directly above the grid, it is coated at an angle. Any object that rises above the grid will result in a 'shadow' area (see *Fig. 16.4*). By knowing the angle and the length of the shadow the height of the object can be calculated.

The metal vapour is generated by using a low voltage arc between two metal electrodes in a vacuum. The metal condenses on the cold surface of the specimen and leaves a deposit.

When a normal electron microscope photomicrograph of a shadowed specimen is viewed, the shadowed area is bright because it is electron transmitting, whilst the coated areas are black (electron dense). This looks odd to the human eye so the final photograph is printed in negative form so that the shadow is dark and the rest of the image is light (see *Fig. 16.5*). This

Figure 16.5
Shadowing. The first image is the one that is usually used and shows a small polystyrene ball shadowed with metal from the top right. This is a negative image. The positive image, which would be seen in the electron microscope, is seen in the centre with an electron-transparent white shadow. The image on the right is a table tennis ball lit in the same way from the top right. Although the left-hand image looks superficially like a three-dimensional photograph it is a false impression since the true three-dimensional image shows a shadow (half-tone shadow) across the ball. This is missing from the electron microscope-shadowed image

gives an impression of three dimensions. Shadowing is also use to give this effect of three-dimensional relief even when direct measurements of height are not needed.

Replica making

The surface texture of specimens is usually not seen with TEM as it usually uses sectioned material but it can be seen by making a mould of the surface using a heavy metal coating. The replica matches the surface exactly and can be removed and examined; this gives a good representation of the surface structures. Coating needs to be very even, unlike the shadowing technique, so the specimen is either placed directly under the electrodes in an evaporation coating chamber or is coated by **sputter coating.** Sputter coating uses a stub of metal (e.g. gold) that is connected to a high-voltage supply (1.25 kV) and the chamber is then filled with argon. Gold ions are discharged from the surface of the stub by the high voltage and are focused and accelerated by a magnetic field. This gives a plasma beam of ions, which coats the specimen evenly. (This technique is widely used as part of the freeze–fracture technique (see *Box 16.6*), which examines the inside of membranes.) Even specimens that are too thick or too bulky to examine in the electron microscope can be examined by making replicas of their surface.

Box 16.6 Freeze–fracture technique

The freeze–fracture technique allows investigation of the inside of membranes. The membranes of cells are double layers of lipid held together by hydrophobic interactions. The centre of the membrane contains no water and will not freeze and the hydrophobic bonds are quite weak. The tissue is first frozen at –196°C and then cut with a razor blade or scalpel. The tissue breaks (fractures) rather than cutting cleanly and the tissue is likely to cleave along the weaker lipid region in the centre of the membrane. A replica of the surface is made and the tissue is dissolved away leaving the replica, which can be examined in the electron microscope. The inside of the membrane shows the presence of structures that span the membrane such as receptors and intercellular junctions.

Negative staining

Staining is usually done by staining the solid material with heavy metals but in negative staining it is the spaces in the specimen that are filled with an electron-dense material giving a silhouette of the objects (see *Fig. 16.6*). It gives information about size, shape, surface structure and groupings of particles but no information about internal detail of the specimen. This is useful with suspensions of viruses, bacteria, etc., but less useful with sections of embedded material that are solid throughout. Typical stains include potassium phosphotungstate, cadmium iodide, sodium tungstate and uranium nitrate.

A mixed suspension of particles (bacteria, viruses, etc.) and the electron-dense stain (e.g. phosphotungstate) is made and thinly spread on a carbon-

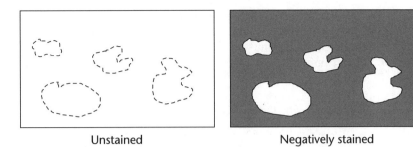

Unstained   Negatively stained

Figure 16.6
Negative staining. The untreated specimens on the left have no contrast but by filling
in the spaces in between, the outline of the objects becomes apparent

coated copper grid and dried. The suspension can be sprayed on or a drop
can be placed on the grid and excess fluid removed after a few moments
using a piece of filter paper.

Electron microscope histochemistry

Histochemical techniques can be applied to electron microscope specimens
but usually involve **block staining** of fresh tissue followed by embedding
and sectioning rather than staining of frozen ultrathin sections on electron
microscope grids. 'Blocks' is a very flexible term in electron microscopy. A
20 μm frozen section cut in a conventional cryostat can be an electron
microscope block since it is large enough to be a complete block for electron
microscopy. A cryostat section can be cut and stained by a suitable histochemical technique and then processed to produce an electron microscope
block.

The final product of the histochemical technique must be electron dense.
This occurs with metal salt methods, e.g. Gomori phosphatase methods, and
some tetrazolium salts are electron dense (e.g. the osmate of TNST, 2,2′,5,5′-
tetra-*p*-nitrophenyl-3,3′-stilbene ditetrazolium chloride). Some reaction
products (e.g. diaminobenzidine product) are **osmiophilic** (i.e. absorb
osmium salts) and so will become stained when the block is fixed with
osmium tetroxide.

Electron microscopy immunotechniques

These are similar to the immunotechniques discussed in Chapter 10 but use
electron-dense labelling instead of fluorescent dyes. Antibodies can be
labelled directly with ferritin (an iron-containing protein) or colloidal gold
spheres that are visible with electron microscopy. Colloidal gold is probably
the most popular since the colloidal gold particles are perfect spheres.
Perfectly spherical objects are rare in sections so positive identification and
localization of the spheres is comparatively easy. By using particles of two
different sizes to label different antibodies, it is possible to identify the sites
of binding of more than one antibody in a single section.

Immunoenzyme techniques are also applicable, e.g. immunoperoxidase, provided the final product can be made electron dense, as is the case with diaminobenzidine used in peroxidase methods, which is osmiophilic as mentioned above. The technique can be done either before or after embedding in plastic.

Paraffin-embedded material in electron microscopy

Although it is usually better to process material directly for electron microscopy (see *Box 16.7*), it is possible to use paraffin-processed material as electron microscope blocks. This can be done either from paraffin blocks or from sections.

One advantage of this is that areas of interest can be identified using light microscopy and only relevant areas are then examined by electron microscopy. Since the size of a typical electron microscope section is <1 mm in diameter, this can greatly reduce the number of blocks needing to be examined, saving much time and work. Wax blocks simply need dewaxing in xylene, transferring to alcohol and treating with osmium tetroxide to increase their contrast. They can then processed as if they were normal tissues.

Using paraffin sections works best with thicker sections than is usual for light microscopy (>7 μm). The best way is to dehydrate the section (to alcohol or acetone) and then invert an embedding capsule containing resin over the area of interest in the section. The resin can permeate the tissue and is then polymerized. The whole thing (glass slide, section and resin capsule) is then cooled in liquid nitrogen and the capsule snapped from the slide. The glass and tissue usually separate very cleanly. The resin block is then trimmed and sectioned.

Preservation of material previously sectioned in wax is adequate rather than good but may be better than tissue stored for several days in routine fixatives. The ability to use sections or blocks is useful in **retrospective studies**. This is where the laboratory has a specimen that could be useful in research in its archives as a paraffin block or section but not as an electron microscope block. Thus, it is possible to do electron microscopy on blocks from many years ago.

Box 16.7 Perfect fixation is not always possible

The preservation of material for the electron microscope is critical to get the best results; however there are occasions when the preservation is poor but it is still worthwhile looking at the material in the electron microscope. In this way, the electron microscope is a useful tool for archaeologists looking at mummified remains or human materials recovered from bogs. The tissue preservation will be extremely poor but since it is not possible to go back thousands of years to get a better specimen you have to do the best you can with what you have. Ensuring that fixation and preservation are done properly will always give better results but we cannot ignore the benefits of any technique just because it cannot be done in a perfect way.

16.2 SCANNING ELECTRON MICROSCOPY

SEM is quite different to TEM and has no direct counterpart in conventional light microscopy. SEM is totally reliant on video technology and the user never directly sees the specimen, as only a video reconstruction of the specimen is seen on the monitor screen. SEM is used mainly for examining the surface of structures, although by fracturing a block of tissue it is possible to study an exposed surface that was originally an internal structure.

SEM can examine relatively massive and dense structures since the electron beam does not need to penetrate right through the specimen. Unlike TEM, SEM is not often used at very high magnifications; indeed, it is often used at magnifications lower than would be possible with light microscopy. The main benefits of SEM are in the way that it visualizes objects as three-dimensional photographic images rather than giving better resolution (see *Box 16.8*).

The examination of the surface by SEM relies on the electrons that are reflected back by the specimen or are emitted from the surface of the specimen when it is irradiated by a beam of electrons. The interaction of electrons with the specimen is illustrated in *Fig. 16.7.*

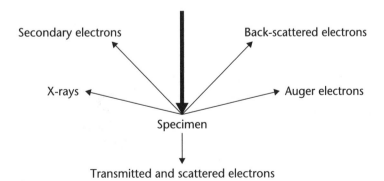

Figure 16.7
Diagram of scattering of the electron beam

Electrons produced from the incident beam

The incident electron beam from the microscope produces several types of electrons and also X-rays. The electrons have different energies and properties and will give different appearances to the specimen if they are used to produce the final image.

Back-scattered electrons have a high energy and are produced by electrons in the beam being deflected when they 'hit' an atom in the specimen (like a ball bouncing back from a wall). The back-scattered electrons are produced within a pear-shaped region (see *Fig. 16.8*) underneath the incident beam and can emerge at quite wide angles. The degree of scattering is partly dependent on the nature of the specimen, i.e. the elements present, so back-scattered electrons give information about the nature of the specimen and not just surface shape.

Secondary electrons have lower energy and are produced by electrons being dislodged by the passage of the main electron beam (like a ball

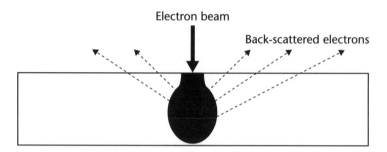

Figure 16.8
Back-scattered electron production. Electrons are dislodged from a pear-shaped area underneath the electron beam and can escape from quite deep in the specimen as they have considerable energy

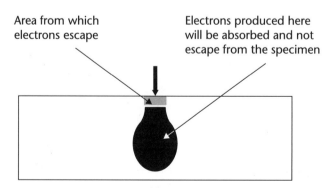

Figure 16.9
Secondary electron production. Electrons are dislodged from atoms quite deep in the object but their low energy prevents them escaping from the specimen

dislodging a brick out of the wall). These low-energy electrons can only escape from the specimen from a relatively thin 'skin' (about 2 nm thick) on the surface of the specimen. These electrons therefore give a good representation of the surface shape (see *Fig. 16.9*). Secondary electrons are less affected by the nature of the material.

Auger electrons are produced by the X-rays interacting with the specimen and have relatively low energy. They are generally not important in SEM.

X-rays and other electromagnetic emissions (cathode luminescence and bremsstrahlung) are also emitted but play little role in SEM. They may be used to identify elements present in the specimen.

Detection of electrons coming back from the specimen

Detection of the electrons in SEM is completely different to TEM. There is no attempt to focus the electrons to form an image and all of the electrons are collected and counted. The image is made by scanning a very narrow illuminating beam of electrons across the specimen. At each point on the specimen as the incident beam of electrons hits atoms in the specimen, some electrons will be emitted. *All* of the electrons are then collected and used to generate an electrical signal. The greater the number of electrons emitted, the greater the electrical signal generated. The electrical signal is then used to feed into a video monitor (essentially a high-resolution TV system), which is scanned in parallel with the electron beam in the electron microscope.

The strength of the signal alters the brightness in the monitor and so an image is built up on the screen, dot by dot, as the SEM beam scans across the specimen and the monitor scans across its screen (see *Fig. 16.10*).

Higher magnifications are achieved not by increasing the power of the lenses but by the electron beam scanning smaller areas of the specimen. The

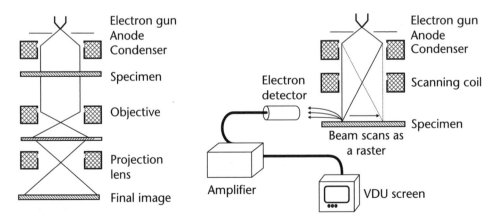

Figure 16.10
Schematic diagram comparing CTEM and SEM

Entry gauze at +300V

Focusing ring

Thin layer of aluminium to allow charging, e.g. +10kV

Perspex light guide going to photomultiplier

Figure 16.11
SEM electron collector (Everhart–Thornley version)

monitor still displays the same sized picture but it now represents a smaller area and this gives greater magnification.

Electron collection system

The electrons are collected by a specialized system such as an Everhart–Thornley collector (see *Fig. 16.11*). Other detectors are also available but the Everhart–Thornley collector is one of the most frequently used.

The actual detector consists of a **scintillating system** that converts the electrons' energy into flashes of light, which are measured by a **photomultiplier** (see *Box 16.9*) and this produces an electrical signal equivalent to the number of electrons entering the detector. The scintillator is kept at a high potential (+10 to +12 kV) so all of the electrons are attracted and accelerated into the scintillant. This accelerating voltage means that electrons are collected from a wide area and have sufficient energy to generate a strong flash of light in the scintillant.

An entry gauze is used to shield the system and this is also held at a voltage; by varying this voltage the type of electrons collected can be controlled. If is held at +300 V, then both back-scattered and secondary electrons will be detected. By altering the voltage from +300 to −100 V, or by switching off the 10 kV high tension, the secondary electrons will no longer be attracted but the higher-energy back-scattered electrons will still be collected.

Box 16.9 Use of photomultipliers in SEM

Scintillation is where electrons emit a pulse of light as they enter certain materials such as Perspex. The light is weak but can be amplified using a photomultiplier. This instrument converts the light back into an electrical signal. It is ironic that the detectors used in electron microscopy are still using optical methods and are not purely electronic. Photomultipliers are one of the most sensitive ways of detecting very weak signals and can detect single photons that are equivalent to single electrons.

The back-scattered image is weaker but gives information about the subsurface

The back-scattered image penetrates further into the specimen and is more dependent on the chemical nature of the specimen, but it is also a much weaker signal as fewer electrons are reflected in this way. As a result there is a lot of noise in the image. For most purposes, SEM is only used to detect the secondary or emitted electrons ('emissive mode'), which gives surface structure rather than penetrating into the specimen. Tilting the specimen can reduce the effect of back-scattered electrons. The incident electron beam glances across the specimen rather than hitting it full on and this minimizes the number of back-scattered electrons.

Secondary or emitted electrons give a surface view

The incident electrons penetrate quite large distances (up to 100 μm) into the specimen but the relatively low energy of the secondary electrons makes them unable to escape from deep inside the specimen. These deep electrons are absorbed and lose energy and so are trapped deep in the specimen. The electrons that can escape are those within 2 nm or so of the surface. If there is an edge or a hole in the specimen, however, then more secondary electrons can escape (see *Fig. 16.12*) and the image is brighter at these points. This gives a 'backlighting' effect that is aesthetically pleasant.

Advantages and disadvantages of SEM

Unlike CTEM, SEM does not focus the electrons coming from the specimen and there are no lenses involved in producing the image so there are no lens aberrations with SEM. Despite the relatively high magnifications used in SEM, there is tremendous depth of field (i.e. the image is in focus at both

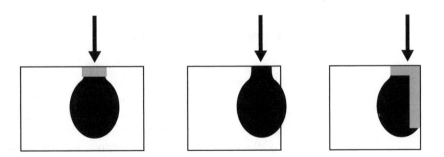

Figure 16.12
Edge effect in SEM. The secondary electrons can only escape from the specimen from a shallow region close to the surface but are produced from a larger pear-shaped region below the point where the electron beam hits the specimen. As the beam scans across, the pear-shaped region overlaps the edge of the object (centre). The region from which electrons can escape is now much larger (right) so there are more electrons escaping and this makes the edges appear brighter in the final image

---

Box 16.10 Depth of field

The depth of field is impressive when compared with light microscopy. SEM can examine quite large specimens such as complete insects or plants or blocks of wood. SEM can show the front and back as acceptably in focus at the same time, even when they are several millimetres apart. The use of a light microscope results in a narrow focus that may be only a few micrometres deep. The only advantage of the light microscope is the use of colour but for monochrome pictures, SEM is better than any of the alternative methods.

---

the front and the back at the same time) and this makes for a very pleasing image (see *Box 16.10*).

Like TEM, the image is only monochrome but many workers colour the image artificially in order to bring out particular features.

Photographs are taken using a high-resolution monitor

Unlike CTEM, it is not possible to use a sheet of film to record the electron image directly and with SEM, photographs are made by photographing the VDU screen. The normal monitor image is relatively coarse so a second high-definition screen is used for making photographs. In this case, the scan is performed very slowly, which gives better definition, but this mode is not useful for direct viewing since only a single dot is visible on the screen and it moves too slowly to allow the human eye to see a complete image. A camera pointed at the screen records all of the dots by using a long exposure and so the photograph appears as a complete image.

As SEM is used mainly for its three-dimensional aspects, it uses whole, intact specimens rather than thin slices or sections of material. Thick sections treated by freeze-etching or freeze–fracture are sometimes used to see the internal detail of specimens but otherwise sections are not used for SEM.

Specimen preparation for SEM

The usual way of preparing specimens is to dry them completely and then coat them with a thin metal or carbon film to protect them and make them electrically conductive. Electrical conductivity is essential to allow static electrical charges to be earthed. If the specimen is not earthed in this way, then as electrons are absorbed by the specimen it becomes highly charged and repels all of the electrons before they can reach the surface of the specimen. In consequence, with an unearthed or uncoated specimen there is no image to be seen.

Specimens are dried and coated for use in SEM

Simple air-drying is not recommended since it is uneven and as the water evaporates there are surface tension effects, which may damage delicate objects or distort the surface. Instead **critical point drying** is used. Critical point drying relies on phase transitions from a fluid to a vapour without evaporation or boiling. The gas occupies the same space as the liquid so there is no dramatic change in pressure. The phase change can be achieved using CO_2. The CO_2 changes from a liquid to a gas by a simple rise in temperature. The critical temperature for CO_2 is 31°C; above this temperature CO_2 cannot be a liquid even at very high pressure and will become a gas.

The specimen can thus be dried without evaporation by putting it into liquid CO_2. Liquid CO_2 is not miscible with water so the specimen is first dehydrated in alcohol or acetone and then transferred into liquid CO_2 in a pressure chamber (commonly called a 'bomb'). The liquid CO_2 is under pressure and kept below its critical temperature until all of the dehydrating agent has been removed. The liquid CO_2 can then be converted to a gas simply by slowly warming it up above 31°C. There is no evaporation – it just turns into a gas instantaneously without alteration in pressure or volume. The gas can then be slowly released. The pressure is dropped gradually to allow the gas to escape from the specimen in a slow and controlled manner. Rapid drops in pressure will result in explosive escapes of gas from pockets trapped in the specimen and are likely to damage the specimen. The specimen is now dry and can be sputter coated with a film of metal. It is then ready to be viewed by SEM.

Box 16.11 Other forms of scanning microscopy

Other forms of electron microscopy and scanning microscopy have also been developed. For example, the scanning transmission electron microscope (STEM), which detects transmitted electrons passing through sections rather than the various types of 'reflected' electrons of SEM but is otherwise similar in its nature to SEM.

The atomic force microscope and scanning tunnelling microscope scan the specimen surface using an extremely fine electrical probe. These are currently used more as research tools for particular applications and are often more useful in non-biological fields such as physics and materials science.

Other SEM techniques

Electron microprobe analysis

The final type of emission from scanning microscopes that can provide information is the X-rays that are released when electrons are dislodged from their atomic orbits. As electrons move back into the hole created by these dislodged electrons they emit X-rays. The electron shells of atoms are characteristic of each element so the X-rays produced by the electrons 'dropping' into empty orbits are of different wavelengths with each element having certain characteristic wavelengths. By irradiating one spot with a thin electron beam, as is done in SEM, and then measuring the wavelength and intensity of the X-rays produced, it is possible to detect any elements present and even to estimate how much of each element is present. This can be done using SEM, STEM or TEM, although the transmission techniques probably give better resolution.

Freeze-etching

In this technique the surface of the tissue is first frozen solid and then dried by sublimation (see Chapter 5). This exposes the structure of the dry material in three dimensions. The surface is very delicate and must be protected by gold coating. The sample is still easily damaged and will not keep. Replicas of the surface can also be prepared for use in CTEM but this technique is mostly used with SEM.

SUGGESTED FURTHER READING

Griffin, R.L. (1990) *Using the Transmission Electron Microscope in the Biological Sciences*. London: Ellis Horwood.

Slayter, E.M. and Slayter, H.S. (1992) *Light and Electron Microscopy*. Cambridge: Cambridge University Press.

Stirling, J. and Woods, A. (2002) Transmission electron microscopy: diagnostic applications. In *Theory and Practice of Histological Techniques*, 5th edn (eds J.D. Bancroft and M. Gamble). Edinburgh: Churchill Livingstone.

Woods, A. and Stirling, J. (2002) Electron microscopy: the preparative techniques. In *Theory and Practice of Histological Techniques*, 5th edn (eds J.D. Bancroft and M. Gamble). Edinburgh: Churchill Livingstone.

SELF-ASSESSMENT QUESTIONS

1. How does CTEM differ from light microscopy?
2. Why do electron microscopy sections need to be embedded in resin rather than wax?
3. Why does SEM not suffer from lens aberrations?
4. What is critical point drying and why is it used in SEM?
5. Why is it necessary to coat SEM specimens with gold?
6. Why is it more difficult in CTEM specimens to identify cellular materials using staining than it is in light microscopy?
7. How can the X-rays produced by the electron beam striking a specimen be used in electron microscopy?

17
Some aspects of the organization of a histology laboratory

Learning objectives
After studying this chapter you should confidently be able to:

■ Describe the organization of a routine histology laboratory.

■ Outline the reasons for storing specimens and data.

■ Understand the problems and regulations associated with the retention of specimens and patient data.

■ Understand the need for safety and where to seek help on safety matters.

There are probably as many different ways of organizing a laboratory to produce histological sections as there are actual laboratories. This is in part a reflection of the differing needs and different services. The organization needed to produce a rapid and reliable service for routine diagnosis is not the same as would be needed to produce large numbers of almost identical sections for teaching. The needs of a research laboratory are to be able to tackle problems that may not have been attempted before and are quite different to the problems encountered by a contract laboratory, which offers a standard level of consistency so that sections will always have the same treatment and a predictable level of quality.

17.1 ORGANIZATION OF A ROUTINE DIAGNOSTIC LABORATORY

There are, however, several features of the organization that are essential and that are common to most, if not all, laboratories, and the organization of a routine diagnostic laboratory will now be considered in more detail to illustrate the way in which laboratories can be organized.

Specimen types and fixation

Specimens can be of several types and widely different sizes. Specimens that are taken from a living patient are **biopsy** specimens. The term is usually

---

Box 17.1 Tissues are removed for therapy as well as for diagnosis

The reasons for removing specimens are often quite varied and only occasionally is the main reason concerned with pathology. Many specimens are removed to treat the patient and a pathology report is a secondary consideration. This means that on some occasions the received specimen is less than ideal for histology. I came across a comment about a specimen in which the report read, 'It is impossible to tell whether the specimen was ruined by a pair of large Spencer Wells or a pair of small Spencer Wells'. Spencer Wells forceps are a type of surgical forceps with serrated jaws. The surgeon had crushed the jaws on to the specimen making it useless for diagnosis. The surgeons providing specimens need to be aware that if they mistreat specimens, then the pathologist may be unable to give an adequate report.

If damage is inevitable during surgery to save the patient's life or health, then it may be justified, but education of surgical staff is needed if they are to provide good-quality specimens for diagnosis.

---

used as an indication that it is a diagnostic investigation that is being carried out. In some cases, the whole lesion is removed as an **excisional biopsy** (for example, a piece of skin with a mole that may be becoming cancerous), so the distinctions are not always clear. Large pieces of tissue may be referred to as **resections** or **amputations**.

Surgical specimens are usually fixed immediately so that post-mortem changes can be avoided. However, they are taken by surgical staff and the staff responsible for fixation are often relatively junior nursing staff. This can mean that tissues may be less well treated after removal (see *Box 17.1*).

Fixation is possibly the most important single part of the processing, yet for most surgical specimens the fixation is done by surgical nursing staff rather than histologists. A badly organized system will cause many problems. Many laboratories simplify the fixation by always fixing everything in formaldehyde so provided specimens are delivered fairly quickly, the laboratory can usually produce good results.

The specimen may still be ruined by insufficient fixative. Very large specimens may be placed in barely adequate containers and then 'topped up' with fixative. Thus, a specimen with a total volume of 700 cm^3 (700 ml) may be placed in a 1 litre container and then 250 ml of fixative added. This would not be enough to fix the specimen completely, but provided the specimen is taken to the laboratory quickly it may be recoverable.

Specimens removed after death are **post-mortem** or **autopsy** specimens. Post-mortem specimens are usually taken several hours after death and so often show artefacts of degeneration (called, not surprisingly, post-mortem artefacts), but as they are taken by pathologists and fixed by post-mortem technicians, who are usually closely associated with the laboratory, they are usually fixed correctly.

Labelling

The lack of proper forms and mislabelling is very dangerous. A couple of small specimens without labels can all too easily be confused. Once tissue is placed in fixative it changes in both colour and shape so deciding which unlabelled specimen is which can be a nightmare. Specimens arriving badly documented should not be accepted. The only thing that should be checked is that the specimen is being fixed correctly, but otherwise it should not be processed until it is labelled correctly.

How the specimen is labelled and the form used will vary with the local system, but for diagnostic hospital specimens it must positively identify the patient and the specimen and should include:

- patient's full name;
- gender;
- patient's hospital number;
- date of birth;
- relevant medical history;
- possible diagnosis;
- examination requested;
- person and department submitting the request;
- date of the request.

On acceptance, the specimen should be logged and, if relevant, given a laboratory number. Laboratories with a high turnover often have automated or semi-automated systems that will print labels; these may include a bar code. Low-throughput laboratories may make do with a hand-written system. Hand-written systems are probably less reliable and need more care but if care is taken they can be satisfactory.

Specimen treatment

Specimens may be of a specialized type, such as a needle biopsy, which may need to be split into separate samples for different treatments (see *Fig. 17.1*). Every laboratory will have slightly different requirements and every specimen type will have different demands so there is no universal system.

Figure 17.1
Needle biopsy. The specimen is split, with the light microscopy (LM) part being fixed in formalin, the piece for frozen sections being left unfixed and the electron microscopy (EM) resin-embedded specimens being fixed in glutaraldehyde

The specimen is allowed to fix for an adequate length of time (12 h or more, depending on size). The specimen is then examined and cut into suitable blocks for processing (sometimes called 'cutting up' or 'grossing') and an accurate description of the whole specimen is made, together with a description of where the individual blocks are taken from specimen. This may be very simple or quite complex. A simple specimen would be a routine vasectomy where only a single block may be needed, whilst a complex or very large specimen may need many blocks and their exact location and orientation may be crucial. Accurate recording of where a specimen was removed from a large piece of tissue may be crucial. If there is an invasive tumour that is spreading through the tissues, the surgeon needs to know whether the tumour has spread beyond the edge of the removed tissue. This means he needs to know exactly where the borders have been crossed. Marking of the borders can be done in several ways (e.g. sewing on of tags, writing with indelible ink) and some laboratories are now using digital cameras, which record the specimen exactly. These cameras do not use film but record the image as computer data so that a picture can be inserted into the final word-processed report.

The blocks are then placed in individual cassettes, which may be colour coded to identify particular types of specimen. The blocks are then processed, usually on an automatic tissue processor. The following day, the blocks are placed into moulds and oriented. At this stage a simple check should be made to confirm that each block corresponds to the description given during the 'grossing'. The blocks are cooled and then sectioned. Some specimens may require more than one section to be taken at differing planes in the block ('levels'). The sections are stained and coverslipped. Once again, larger laboratories may have a degree of automation to all of this, whilst smaller laboratories will be more reliant on manual techniques. Some special stains may be done automatically. Each laboratory, and indeed an individual pathologist within a laboratory, may have different requirements for the number of levels in a block and the type and number of special stains done routinely so it is difficult to give a single description of the usual procedures.

The stained sections should be checked for quality. It is difficult to diagnose accurately from a poor-quality section. If the sections are suitable, then they are passed to the pathologist for diagnosis.

Diagnosis

The diagnosis may be simple and quick, but if there is a problem the pathologist may need to use further special stains, histochemistry, immunohistochemistry or electron microscopy to help him in the final diagnosis. It may even be necessary to consult with other pathologists in a few difficult or unusual cases. Sections may need to be prepared and sent to a distant laboratory where there is an expert in some particular field of pathology. The Internet is now being harnessed to speed up this process by using digitized images from the microscope and video-conferencing facilities. These facilities are currently more widely used in radiography than in pathology, but are likely to become more widespread as the technology becomes more accessible and familiar.

The final diagnosis is then entered into the computer records and also sent to the clinician requesting the result. Some computerized systems do this automatically, but other places still rely on paper copies to be sent to the ward or GP.

Box 17.2 Work rates

The workload in laboratories is quite variable but a few ideas of the rates of work are given here.

For a person working effectively with no distractions, then blocking out into a mould takes about 30–90 s. To cut the block takes about 1–4 min assuming there are no significant problems. Staining is usually quite variable as it depends on whether it is automated, what stain is being done and how many slides are having the same treatment. A single slide needing a special stain might take a couple of hours, but the biomedical scientist would probably do other jobs at the same time.

Most laboratories try to have the routine tasks of cutting and staining done by lunch time and many use one or more staff on an early start to get the embedding done ready for the main start of the day so that cutting can begin immediately. The afternoon is then used for routine maintenance, preparing reagents, grossing for the following day and doing any special stains requested by the pathologist.

The typical output from a single competent histologist can be up to about 50 slides per day, assuming that they have to do everything concerned with the preparation. This corresponds to about 12,000 slides per year.

Record keeping

The final stages in the laboratory are to file the slides and blocks and dispose of tissues that are no longer needed. Tissues, blocks and sections can be retained for several purposes. The retention of tissues/slides is more useful than keeping only the report as it is sometimes possible at a later date to check on the tissue in a way that was not possible at the time of the original examination. For example, it is now possible to perform DNA analysis on 50-year-old blocks; 50 years ago such analysis was impossible as the structure of DNA was not known. Paper records can only show what was known at the time.

Archived specimens of tissue and blocks may be needed for:

■ Further diagnosis and clinical management of the patient at a later date. This allows the progress of the patient to be monitored. If the patient's condition changes, it may be possible with hindsight to re-examine the specimen and find early signs of the change that it was not possible to recognize at the time.

■ Teaching purposes. Good examples of particular diseases are often used in teaching and observation of the actual tissues is the best way to illustrate the condition.

■ Use in research. A good archive of tissues can be an invaluable resource. Some diseases are very rare and the accumulated total of many years of cases is often the only way of collecting enough samples to give a reasonable coverage of the disease. Also, some diseases have only become recognized recently, so it seems likely that there are further diseases of which we are currently unaware but which may become important later. The availability of historical samples allows researchers to find out when the disease first appeared, even though it was not recognized or even known at the time. This has occurred with AIDS, where evidence of

---

Box 17.3 Return of tissues may be hazardous

The return of specimens may involve dangers to the recipients if there is a risk of infection. Even fixation in formaldehyde does not guarantee safety as the infective agent in Creutzfeldt–Jakob disease and BSE ('mad cow disease') can still be infective. Also, the materials used to preserve the specimens may be a hazard. Nineteen objects from the Indian Arts Research Centre due to be returned to the Hopi Indians who considered them sacred were found to be contaminated with arsenic.

---

human immunodeficiency virus infection can be found in samples taken before the disease was recognized. The situation is similar for bovine spongiform encephalopathy (BSE) and Creutzfeldt–Jakob disease.

■ Evidence in legal cases. This occurs where the patient alleges incorrect diagnosis or treatment.

Storage and disposal of records and specimens

Paper or computer records that relate directly to the patient's diagnosis are normally kept for at least the lifetime of the patient and in most cases are kept permanently. Paper records of laboratory procedures (servicing records, quality control records, day books) may be kept for between 2 and 10 years but often are retained permanently. Specific recommendations have been made by the Royal College of Pathologists and these give details of how long to store each individual type of record.

Paraffin blocks and sections are stored permanently whenever possible and as a minimum for the lifetime of the patient. Wet tissue is normally kept for at least 4 weeks after the final report. The Royal College of Pathologists again has guidelines that give details for different specimen types.

The use of tissue samples has become more complex in recent years and is now regulated by law. The Human Tissue Act 2004 regulates the holding of tissue and was initiated by events at Bristol Royal Infirmary and Alder Hey Children's Hospital in Liverpool in 1999–2000. In the past, small amounts of unwanted tissue left from clinical diagnosis were used for medical research or for quality control within the laboratory without specific consent. This had long been held to be ethical and justified by long-standing consensus. This has now changed and any use not directly related to the patient's diagnosis must be specifically sanctioned.

Disposal of unwanted material is a problem since it is personal to the patient and socially sensitive. Strictly speaking, following surgery the tissue still belongs to the patient and they may ask for the material to be disposed of in a particular way or even ask for the return of the material. It is normally considered reasonable to comply with such a request provided there is no obvious reason to refuse (such as a serious risk of infection for example; see *Box 17.3*). In the absence of a direct request, the material should be disposed of carefully, e.g. by incineration, taking care to avoid any specimen being identifiable.

Box 17.4 Professional responsibility

Whatever grade of staff a person is employed as, they are expected to behave responsibly towards patients and the information about patients. The Institute of Biomedical Sciences suggests that professional staff should:

1. Exercise their professional judgement, skill and care to the best of their ability.
2. Fulfil their professional role with integrity, refraining from its misuse to the detriment of patients, employers or professional colleagues.
3. Seek to safeguard patients and others, particularly in relation to health and safety.
4. Treat with discretion all confidential and other information requiring protection and avoid disclosing to any unauthorized person the result of any investigation or other information of a personal or confidential nature gained in the practise of their profession.
5. Act in good faith towards those with whom they stand in professional relationship and conduct themselves so as to uphold the reputation of their profession.
6. Strive to maintain, improve and update their professional knowledge and skill.
7. Promote the study and development of biomedical science and the education and training of biomedical scientists.

Post-mortem tissue is similarly a problem but is slightly more complicated. The deceased person may have made known their wishes, in which case they should be respected, as for a surgical case, but a surviving spouse or relative may also make a similar request, even though there is no record of the deceased person themselves having made such a request. Normally such requests are followed. The exception may be a coroner's post mortem where foul play may be a possibility. In such cases, requests to destroy the tissue rather than storing it could be an attempt to destroy evidence so the coroner's permission is needed for any disposal.

Electron microscopy laboratories

Electron microscopy laboratories tend to be a much smaller set-up. There are far fewer electron microscopy laboratories and often only the very large hospitals have a histological electron microscopy unit and these are more heavily involved in research than a typical histology laboratory. They are more often organized with a particular person following a specimen from start to finish rather than specimens being passed from one person to another at each step.

Research laboratories

These are organized for a different purpose, so the organization tends to be slightly different. The need to investigate one particular problem in depth often means a small team including senior academic staff, post-graduate students and technical support staff who will follow an organized programme of research and may well need to call in expertise and facilities not available 'in house'. This means that collaboration is crucial. In research, the results are the main criterion of success so quality is essential. This means choosing the appropriate methods and applying them skilfully. Most things are non-routine and speed is secondary to quality. There is likely to be a much greater variety of techniques used, a greater diversity of methods and a less predictable working schedule.

Every histology laboratory I have ever walked into has been organized slightly differently. To make an analogy with kitchens, some are large with lots of staff, plenty of specialist equipment and can produce hundreds of meals at a time, whilst others are small, fairly basic in their equipment and only produce a few meals. Provided the food is good, then who really cares how the kitchen is organized? The same applies to histology laboratories. Provided they work effectively and produce good sections reliably, then the details of the laboratory are of less importance.

17.2 QUALITY CONTROL

It is now expected that every laboratory will maintain at least a minimum level of satisfactory quality. If this standard is reached in the UK, then the laboratory can become accredited by Clinical Pathology Accreditation Ltd. In the USA, there is a similar system operated by the College of American Pathologists. This includes several aspects of quality. Many of these relate to management including aspects such as administration, staffing, facilities (buildings and equipment), staff development, record keeping, ethics and confidentiality. Detailed consideration of these aspects is beyond the scope of this book.

One aspect is more relevant to the science of cellular pathology and this is the quality of the preparations. In the past, quality was maintained internally by direct visual assessment by senior staff. In the UK, an external quality audit has been introduced under the UK National External Quality Assurance Scheme. In this scheme, each laboratory submits a series of stained preparations, which are assessed by a panel of competent judges against a list of predefined standards. Each of the assessors assigns a mark for each preparation and the scores given are aggregated into a single final figure for each preparation. The laboratory receives a set of marks (out of 10) for each of the submitted preparations plus a bar chart indicating the performance of all of the other laboratories. This allows the laboratory to take remedial action if a low standard of quality is achieved. A mark below 6 is considered unsatisfactory. Consistently low marks will be noted by regional organizers of the scheme who will then make assistance available to improve performance.

17.3 SAFETY IN THE HISTOLOGY LABORATORY

The safety of staff has become a much greater issue in the management of UK laboratories since the introduction of the Control of Substances

Hazardous to Health regulations in 2004. Safety is an area that involves not only management but every person in the workplace and has implications for the wider public and the environment.

Help can be obtained from the Health and Safety Executive who maintain a useful website and produce numerous publications to help staff comply with current UK regulations.

Every aspect of the running of a laboratory should undergo a risk assessment but particularly any procedures that involve an obvious hazard. The assessment will indicate how risks can be reduced but it is probably impossible to eliminate every hazard completely, so the regulations say that risks should be reduced 'so far as is reasonably practicable'.

Hazard assessment

The term 'hazard' includes anything capable of causing harm such as chemicals, electrical equipment and machinery, whilst 'risk' is used in the sense of probability or chance that somebody will be harmed by that hazard.

It is suggested that the assessment should include five steps:

1. Look for possible hazards.
2. Identify the people at risk from each hazard and how the harm might occur. This may involve suggesting that a particular group of people should not work on particular tasks (e.g. pregnant women need to avoid some chemicals and sources of ionizing radiation).
3. Determine the risk, whether the current working practices are safe and how frequently an accident or incident may occur. Consider whether better precautions can be implemented to reduce the risk further. For any particular hazard, this may involve considering whether the hazard can be avoided completely, whether the hazard and risk can be safely controlled or whether serious incidents can be prevented.
4. Keep a clear and accessible written account of the assessment so that anyone can refer easily to the conclusions.
5. Review the assessment periodically and revise it when necessary.

Hazardous chemicals

Many of the risks in a laboratory will relate to chemical hazards. Each chemical needs to be considered carefully but this is relatively straightforward since the manufacturers will provide data hazard sheets with their products. In the risk assessment, it should be standard to identify how the material should be stored safely and how it can be used safely, including such precautions as using fume hoods and protective clothing and the safe disposal of the materials when they are no longer required. It should also include the steps to be taken if the precautions fail or there is an accident resulting in an emergency situation, including the medical treatment of the affected person.

Box 17.5 Categories of hazardous chemicals

Irritants cause inflammation and this is usually reversible. **Corrosive chemicals** cause irreversible destruction of living tissues. **Sensitizers** cause allergic reactions. This is usually only specified if a significant proportion of the population would develop an allergy if they were exposed to the agent. A much wider range of chemicals may cause allergies in a small proportion of people exposed. **Carcinogens** cause tumours in animals but the dosage is often critical. **Toxic** infers that the chemical can result in death if ingested, inhaled or absorbed through the skin in a large enough dose.

Chemical exposure has two dimensions, both of which need to be considered. One is concentration – the more concentrated a toxic material is, the more likely it is to cause damage. This is particularly the case with volatile materials that can be breathed in. The use of effective fume hoods is one way of limiting exposure to such air-borne risks. The second aspect of respiratory toxicity is the length of exposure. The hazards are usually specified by manufacturers on the packaging or in their literature but can be in a variety of forms. They may be relatively non-specific with such terms as **toxic** or **irritant** (see *Box 17.5*) without giving precise details of the dosages causing these effects. They may be in coded form with a defined list of meanings; thus, R45 means the compound 'may cause cancer' and S20 indicates the precaution 'When using, do not eat or drink.' More precise information is given in occupational exposure levels, which are often legally mandatory. The exposure is related to time; thus, **time-weighted average** (TWA) levels indicate the maximum concentration averaged over a complete working day (this may allow higher levels for short periods of time provided they are balanced by lower levels at other times); the **short-term exposure limit** (STEL) indicates the time-weighted average for a 15 min period, which controls the levels during the peak times; and the **ceiling limit** or **ceiling exposure value** gives a value that must never be exceeded, even for a brief period of time. These phrases and codes are often specific to one

---

Box 17.6 Fire hazards

Fire hazards have their own nomenclature problems. The simplest description is anything that will burn or cause a fire, but things are not quite that simple. Materials may be described as explosive, an oxidizer, combustible, flammable or even inflammable. They also have a defined flashpoint, which indicates the ease with which they ignite.

   Explosive materials may be caused to explode by a variety of mechanisms. Some may explode if simply shaken (which need not necessarily be vigorous shaking), or if they are exposed to electrical currents or raised temperatures. The explosion may also cause a fire. **Oxidizers** do not burn directly but may promote or initiate fires in other chemicals. A **combustible** material is defined as having a flash point above a specified level. The specified level will vary depending on the regulatory authority (in the USA it is set at 100°F/37.8°C by the Occupational Safety and Health Administration and 141°F/60.5°C by the Department of Transportation). A **flammable** material is defined as having a flash point below the specified threshold. Despite the apparent negative prefix, the term inflammable means exactly the same as flammable and is now discouraged as a safety term.

country or even one regulatory authority within a country, so other terms may found such as **threshold limit value, permissible exposure limits** and **maximum allowable concentration.**

Safety personnel

Safety needs to have someone who is identifiably responsible. This may be a supervisor or a designated safety officer. This person should not only prepare the assessment but should monitor its implementation – a good safety protocol is useless unless everyone adheres it to. There should also be appropriate monitoring of the health of the people performing the task. Monitoring may be relatively simple involving noting whether a member of staff suffers from obvious effects such as recurrent dermatitis or respiratory problems, but if appropriate may mean specific tests, for example, for liver function or early signs of chronic effects.

Safety is a state of mind

Although safe working requires clear specific precautions such as wearing rubber gloves and protective goggles, such precautions are best considered as an additional means of protection and not treated as a replacement for other control measures. The best protection is probably an awareness of danger and a personal commitment to safety. If the laboratory can instil an ethos of caution and care, then it will be better protected than relying on a few prescriptive safety measures.

A concept known as Murphy's or Sod's Law states that 'If anything can go wrong, it will,' with an addendum that 'If something can go wrong in more than one way, it will go wrong in the way that will cause the most damage.' This seems at first to be a cynical and pessimistic outlook but despite its jokiness it is a good basis for safety. When assessing hazards and risk, the worst-case scenario should always be considered.

Assessment of risk is not always just considering the obvious. For example, the use of liquid nitrogen, e.g. in frozen sections, may require the material to be transported between floors of a building. With liquid nitrogen, the very low temperature is the main hazard. Thus, carrying it by hand in a Dewar flask, especially in large quantities, is a risk if it is dropped or spilt on to clothing or living flesh. A safer alternative is a specially designed

---

Box 17.7 Be aware of the less obvious hazards

Hazards are not always obvious. In microtomy, for example, the dangers of the ultrasharp knives are usually well recognized. I have personally worked in histology for many years and have suffered only three minor cuts from microtome knives. However, in the same period I had many minor cuts from slides, coverslips and even paper – these seem less dangerous and threatening so fewer precautions are taken.

wheeled trolley incorporating a secure damage-resistant flask. Unfortunately, wheeled trolleys are difficult to manoeuvre on stairs and require an lift. However, although liquid nitrogen is not directly toxic (80% of the air we breathe is nitrogen), it is suffocating if it evaporates and replaces the oxygen in air. Thus, when liquid nitrogen is transported in a lift it should not be accompanied in person in case the lift breaks down. This would mean the person would be in an enclosed space with the consequent risk of suffocation, as the cold nitrogen gas evaporating would replace the air in the elevator. In 1999, a technician died in this way resulting in the prosecution of the Medical Research Council who employed him. However, putting liquid nitrogen in an elevator unsupervised would be a risk to unaware passengers boarding at intermediate floors, so further precautions are needed, such as supervision of intermediate floors during the transport. Consideration of worst-case scenarios and Murphy's Law is needed to identify and control such risks.

SUGGESTED FURTHER READING

Banks, I. and Gamble, M. (2002) Managing the laboratory. In *Theory and Practice of Histological Techniques*, 5th edn (eds J.D. Bancroft and M. Gamble). Edinburgh: Churchill Livingstone.

Dapson, R.W. (2002) Safety in the laboratory. In *Theory and Practice of Histological Techniques*, 5th edn (eds J.D. Bancroft and M. Gamble). Edinburgh: Churchill Livingstone.

Furness, P.N. (2002) An overview of quality control. In *Theory and Practice of Histological Techniques*, 5th edn (eds J.D. Bancroft and M. Gamble). Edinburgh: Churchill Livingstone.

Health and Safety Executive (2002) *COSHH: a Brief Guide to the Regulations*. Available from: http://www.hse.gov.uk/pubns/leaflets.htm

Health and Safety Executive (2003) *Health and Safety Regulation...a Short Guide*. Available from: http://www.hse.gov.uk/pubns/leaflets.htm

Institute of Biomedical Science (1996) *Code of Professional Conduct and Code of Practice for Biomedical Science Laboratories*. London: Institute of Biomedical Science.

Report of the Working Party of the Royal College of Pathologists (1995) *Retention and Storage of Pathological Records and Archives*. London: Royal College of Pathologists.

Report of the Advisory Committee on Histopathology of the Royal College of Pathologists (2002) *Interim Guidelines for the Disposal of Tissue, Blocks and Slides from Biopsies and Surgical Resections*.

Report of the Ethics Committee of the Royal College of Pathologists (2005) *Interim Guidance on the Use of Clinical Samples Retained in the Pathology Laboratory*. London: Royal College of Pathologists.

The Human Tissue Act (2004) Available from: www.parliament.the-stationery-office.co.uk/

The Retained Organs Commission (2004) *Good Practice Guidance*, March.

Answers to self-assessment questions

Chapter 1

1. An artefact is an alteration in tissues brought about by the treatment of the tissue following its removal from the body.
2. (a) Materials normally present in cells can be lost from tissues during processing, e.g. glucose. (b) Materials that were not present in life can be added to the tissues, e.g. fixation pigments. (c) Tissues can be distorted by processing, e.g. shrinkage of cells.
3. Glycogen is probably present in the cells because the two different preparative techniques show the presence of glycogen. The distribution of glycogen within the cells cannot be determined with any certainty from these sections because the two techniques give conflicting results. One, or both, techniques have introduced an artefact and further techniques are needed to resolve the problem.
4. No single technique is perfect for every specimen and every investigation. Different people have different requirements and each person will choose the method that best matches their needs. Thus, frozen sections are good for demonstrating lipids but are not ideal for most routine applications as the tissue cannot be stored easily.

Chapter 2

1. Tissues removed from the body may change by autolysis, where the cell's lysosomal enzymes break down the structure of the cells. Tissues may also change by putrefaction, where bacterial or fungal contaminants break down the tissue structure. Tissues may change if the cells remain alive after removal from the body as they will respire anaerobically. Cells will deplete their nutrient reserves and the accumulation of waste products may alter the tissue's structure.
2. Post-mortem changes can be prevented by

stopping enzyme activity. Enzyme activity can be halted by chemicals or heat. Chemical fixation is most common and requires the cells to be treated with a large excess of fixative as quickly as possible. Perfusion of the fixative through the blood vessels or slicing of the tissue may be needed to ensure rapid penetration to all cells.
3. A good fixative has the following properties:
   - Penetrates tissues quickly and evenly.
   - Kills cells quickly and evenly; the killing stops abnormal metabolism.
   - Prevents autolysis.
   - Prevents putrefaction.
   - Does not add any extraneous material to the tissue.
   - Does not swell or shrink the tissue.
   - Prepares the tissue for later treatments such as staining and does not prevent any later investigation that might be needed.
   - Prevents desiccation and drying of tissue, which would cause shrinkage and distortion.
   - Safe to use (non-toxic, non-flammable).
   - Reasonably priced.
   - Convenient to use (shelf life, storage, etc.).
4. Dettol is not a good fixative, despite killing bacteria and thus stopping putrefaction. The prevention of putrefaction is only one of the three types of change that need to be inhibited. Only if the chemical also stops autolysis and cellular metabolism without damaging the tissues will it be a useful fixative. Dettol is an antiseptic and can be used on open wounds without killing the tissues. It will not stop normal tissue enzymes so it is not a good fixative.
5. Formaldehyde is readily washed out of tissues and leaves no residual aldehyde groups. Glutaraldehyde is a bifunctional aldehyde and is not easily washed out of tissues so there will be aldehydes from the glutaraldehyde left in the tissues following fixation and these will give a non-specific background reaction with Schiff's method for aldehydes.

6. Fixatives are intended to kill tissues so they are all toxic chemicals. Some are extremely nasty substances and may cause specific problems such as inducing allergies or predisposing to cancer.

Chapter 3

1. Wax embedding is used to support the tissues during the cutting of sections. In the absence of a support medium, the sections will collapse and the structure of the cells and tissues will be lost. Wax is the commonest embedding medium as it is cheap and allows good sections to be prepared.
2. Fixation (to preserve the tissues), dehydration (to remove the water and replace it with alcohol), clearing (to remove the alcohol and replace it with a solvent miscible with wax), wax impregnation (to replace the clearing agent with molten wax), blocking out (to set the tissues in a mould with fresh wax) and finally solidification of the wax to form the wax block. Other steps such as decalcification (needed with mineralized tissues) and vacuum impregnation (not absolutely essential but useful) could also be included in the list.
3. A graded series of any reagent, including alcohol, is a series of baths of gradually increasing strength. The purpose is to remove the water more gently to minimize tissue damage. If tissues are placed directly into 100% alcohol, it can cause more hardening and distortion of the tissues than a slower removal using baths of increasing strength. An example of a graded series would be 50%, 70%, 90% and 100% alcohol. Alternatives to alcohol might be acetone, propylene oxide or Cellosolve.
4. Clearing agents were so called because they rendered the tissue transparent. This is not true of all reagents but the name has been retained.
5. (a) Benzene gives good results but is carcinogenic and is no longer used routinely. (b) Xylene is less of a health problem than benzene; it clears tissues rapidly but hardens the tissues and is more useful for clearing sections after cutting than for preparing blocks of tissues. (c) Cedarwood oil is slow and expensive but gives good results. (d) Petrol hydrocarbons are considered safer than many other materials and give acceptable results.
6. Vacuum embedding is the reduction of pressure in the wax bath during wax impregnation and is used to remove air bubbles and help to remove the clearing agent.
7. Mineralized bone can be softened using acids or chelating agents to remove the calcium salts.
8. Undecalcified sections can be prepared by embedding the tissue in a hard embedding medium such as plastic and then sectioning with a hardened tungsten knife or by preparing a ground section in which most of the bone is ground away leaving a single thin section.
9. The bone marrow fragments would have lost any mineralized material during fixation, as acetic acid is also an effective decalcifying agent. Thus, there is no way to be sure whether the patient's bones were fully mineralized or whether the patient suffered from osteomalacia. (If osteomalacia is suspected, then the bone must be protected from acids during processing.)
10. Tungsten knives are harder and can be used for hard and difficult tissues such as bone. They become blunt less quickly than steel knives. Disposable knives are thinner and sharper than solid knives but their thinness makes them less rigid and they are not as good for hard materials. Disposable knives are more easily replaced, as individual knives are much cheaper so it is easier always to have a sharp knife. Plano-concave knives have a thin edge profile and are good for cutting soft tissues.

Chapter 4

1. Plastics are harder than most other embedding media and so can be used to cut thinner sections (including sections for electron microscopy). They can also be used to cut sections from hard tissues like bone. Preservation of plastic-embedded tissue can be better than with wax embedding since plastic embedding involves fewer reagents and does not overheat the tissue.
2. The epoxy resins are preferred for electron microscopy since they are stable in the electron beam of an electron microscope unlike wax and methacrylates.
3. Epoxy resins can form bonds with active groups in the tissues (e.g. amines). This prevents dyes binding to the groups and reduces staining. Also, the resins cannot easily be removed from the tissues without destroying the tissues, so dyes cannot penetrate into the sections and this reduces staining intensity. Neither wax nor methacrylates directly react with tissue groups and can easily be removed, allowing dyes to access all stainable groups.
4. The usual way to flatten sections and remove wrinkles from sections is to float them on warm water. Water-soluble waxes cannot be floated on to water as they will dissolve, allowing the section to disintegrate.

Chapter 5

1. Slow freezing allows large ice crystals to grow and these can mechanically damage the tissues. Slow freezing also causes concentration of tissue fluids,

as it is pure water that freezes first. The hypertonic tissue fluids may cause cell shrinkage by osmosis.

2. (a) Frozen sections are used to diagnose malignancy because of the need for an urgent diagnosis. Stained frozen sections can be available within a few minutes of the tissue being removed from the patient. (b) Frozen sections are used for lipid demonstration, since the tissues are cut without needing to be embedded or processed. Most lipids are lost if the tissues are processed using organic solvents. (c) Frozen sections are used for enzyme techniques, as they can be cut without the need to fix or process sections. Fixation will destroy most enzyme activity.

3. In the cryostat sectioning technique, everything (tissue, knife and microtome) is kept below freezing so neither the block nor the section thaws during sectioning. In the freezing microtome technique, it is only the block that is kept frozen and sections usually thaw during sectioning. The cryostat is better for most purposes but the freezing microtome has some advantages for large blocks or when thick sections are needed.

4. The boiling of liquid nitrogen when it contacts warm tissue may slow down the rate of cooling by producing a layer of insulating gas around the block. The use of isopentane cooled with liquid nitrogen avoids the boiling problem. The boiling effect does help to prevent minor splashes causing freezing burns to the histologist using the liquid nitrogen.

5. Ice is not completely stable at −20°C and will gradually recrystallize and cause tissue damage.

Chapter 6

1. Chromophores are groups that bring colour to a dye structure. Without a chromophore group, organic compounds are colourless. Auxochrome groups allow dyes to bind to the tissues. Auxochromes are usually ionizable groups that allow the dye to dissociate into charged ions.

2. Basic and acidic dyes bind to ionized groups in the tissues. Basic (cationic) dyes will bind to acid groups in the tissues such as nucleic acids. Acid (anionic) dyes will bind to basic proteins in the cytoplasm and connective tissues. If the two dyes have contrasting colours, they will show the nucleus in one colour and the cytoplasm and connective tissues in the contrasting colour. For example, methylene blue is a basic dye and will stain the nucleus blue, whilst eosin is an acid dye and will stain the cytoplasm pink.

3. Altering the pH of a dye solution will alter the ionization of the tissue. If the tissue groups are not ionized, then no staining will occur. A high pH will favour staining by basic dyes and a low pH will favour staining by acid dyes. Salts also affect the staining by altering the ionization and charge on the tissues. At low salt concentrations, the ions may help dyes to bind by masking surface charges that would otherwise repel the charged dye molecule. High concentrations of salt, however, are inhibitory to staining, as the salt ions will compete with the dye ions for the tissue-binding sites. Thus, low concentrations increase dye binding ('salting on'), whilst high concentrations decrease staining ('salting off').

4. With mordanted dyes, the mordant acts as a bridge between the tissue and the dye, allowing binding. In the absence of the mordant, staining will not occur. If a small amount of mordant is added, it will bind to the dye forming a dye lake and this dye lake will then bind to the tissues colouring them. If, however, there is more mordant than dye, there will be a lot of mordant without any dye attached. This unattached mordant will compete for the tissue-binding sites and inhibit binding of the dye lake (mordant with attached dye) and so reduce staining.

5. It is the mordant that binds to the tissue and so it is the mordant that determines where the dye will bind. Aluminium salts bind to the nucleus most strongly, whilst other metals will bind to elastic fibres or muscle proteins.

6. The name of the phenomenon is metachromasia. The colour change is believed to be due to polymerization of the dye on the surface of the tissue component.

7. An example of a red nuclear stain is neutral red and an example of a blue nuclear stain is methylene blue. A red nuclear stain is used when the main staining reaction produces a green or blue colour, and a blue nuclear stain would be used to contrast with a method producing a red primary reaction.

8. Haematoxylin itself is not a dye and must be oxidized to haematein to stain effectively. The dye solution will improve as atmospheric oxygen converts the haematoxylin to haematein; this is called ripening. The haematein can be further oxidized to a colourless product, which cannot act as a dye. Thus, a haematoxylin solution will begin to deteriorate when there is more haematein being overoxidized than there is haematoxylin being oxidized to haematein.

9. Dyes differ in their molecular size and their ability to penetrate is dependent on this size. Small molecules will penetrate more readily than larger dyes. When in direct competition, the larger dyes will tend to displace or mask the smaller, paler dyes. Tissues differ in their permeability, with red

blood cells being very dense, most cytoplasm being intermediate and collagen being very permeable. Using a small yellow or orange dye, an intermediate-sized red dye and a large blue dye, it is possible to have conditions such that only the smallest dye will stain the dense red cells and they will stain yellow or orange. The medium dye and small dye will both be able to penetrate and stain the general cell cytoplasm, but the larger red dye will displace or mask the yellow dye and so the cytoplasm will appear red. Although all three dyes will be able to penetrate the permeable collagen, the largest and densest dye will prevail, so the collagen will stain blue.

10. Argentaffin reactions occur when there is sufficient reducing strength in the tissues to give a visible silver deposit without using any extra reducing agent. The argyrophil reaction produces submicroscopic silver deposits, which can be enlarged and made visible using extra reducing agents such as quinol or formaldehyde.

11. Silver is the best material for metallic impregnations as its salts are easily reduced and small deposits of silver catalyse the reduction of more silver. The deposit is also stable and is a very dense black colour, which gives a good contrast.

12. DPX mounting medium requires tissues to be dehydrated with alcohol and cleared in xylene. These reagents will dissolve most lipids, so the staining would be lost in the processing. Water-based mounting media do not require this processing and tissues are mounted directly from water.

13. Resinous mounting media give greater clarity to the specimen, as they have a higher refractive index than most water-based mounting media. Resinous mounting media also usually set or dry firmly and remain clear for longer. This means that most resinous mounting media can be considered as a permanent mount and stored indefinitely, whilst water-based mounting media are usually best considered as temporary mounts.

Chapter 7

1. Histochemical methods must produce a final product that is insoluble and highly coloured to ensure that the location of the reaction is accurate and visible. Biochemical techniques are less restricted and can use reaction products that absorb in the UV region and can employ products that are soluble. Histochemical tests need to ensure that the material does not relocate but remains *in situ*.

2. The PAS reaction detects glycols (hydroxyls on adjacent carbon atoms, R-COH-COH-R) or some

derivatives of this group such as the amino and alkyl amino derivatives. The main materials found in tissues that have this arrangement are carbohydrates and proteins that have carbohydrate attached (glycoproteins and proteoglycans).

3. Periodic acid readily oxidizes the glycol groups to aldehydes, which can be detected with Schiff's reagent, but has less tendency than potassium permanganate to oxidize the aldehydes to acids.

4. The biggest division is into neutral mucins and acidic mucins. The acidic mucins can be subdivided further into sulphated and non-sulphated mucins. Sulphated mucins are subdivided again into strongly and weakly sulphated mucins. The non-sulphated or carboxylated mucins can be subdivided into sialic-containing and uronic-containing mucins.

5. Alcian blue will stain acidic mucins blue, but this is sensitive to pH and salt concentration. By using several strengths of salt (e.g. magnesium chloride), it is possible to selectively stain and therefore identify different groups of mucins. The critical concentration of the salt is the one that will completely inhibit one group of mucins but allow more strongly acidic mucins to stain.

6. Hyaluronic acid- and sialic acid-containing mucins can be distinguished using enzyme digestion with hyaluronidase or sialidase. The enzymes will selectively remove the reactive groups and so prevent them from staining with alcian blue.

7. Lipid techniques are often unpopular, since lipids are difficult to fix and are easily dissolved or relocated. This means that the more usual preparative techniques are not appropriate, so lipids require special techniques, which are more trouble to the histologist.

8. The dye will dissolve more readily in the lipid than in the solvent, so the lipid becomes highly coloured whilst the remainder of the section remains uncoloured. This is an application of the partition effect.

9. Only osmium tetroxide fixes lipids, although potassium dichromate may have some fixative action on phospholipids.

10. During the degeneration process, the phospholipid of the myelin becomes degraded and forms neutral lipids. This is a change from an amphipathic lipid to a hydrophobic lipid and this alters its staining properties.

Chapter 8

1. Basophilic staining for DNA can be controlled using enzyme digestion with deoxyribonuclease. The enzyme will destroy the DNA but leave RNA and basophilic mucins unaffected. By using two

adjacent sections, one of which is treated with deoxyribonuclease before staining, it is possible to identify the basophilic materials that have been destroyed by the enzyme and these will be the sites of DNA.

2. Intercalation is the insertion of a molecule into the slot between adjacent pairs of bases in the DNA helix.

3. The Feulgen technique uses acid hydrolysis to produce aldehydes from DNA and these aldehydes are then detected using Schiff's reagent.

4. Proteins can be stained using simple dyeing with acid dyes such as eosin. This is not very selective or specific. Most, but not all, proteins will stain to some extent but some other materials may also stain. Proteins can be stained using specific amino acid tests, e.g. Millon's test for tyrosine. These are more selective in that only proteins or free amino acids will react, but since free amino acids are usually lost during processing the method is quite selective; however, it is more difficult than simple staining.

5. The enzyme may be lost by simply diffusing out of the section into the substrate solution or the activity may be diminished by fixatives or other chemicals.

6. Cyanide is used in dehydrogenase reactions to poison the electron transport enzymes in the mitochondria. This should prevent any reduced NAD being processed by the electron transport chain where the hydrogen would be converted to water. In the absence of the electron transport chain reactions, all of the hydrogen generated by the dehydrogenase reaction will then be available to reduce the tetrazolium salt and give a visible reaction.

7. The α-naphthol method can be used to demonstrate any hydrolase enzyme provided an artificial substrate can be prepared that the enzyme can hydrolyse to release α-naphthol. The α-naphthol can then be trapped and visualized using an azo-coupling reaction.

8. Biochemical measurement is easier to control. For histochemical measurement, the section thickness is crucial for accurate measurement but is very difficult to control or measure accurately. The reaction may not follow the Beer–Lambert relationship in sections and may give a false quantification.

Chapter 9

1. Carbon, asbestos and silica.
2. Lipofuscin gradually accumulates with age.
3. Haemosiderin and asbestos bodies are both positive with the Perls technique.

4. Melanin, lipofuscin, argentaffin and chromaffin pigments are all positive with the Schmorl's technique.

5. APUD cells secrete amine neurotransmitters and peptide hormones.

6. Haemosiderosis and haemochromatosis.

7. Insoluble calcium salts can be demonstrated using alizarin red. The von Kossa technique will demonstrate mineralization, which usually involves mainly insoluble calcium salts. Xylenol orange, tetracycline and alizarin can be used *in vitro* to show the deposition of calcium during bone growth and remodelling. Soluble calcium salts can only be demonstrated in intact living cells using ion-selective dyes.

8. Copper accumulates in Wilson's disease and can be demonstrated using rubeanic acid.

9. Ratiometric fluorescence measures the concentration of an ion by comparing the intensity of fluorescence at two wavelengths. Ratiometric measurements are independent of the concentration of the dye. Single-wavelength measurements use the change in intensity at a single wavelength to measure the concentration and are dependent on dye concentration. The single-wavelength methods use an ionophore and ionic buffer to calibrate the amount of dye present within the cell.

Chapter 10

1. An antibody is a soluble protein produced as part of the immune response to the presence in the body of a foreign material. An antigen is a material capable of eliciting the production of an antibody when introduced into the body. Antibodies are good histological reagents as they can be highly specific and very sensitive in the detection of their specific antigen.

2. Fluorescein isothiocyanate (FITC) is a derivative of fluorescein and can react with proteins to form a conjugate. This conjugate is stable and will not dissociate spontaneously from the dye. The labelling process involves a simple reaction between FITC and the protein followed by purification of the conjugate to remove unreacted FITC.

3. Immunofluorescence techniques suffer from several disadvantages compared with enzyme-labelling methods. Immunofluorescence requires a fluorescent microscope and not just a routine light microscope. The fluorescence can be quite faint and needs a darkened room to allow the eyes to become dark-adjusted. The fluorescence fades quite rapidly, so specimens can only be considered temporary. It is difficult to counterstain the

specimen effectively without interfering with the fluorescence of the fluorescein.

4. Alkaline phosphatase and horseradish peroxidase are two enzymes used in immunocytochemistry.

5. For the peroxidase–anti-peroxidase (PAP) method, the following steps are needed:
   (a) Bring the test sections to water.
   (b) Treat with diluted primary antibody.
   (c) Wash well to remove excess antibody.
   (d) Treat with bridging antibody.
   (e) Wash well to remove excess bridging antibody.
   (f) Treat with PAP reagent.
   (g) Wash well to remove excess PAP.
   (h) Incubate in enzyme substrate solution to detect sites of binding.
   (i) Counterstain.
   (j) Mount the sections.
   In addition to these steps, it may be necessary to destroy any endogenous peroxidase activity and to prevent non-specific binding by blocking with normal (non-immune) sera. It may also be necessary to unmask antigens. These three extra steps would normally be done before step (b).

6. The final product of the PAP technique is the brown deposit from diaminobenzidine and this can be treated with osmium tetroxide, which makes it visible with the electron microscope.

7. Antigen retrieval is the treatment of sections to make the antigens available to the antibody. This may be needed after some fixation and processing schedules. Antigen retrieval can be done using proteolytic enzymes, microwave heating or heating in a pressure cooker.

8. Lectins can be labelled using fluorescein, enzymes, gold particles, etc. in the same way as antibodies. Lectins will bind to specific carbohydrates in tissue and can be visualized in the same way as for antibodies.

9. It is mainly used in electron microscopy where the colloidal gold particles are easily recognizable.

10. Avidin is a high-affinity binding agent for biotin. Avidin can be used to form a bridge between biotin-labelled antibodies and biotin-labelled enzymes.

Chapter 11

1. Autoradiography uses chemicals labelled with radioisotopes. The position of the radioisotopes can be determined using a photographic emulsion. When the radioisotopes decay, the ionizing radiations affect the film. After development, the areas of the emulsion exposed to the ionizing radiations show up as black and this locates the radioisotopes.

2. The prostaglandin will be removed by hydrophobic solvents but as it will be bound to a receptor and has a low solubility in water, it is likely to withstand freezing and thawing without being displaced. Therefore, the tissue can be cut as unfixed cryostat sections, which can be air-dried. The dry sections can then be coated in emulsion. Following successful exposure and development of the emulsion, the slide could be stained with a standard haematoxylin and eosin stain.

3. (a) There are two possibilities using ^{14}C (^{14}C$_2$H$_5$OH) or ^{3}H (C$_2$^{3}H$_5$OH). (b) The labelling could be on the sulphur ^{35}S (H^{35}SCH$_2$CH(NH$_2$)CO$_2$H) or any of the carbons could be labelled with ^{14}C, or using tritium it would be reasonable to label the three hydrogens directly attached to a carbon (HSC^{3}H$_2$C^{3}H(NH$_2$)CO$_2$H). (c) Labelling here is not very reliable with any atoms. Oxygen has no suitable radioisotopes and labelling the hydrogen with tritium is not likely to be stable, so autoradiography is possibly not the best technique. (d) Only the phosphorus is suitable (H$_3$^{32}PO$_4$).

4. Fogging is the blackening of the film at a point not affected by the radioisotopes used in the experiment. This non-specific blackening can be due to chemical contamination, exposure to light, stray radiation from another source (e.g. cosmic rays) or pressure on the film.

Chapter 12

1. Any method used for screening must not have any serious risk for the patient, it must not be painful for the patient and it must be reasonably inexpensive. Exfoliative cytology uses only cells being shed naturally from the body and so does not seriously damage the patient. Cervical cytology sampling should not be painful although patients may consider it uncomfortable or embarrassing. It is not too expensive as it can be performed by GPs or nurses without the need for a hospital appointment or full surgery.

2. The main method of staining gynaecological smears is the Papanicolaou method. This method gives good nuclear detail, transparent cytoplasm and good cytoplasmic differentiation between the different cell layers. Other methods do not have this range of properties although they may be useful in more specific cases.

3. (a) Superficial cells are normal constituents of smears. (b) Parabasal cells are unusual but not abnormal constituents of smears and are more common when oestrogen levels are lowered. (c) *Trichomonas vaginalis* is a pathogenic organism although in some patients it may not cause any

symptoms. (d) Dyskaryotic cells are abnormal although mild dyskaryosis may revert to normal. (e) Koilocytes are indicative of viral infection and are not normal. (f) Erythrocytes are normal at around menstruation but at other times they indicate a haemorrhage. (g) Plasma cells are uncommon in normal smears and usually indicate a chronic inflammation.

4. A navicular cell is elongated with curling edges giving a boat-shaped cell with an eccentric nucleus. This is usually found in pregnancy.

5. The best stages at which to take smears are around ovulation, i.e. late proliferative phase, ovulatory phase and early secretory phase. Smears taken around menstruation are unsuitable.

6. Acute inflammation will typically show a large increase in the number of neutrophils present, possibly with more mucin and sometimes the presence of fibrin and red blood cells from a haemorrhage. If there is an infection, characteristic organisms may be seen and the cells may show signs of degeneration. Chronic inflammation will typically show an increase in the number of macrophages and lymphocytes rather than neutrophil leukocytosis.

7. *Trichomonas vaginalis, Candida albicans,* herpes virus and human papilloma virus.

8. Cervical intraepithelial neoplasia.

9. Too few cells in the smear, the presence of red cells obscuring detail, the presence of pus obscuring detail, and the presence of artefacts caused by air-drying or inadequate fixation.

Chapter 13

1. Cytogenetics is the study of changes in chromosome number or structure that can be seen by microscopy.

2. Cytogenetics can diagnose syndromes associated with chromosomal changes before and after birth. Although diagnosis in children and adults cannot lead to the disease being cured (the abnormalities are currently not curable), the recognition of a genetic abnormality will allow treatment of the symptoms and save the need for further diagnostic investigation. Prenatal diagnosis allows the possibility of termination of the pregnancy to avoid the birth of a severely affected child. Cytogenetics can also be of help in diagnosing somatic diseases such as leukaemia where there may be characteristic chromosomal changes in the diseased cells.

3. Cells are taken from the patient (blood cells, chorionic villus cells or amniocentesis cell samples) and grown in culture. Cells may need to be stimulated to divide in some cases and cells may be treated with colchicine to accumulate mitotic cells. Cells are then treated with hypotonic solutions, fixed and spread on to a slide and finally stained to show banding. The hypotonic solution causes the cells to absorb water by osmosis and this inflates the cells and causes chromosomes to separate.

4. The banding patterns can be stained using fluorescent dyes such as quinacrine or by Giemsa staining following digestion of the cells.

5. A normal female has the constitution 46XX. 47 XY, +21 would indicate a male Down's syndrome patient.

6. At conception it is estimated that up to 1 in 12 (~8%) human conceptions are chromosomally abnormal and this falls to about 1 in 200 at birth (0.5%) due to spontaneous abortions.

7. The Y chromosome is small and contains only genes needed to produce a male foetus. Thus, the absence of a Y chromosome simply results in the female phenotype being produced. The presence of an extra Y chromosome results in only a few extra genes and seems to cause only minor physiological consequences. The cells have a mechanism to switch off any X chromosomes in excess of the single X found in males to maintain the chromosome balance between the different sexes. This means that supernumerary X chromosomes do not cause the severe abnormalities seen with comparably sized autosomes.

8. In translocation Down's syndrome, there is a single large chromosome, which corresponds to the long arm of chromosome 21 attached to the long arm of another chromosome (commonly chromosome 14). This translocation chromosome can be seen in chromosome spreads. Translocation Down's syndrome-affected patients have only 46 chromosomes, not the 47 found in the commoner form of Down's syndrome. Translocation Down's syndrome shows a familial pattern of inheritance with the presence of carriers who are themselves unaffected by Down's syndrome but who have an increased chance of passing it to their children. Translocation Down's syndrome is independent of maternal age.

9. A pericentric inversion occurs when there is an inverted piece of chromosome that includes the centromere. The inversion is symptomless until meiosis occurs, when it can result in the death of the cells if a crossover occurs in the inverted region.

10. *In situ* hybridization is achieved by first separating the strands of DNA by high-temperature melting. Labelled DNA probe (e.g. biotin-labelled DNA) is then added and the conditions are adjusted to allow annealing of the DNA. The labelled probe can hybridize with the cell's own

DNA if the two sequences match. The label can then be visualized (e.g. using avidin and an enzyme). *In situ* hybridization can be used to identify and locate specific DNA sequences inside cells, e.g. it can be used to identify which cells are infected with a virus.

Chapter 14

1. Specimens for microbiology are living bacteria that allow cultures to be grown and biochemical and sensitivity tests can be carried out using these cultures. Paraffin wax sections only contain dead cells, which limits the investigation to staining and serology. Cultural and biochemical tests are more flexible and can identify a wider range of organisms.
2. Staining methods, e.g. Gram staining, can be used to identify the organism as Gram-positive or -negative. Immunological methods and *in situ* hybridization can be used to confirm the type of bacteria. Careful observation of the morphological changes in the tissue may help to identify the causative organisms.
3. Viruses (e.g. herpes virus), bacteria (e.g. *Staphylococcus aureus*), fungi (e.g. *Aspergillus fumigatus*) and protozoa (e.g. *Entamoeba histolytica*) can all appear in sections.
4. Amyloid is an abnormal protein with a β-pleated sheet conformation that accumulates in certain pathological conditions. Amyloid is resistant to most proteolytic enzymes because of the unusual β-pleated sheet conformation.
5. See table below.

Chapter 15

1. The numerical aperture is related to the resolving power of the lens, which is one of the most important characteristics of any microscope lens. Numerical aperture is also related to the depth of field of the lens and determines how much depth of a specimen is in focus at any one time.
2. Empty magnification is where the image is enlarged but with no increase in detail. Empty magnification may even result in less detail being observable than at a lower but more useful magnification. The useful magnification is approximately 1000 times the numerical aperture of the objective.
3. An achromatic lens is a lens that has been partially corrected for chromatic aberration. The colour fringing (a spectrum of light produced by the lens) is greatly reduced but not totally eliminated.
4. The darkground microscope uses oblique illumination in the form of a hollow cone of light. None of the direct light can enter the objective so the field of view appears dark. Objects that can bend the light by diffraction or refraction will appear bright against this dark background.

Amyloid type	Diseases with which the amyloid is associated
AL Amyloid light chain immune-associated amyloid	Multiple myeloma, Waldenström's disease
AA Reactive amyloid	Rheumatoid arthritis, tuberculosis, Hodgkin's disease, familial Mediterranean fever
AE Endocrine-related amyloid	Insulinomas, medullary carcinoma of the thyroid
β-Amyloid	Alzheimer's disease
AS Senile amyloid	Old age (80+)
AF Familial amyloid	Familial amyloidosis
AD Dermal amyloid	Lichen amyloidosis
AH Haemodialysis-associated amyloid	Renal failure with haemodialysis

5. In the polarizing microscope, two polarizing filters are used, with the first filter between the light source and the specimen and the second between the specimen and the eye. The first filter produces plane-polarized light and the second polarizing filter is rotated or 'crossed' so that in the absence of a specimen no direct illumination is seen. Urea crystals are birefringent and rotate the plane of polarization allowing some light to pass through the second polarizing filter so that the crystals appear bright against a dark background.

6. Two filters are used in a conventional fluorescent microscope. The first filter is placed between the light source and the specimen and this allows only short-wavelength light to pass. The second filter is placed between the specimen and the eye and allows only long-wavelength light to pass. Only fluorescent light that has been emitted by the specimen will be seen with this arrangement.

7. The human eye can be fooled by optical illusions and apparent size is a subjective assessment by the eye and the brain and not an absolute measurement.

8. 0.55 or 55% (area proportion is 110/200 = 0.55).

9. The density is not necessarily homogeneous. The amount of light passing through the lightly stained areas will be disproportionate to the amount of light coming through the darker areas and the amount of material will be underestimated.

Chapter 16

1. CTEM differs from light microscopy by using electrons instead of light. It has a better resolving ability since electrons can have much shorter wavelengths than light. The lenses in the electron microscope are electromagnetic, not glass, and magnification is changed by altering the magnetic strength of the lens rather than changing lenses as in the light microscope. The electron microscope must work in a vacuum and this prevents the examination of living specimens. The electron microscope needs thinner sections and they need better support than in light microscopy, so specimens are mounted on copper grids not glass slides. The image cannot be viewed directly in the electron microscope but must use either a phosphorescent screen or a camera to take a photograph. The image in the electron microscope is always monochrome, whilst the light microscope image can be multicoloured. Contrast is achieved in the electron microscope using heavy metal salts rather than the dyes used in light microscopy.

2. Resin or plastic embedding is needed to give better support to the specimen and allow thinner sections to be cut. The plastics are also more stable than wax when subjected to a high vacuum and an electron beam, so they support the tissue better during examination.

3. There are no lenses used in SEM to image the specimen so there are no lens aberrations. The condenser lenses used to focus the electron beam on to the specimen play no direct part in producing the image.

4. Critical point drying is the use of a liquid that has a critical temperature and pressure at which there is no distinction between the gaseous phase and the liquid phase. At this critical point, the gas and liquid have exactly the same density. One such liquid is CO_2. By dehydrating the tissues and then replacing the water with liquid CO_2, it is possible to remove the CO_2 without evaporation simply by warming it to above its critical temperature. The liquid becomes a gas without boiling or evaporating and can be allowed to escape gently without damaging the tissue.

5. It is necessary to coat SEM specimens to make them electrically conductive and gold is the best metal for this purpose. The electrical conductivity is needed to earth any static electrical charge, which would otherwise interfere with the image.

6. The positive identification of a material in the light microscope is easier because there is a wide range of available dyes, which can be quite selective in their staining and which have a wide range of contrasting colours. In electron microscopy, there are only a few heavy metal ions available for use. These are less selective in their staining properties and will react with a wider range of materials. Finally, the electron microscope image is only in shades of grey so there is less distinction between materials.

7. The X-rays produced in the electron microscope will have wavelengths characteristic of the elements within the specimen, so examining the spectrum of X-rays allows determination of which elements are present in the specimen.

Index